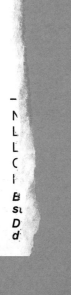

The Ultimate Natural Beauty Bible

SARAH STACEY is an award-winning beauty and health writer, and currently Health Editor of the *Mail on Sunday YOU* magazine. She has written for many leading newspapers and magazines in the UK and abroad. In 1994, she was elected the first Honorary Chair of the Guild of Health Writers UK and later co-founded the food labelling campaign FLAG. She is married and lives partly in London with a lot of driving up and down the A303 to west Dorset to see her much-loved and and rather large horses.

JOSEPHINE FAIRLEY is a Contributing Editor to the *Mail on Sunday's YOU* magazine, writing on beauty and organic living. She contributes to a very wide range of publications including *Psychologies*, *Green Magazine*, *Waitrose Kitchen* and *Healthy*, and has her own fragrance blog www.thescentcritic.com. Jo is also founding partner of Green & Black's Organic Chocolate. She lives in East Sussex with her husband Craig Sams, her co-founder in Green & Black's.
(For more info see www.josephinefairley.com)

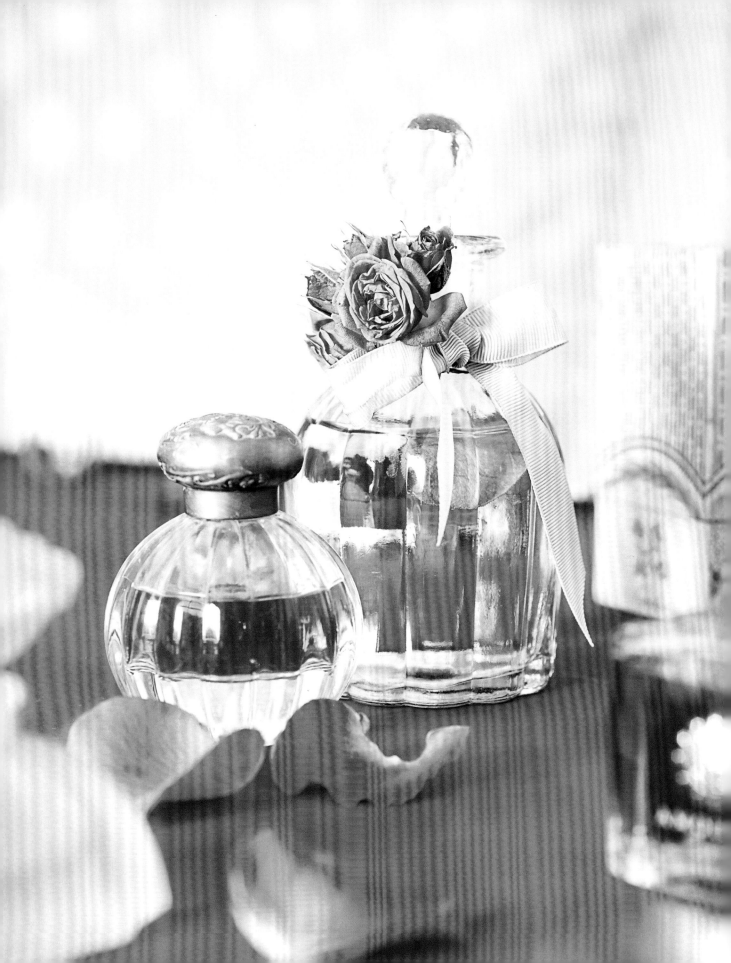

The Ultimate Natural Beauty Bible

Sarah Stacey & Josephine Fairley

Photography by Claire Richardson

Illustrations by Yoco Nagamiya

KYLE BOOKS

CONTENTS

THE ULTIMATE NATURAL BEAUTY BIBLE

Of the 18,000 women (and counting) who we've been in touch with since we began our *Beauty Bible* series of books, the vast majority tell us: 'I'd like to be a natural beauty.' That doesn't mean going barefaced: far from it. It means having the best possible skin, for a start. So: botanical ingredients have a time-honoured tradition of beautifying skin – but the good news is that nowadays they're being formulated into ever-more-effective lotions, potions and creams, alongside a serious pleasure factor. Today, being a 'natural beauty' doesn't mean compromising on texture, fragrance or performance. Not for a moment. Natural beauty has definitely moved on from the time it was all about balms and oils (often mixed on the kitchen table). As we know from the trials for this book, plenty of natural (and mostly natural) products rival their synthetic/rocket-science counterparts. (Indeed, leading natural brands – such as Melvita – are carrying out in-depth research into promising ingredients and finished products that rival anything in 'mainstream' beauty.)

But there are other reasons we're increasingly interested in going *au naturel*. There are some serious beauty issues, which the world of natural, organic (and 'greener') skincare touches on. Animal testing, for instance. (The dawn of China as a major market for cosmetics put the clock back on this, although things may be changing.) Allergic reactions to synthetic chemicals, such as the preservative MI, which has caused a new 'epidemic' (the scientists' word, not ours) of contact eczema. Nanotechnology: there are some suggestions that, long term, the use of products based on this super-high-tech science might potentially have health implications; the jury is still out. Ditto hair colouring: there are still concerns about its safety, and plenty of confusion. According to a recent survey from natural beauty brand Evolve, over 90 per cent of customers are concerned, or moderately concerned, about 'toxins' in beauty products. And then there's organic and Fairtrade: increasing numbers of consumers are looking for cosmetics that reflect positive lifestyle choices.

We like to think we're known for our no-nonsense, down-to-earth, practical approach to the celebration of beauty – helping real women to understand issues like these (if you are interested). We appreciate it's hard to get your head round what's natural, ethical, organic – and what's not. So all the products that feature in this book have a 'daisy rating': our own 'naturalness' assessment (which you can read more about, right).

But the very best way to ensure you know exactly what you're putting on your skin – rather like making a meal at home – is to create products from scratch. It's surprisingly easy. It's really fun. (The teenagers in our lives love getting involved.) And the results can be really effective. So in *The Ultimate Natural Beauty Bible* you'll also find recipes for making skin- and haircare products – even the occasional make-up item – from simple-to-find ingredients.

Our own philosophy is to aim for balance. We're not about scaremongering headlines (although we do warn you of, for instance, potential skin irritants). We're all about getting things into proportion, and 'positive health': living healthily, eating well, exercising – and building up natural resilience to our modern world, its threats and toxins, as well as appreciating its wonders, big and small. That's the path to true wellbeing.

And what we've seen with our own eyes, time and again, is that the women who take care of themselves naturally radiate beauty, grace and ease – what the French call '*être bien dans sa peau*', or feeling comfortable in your skin. Which also means getting your appearance into proportion. After hundreds of (anti-ageing) consultations with real women in stores and at reader events, we've met so many women who fixate on a flaw that is literally invisible to the naked eye. We say: ditch the magnifying mirror. Never flip open the one in the car, either: it's surely enough to make Elle Macpherson feel ancient and flawed. Instead, try to see yourself as others see you. They look at your clothes and notice that nice blue scarf or those silver earrings. Note how great your hair's looking, maybe. And (most importantly) hear your laughter, see your smile (the fastest way for anyone to drop a decade) – and look into your eyes, to your soul. Trust us: they're not sitting

THE DAISY RATING

Are the products in this book 99 per cent – or even totally – natural? In some cases, yes. In others, they're mostly natural with a high percentage of botanicals. We make no apology for including these latter because the feedback is that all-natural products don't always live up to women's beauty expectations (although some exceed them) – and we know many, many women who will happily opt for that 'mostly natural' category, if it means better performance.

The bottom line is that – as with everything in life – it's about choice. So to help you identify which products are all natural, which are natural and organic, and which just feature lashings of beautifying botanicals, we're sharing with you the 'daisy rating' we came up with a few years ago. (We were asked recently if we might launch this as an easy-to-understand industry standard – but we're not up for another career.)

✳ **ONE DAISY** Mostly natural with a small percentage of synthetic and/or petrochemical ingredients.
✳ ✳ **TWO DAISIES** Botanically derived with no synthetics or petrochemicals.
✳ ✳ ✳ **THREE DAISIES** Certified organic by one of the leading international certification bodies, such as USDA, Ecocert, and Soil Association.

there making a mental tally of wrinkles, age spots and the bags under your eyes.

So: you want to look beautiful, and feel fantastic? Naturally, you do. And as ever, we're here to light the way...

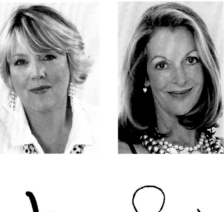

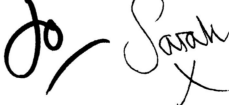

What sort of NATURAL BEAUTY *are you?*

There are many different reasons why *Beauty Bible* readers are drawn to botanical, organic and 'greener' products, we find. Feedback tells us that some of you simply prefer the power of plants to sort out your skin and hair, rather than the sort of Nobel-prize-winning high-tech molecules that feature in a lot of 21st century skincare. For some, it's concern about chemical ingredients, while others want to tread a little more lightly on the planet, choosing organic ingredients in their cosmetics – and perhaps certified products – because they eat organic and support a more sustainable way of farming. Or maybe it's a mix of all three!

If you want to take a shortcut to the products in this book that fit with your personal natural beauty philosophy, just ask yourself a few questions – and then let our 'daisy rating' (see the previous page) steer you to the choices that best match that.

ARE YOU 'HIGH-TECH NATURAL'?

Maybe you believe that, yes, natural beauty ingredients have been around for thousands of years – but that doesn't mean they can't be improved upon. Do you sometimes shop from brands that use the phrase 'science-meets-nature' in their marketing?

Let's get one thing straight: there aren't any whizz-bang, 100 per cent high-tech products in this book (although there are plenty of those in our 'sister' volume, *The Anti-Ageing Beauty Bible*, which is awash with breakthrough molecules!). Nobody's going to win a Nobel prize off the back of anything in *The Ultimate Natural Beauty Bible*. However, that doesn't mean to say that, in some cases, there hasn't been a deal of research to back up the claims for the botanicals that feature in the products.

All the 'one daisy' products in this book feature high levels of botanicals, often near the top of the ingredients lists. But there are also some synthetics in there – the 'science' bit – used by the brands to create a more familiar texture, perhaps a product that feels more like something from the mainstream. If you're being drawn towards more natural beauty after using high-tech brands, the one-daisy products may fit best with your expectations at first, as you begin to explore the natural beauty universe.

ARE YOU 'SORT OF NATURAL'?

Are you the type of beauty-hound who knows that botanicals have benefits? Do you live a 'more natural' lifestyle, and feel more grounded in this high-tech world by being more closely in touch with nature – even if it's via a beauty product?

Plenty of women fall into this category. 'Natural', for you, means lashings of botanicals – which, of course, have been known for their beautifying powers since the era when every community had its own 'wise woman', and back into the mists of time. (We thank our lucky stars, personally, to have been born at a time when we're not at risk of being burned at the stake for believing that calendula can soothe touchy skin, lavender relax a chattering brain or rosemary awaken the senses!)

If it's serious plant-power that you're after – to soothe, smooth, soften, brighten and more – then any two-daisy (and above) product in this book will fit with your 'sort of natural' beauty thinking.

ARE YOU 'SUPER NATURAL'?

Do you eat organically, recycle, and long for a beauty bag stocked with eco-conscious, maybe even Fairtrade products that fit in with your 'greener' lifestyle?

We fall into this category ourselves, actually. We seek out organic food (and grow quite a lot of our own), we walk or hop on to public transport rather than drive whenever we can, and probably hang on to favourite clothes longer than is decent, feeling rather proud when something's just too threadbare to be rescued one last time. And frankly, we'd rather not have petroleum-derived ingredients in our beauty products when there are sustainably farmed alternatives to ingredients like mineral oil.

If you're like us, you may well find the sort of products that you're looking for in a natural food store (though beauty halls and supermarkets are increasingly stocking them too). You'll probably want to look out for an organic symbol on the packaging, too, which shows the commitment of the brands you buy to an environmentally friendlier lifestyle. (Brands that jump through the hoops to prove their organic credentials through certification often think more deeply about issues like packaging and recycling, in our experience, as well as corporate sustainability initiatives.)

Any product that has been officially certified as organic gets three daisies (and a resounding Hoorah! from us) in this book. There are fewest of these three-daisy products across the book – but a respectable quota, well up on previous books. The 'next-best' category is the all-natural, two-daisy ranking. You'll find plenty to love, we promise.

ARE YOU 'CONCERNED NATURAL'?

Do you have health concerns about toxins and ingredients to which the word 'carcinogen' is sometimes attached?

Well, first of all, we do counsel balance here. Yes, there are ingredients that may be of concern to some (see page 152). But very few single ingredients, used in the tiny quantities found in beauty products, are going to have as much negative impact on your overall wellbeing as a healthy diet, exercise and lifestyle will confer on the positive side.

It's your personal choice if you decide to avoid what you consider to be 'questionable' ingredients. We respect that so we suggest you look for products in the book that have two or more daisies, in which those 'questionable' ingredients do not feature – and which have lots of glorious, nurturing plant elements to feed your skin and your soul.

There are a teeny number of people who still hand-make cosmetics (so look locally) but in most cases, even if an ingredient started as a plant, synthetic chemicals may be used to process the extracts or derivatives somewhere along the line. In many cases, not a trace of those chemicals remain in the finished product – but the only way to be 100 per cent, totally certain about the naturalness of what you're putting on your face, body and hair is to make products yourself from scratch. And if that fits with your natural way of thinking – well, we have plenty of ideas for D-I-Y gorgeousness in this book, especially for you.

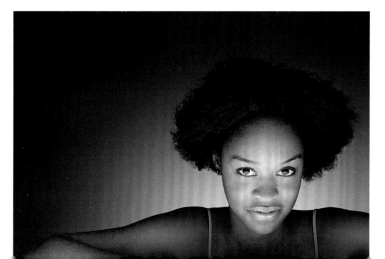

HOW TO READ A LABEL

How much can you trust the labels on your 'natural' beauty buys? The packaging can be misleading and then there's often an endless list of Latin ingredients to decode. Here's our foolproof guide

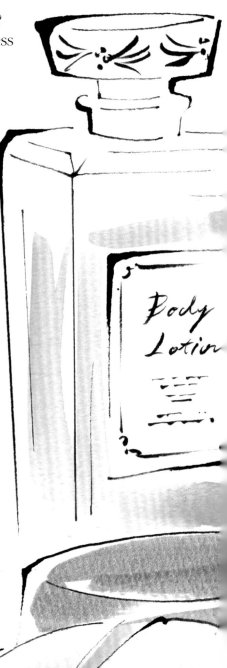

First, get yourself a magnifying glass. This is no joke. We went half-blind reading cosmetics ingredients lists before we invested in a lightweight magnifying glass that fits into a handbag. So, pop it in your bag to have at the ready.

Be aware that there is no legal definition of natural. Or indeed organic. The fact that the label trumpets either or both doesn't mean the ingredients are. Equally, pretty pictures of herbs and flowers don't mean the product is based on more than a waft or whiff.

If you are shopping for an organic product, look for an official certification symbol. USDA (USA), Soil Association (UK), Ecocert, Cosmebio (both France), COSMOS (Europe-wide) and NASAA (Australia) are the best-known bodies certifying organic cosmetics. (Our website, beautybible.com, has a rundown of the different symbols and their annoyingly slightly differing standards.) A symbol is your only real assurance of true organic (and thus natural) status.

Read the ingredients list. (That's where the magnifying glass comes in.) Although it will never tell you the amount of each ingredient (for reasons of commercial confidentiality) the list is in descending order of quantity so you have some sort of notion of the biggest ingredients. (Very often you will find water at the top of the list.)

RED ALERT

If you have sensitive skin, the following ingredients may cause problems. If you do have a reaction, ask your doctor for a patch test to determine the cause.

MI and MCI: the preservatives methylisothiazolinone and methylchloroisothiazolinone have caused a rapid rise in facial eczema with red, swollen, itchy, blistery skin appearing a day or so after use.

Sulphates: foaming agents sodium lauryl sulphate (SLS) and sodium laureth sulphate (SLES) irritate eczema sufferers and some people with healthy skin. They are also linked to mouth ulcers, via toothpaste.

Fragrance, colourings, formaldehyde, parabens, lanolin and benzoyl peroxide may all cause allergic reactions. Paraphenylenediamine (PPD), an ingredient in dark hair colours, can also affect some sensitive people.

'You want botanicals to feature at the top of the list, and any synthetic chemicals to languish down the bottom'

Be aware that many natural ingredients read like synthetics when they are translated into Latin – which they must be by law in many countries. For a list of the ingredients that we really, really don't want to find in natural skincare, though, see pages 152–153. Sometimes manufacturers put the English translations beside the Latin, which makes life easier. You want botanicals to feature at the top of the list, and any synthetic chemicals (or petrochemicals, see box opposite) to languish down the bottom (if at all).

If you see the words paraffinum liquidum, or mineral oil, on a label, that means petroleum-based. That doesn't mean they're harmful to you (although there are issues about how good these ingredients are for some skins), but there are many sustainably produced natural alternatives to choose from. (See our daisy rating on page 7.)

New EU regulations mean that nano-sized compounds must have the word 'nano' after them in the ingredients list. This is something that campaigners have lobbied for after years of weasel wording.

But please: don't be paranoid. Tiny quantities of even 'questionable' ingredients will not have a major health impact on most people.

NB We can't list every ingredient in every product in this book, but an A–Z of many can be found in the *Green Pages* section of www.beautybible.com.

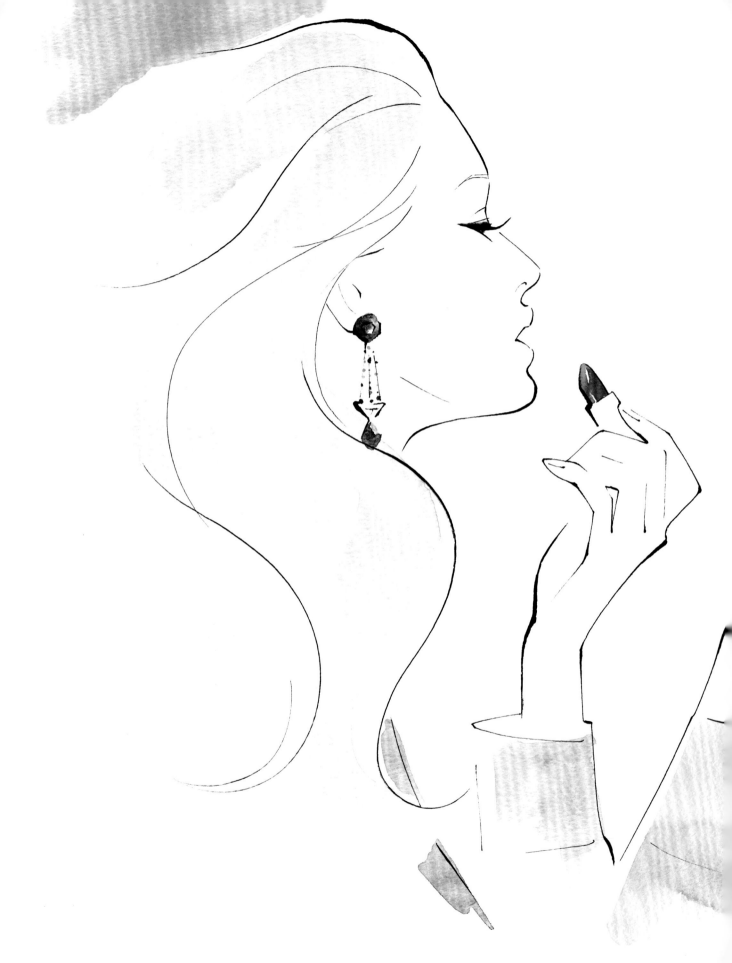

Naturally radiant
MAKE-UP

In reality, most women we know don't want to be
barefaced. So here are the make-up products
(and tips) to help you bring out your own
natural beauty

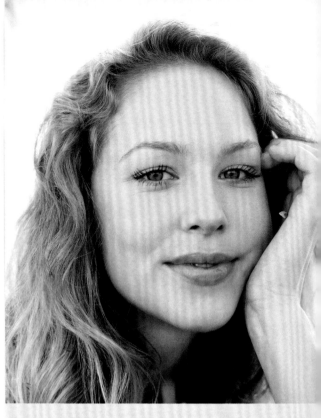

SHAKE UP YOUR MAKE-UP

Six lipsticks (four that don't really suit us), three mascaras (one gummy, another that gives us panda eyes by lunch), four foundations (none quite the right shade/texture) – and so on. That's just some of what we found when we dejunked our make-up stash. Like most women, we can accumulate a small landmass of make-up that doesn't live up to the job description, ie, making us look like ourselves but prettier.

So we say: it's time to de-junk your make-up and focus on the products that make the most difference to your individual appearance. And in our experience, you only need a handful to look gorgeous (well, maybe a double handful for day and evening). The key is to get the right ones.

MAKE-UP FOR DIFFERENT COLOUR TYPES

BLONDES

You often have lovely skin, so the trick here is to subtly emphasise pale complexions, lashes and brows.

EVERYDAY ESSENTIALS:
- **Brow pencil/powder:** choose grey/taupey shades
- **Mascara:** brown not black
- **Eyeliner:** brown/black (otherwise eyes tend to disappear)
- **Concealer:** a touch to even out skin tone if you need
- **Blusher:** gives a 'pop' of colour to pale skins, but be careful if you are prone to flushing or high colour
- **Lip colour:** a slick of something sheer, or tinted lip gloss may be all you need for day

FOR EVENING ADD IN:
- **Eyeshadow**
- **Foundation**
- **Lip pencil, lipstick and lip gloss**

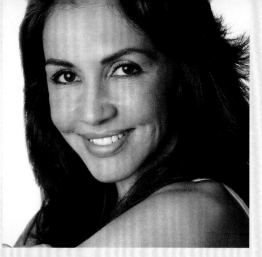

BRUNETTES

Focus on creating dewy natural skin
and making the most of your more
dramatic colouring.

EVERYDAY ESSENTIALS:
- **Tinted moisturiser:** often all you need,
especially in summer
- **Foundation:** if you need more coverage –
do try mineral make-up (see pages 20–21)
- **Concealer:** for dark shadows or small flaws
eg, thread veins, dark circles, little scars etc
- **Blusher or bronzer:** to accentuate cheeks
(and see the effect on your eyes, too) and add
a glow
- **Tinted lip gloss**

FOR EVENING ADD IN:
- **Mascara**
- **Brow pencil** – if necessary
- **Eyeshadow**
- **Lipstick and lip gloss**

REDHEADS

Adding definition to lashes and brows and softly
warming ivory skin will transform you in a flash.

EVERYDAY ESSENTIALS:
- **Brown mascara**
- **Brow pencil:** like blondes, redheads
often lack definition round the eyes, so
mascara (top and bottom) and brow pencil
make a huge difference
- **Bronzer:** to prevent a washed-out look or…
- **Blusher:** peachy, nutmeg tones work well
for redheads

FOR EVENING ADD IN:
- **Mineral foundation:** good for freckled
skins, covering lightly without creating a
'mask' look
- **Eyeshadow**
- **Lipstick and lip gloss**

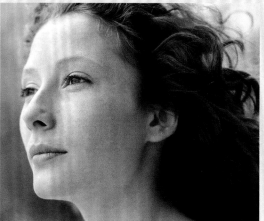

COLOURED SKIN

Lucky you: your natural colouring has such
impact, you need the fewest products

EVERYDAY ESSENTIALS:
- **Eyeshadow**
- **Lipstick:** choose a bright colour – shades of
purple look wonderful on dark skins

FOR EVENING ADD IN:
- **Mineral foundation**
- **Highlighter:** a gleam of gold looks
wonderful swept across cheekbones
- **Mascara:** to extend and thicken rather than
add colour
- **Brow pencil:** if needed to define shape
- **Lip gloss**

TINTED MOISTURISERS
our award winners

We hoped to include some BB (or even CC) creams here but none of the natural versions made the grade. And actually, tinted moisturisers are quite similar to BB products in that they are hydrating, add colour, a little coverage, plus SPF

AVEDA INNER LIGHT MINERAL TINTED MOISTURISER SPF15
✳

SCORE: 8.64/10
This is suitable for men and women, Aveda tell us. You'll be sharing a lightweight but nourishing moisturiser, complete with oil-free hydration from coconut and jojoba seed, plus mega-antioxidant resveratrol from Japanese knotweed – at last, a use for it! Tourmaline, a gemstone, gives the cream a natural radiance, while lavender, bergamot and rose add an aromatic (unisex) scent. It's offered in seven shades: Sweet Tea, a mid-tone, was ours.
COMMENTS: 'Very easy to blend, goes on evenly every time' • 'if you add another coat it becomes more of a sheer foundation – I like that' • 'I didn't need to use a moisturiser under this product which (ironically) I do with quite a few tinted creams' • 'I loved using this and found it gave great results – smooths in easily, and fine lines round my lips appeared much softer' • 'gives sheer coverage with a satin finish, which hydrates very well – yet the light formula makes you feel like you're not wearing any make-up. Love it!' • 'it was hard to tell I was wearing any make-up, yet my skin looked healthier and felt nourished' • 'everyone seems to think I've lost years since using this!'

WILD ABOUT BEAUTY SHEER GLOW MOISTURE TINT
✳

SCORE: 7.75/10
Another excellent performance from newish brand Wild About Beauty who feature quite widely in our make-up categories. This long, slim, nozzled tube delivers a can't-tell-it-from-real healthy glow with a choice of three shades (we tried Beige). It contains a couple of skin-caring

THESE WINNERS ALL BLEND BOTANICALS WITH SOME SYNTHETICS; OTHERS SIMPLY DIDN'T COME UP TO SCRATCH

ingredients: anti-inflammatory winter cherry and skin-conditioning vitamin E, and offers SPF20 – a slightly higher level than Aveda's. However, we advise that none of these three winners offers enough UV protection for anything more than a cloudy day.
COMMENTS: 'Skin definitely looks 100 per cent better with this on' • 'went on incredibly smoothly, and is as good as any moisturiser – loved it; I was sceptical at first but once on my face it seems to glow (in a good way) and I look as though I've been away for a weekend break' • 'nice and velvety, easy to apply – I've loved this and it gives a youthful glow to my skin' • 'complexion looks radiant and plumper – a great piece of kit for the make-up bag' • 'made me look more "awake" and healthy'.

PÜR MINERALS 4-IN-1 MINERAL TINTED MOISTURISER
✳

SCORE: 7.3/10
The '4-in-1' refers to the fact that this multitasks as a moisturiser, primer, foundation and SPF (it's SPF20, but see our note about sun protection above). Four shades are available: our testers smoothed in Light, the palest shade of this antioxidant-rich lightweight cream – which features plenty of radiance-enhancing particles.
COMMENTS: 'I was sceptical about this as I couldn't see how it would provide coverage and moisturise without needing to use another product but it absolutely delivered, and looked natural – love it!' • 'a good tinted moisturiser with more coverage than most' • 'lovely velvety feel' • '4-in-1 is a big ask of a product, but this one does very well – skin looks healthy and natural when I put it on – as if I'm not wearing anything; and it stays fresh all day' • 'my skin still looks good after 12 hours of wearing this'.

LIQUID FOUNDATIONS
our award winners

It was a struggle in previous books to find all-natural – or 'more natural' – liquid foundations that could rival the mainstream brands, but this bunch were a revelation, delighting testers with their light, dewy coverage

LIVING NATURE FOUNDATION
✸✸✸
SCORE: 8.43/10

This is the highest score for a natural foundation in our books – an impressive achievement for the New Zealand brand's 100-per-cent natural formulation. Five shades are available in this product, which features earth minerals, vitamins and antimicrobial manuka oil – making it a good choice for problem skins and rosacea. We sent out Pure Taupe to testers.

COMMENTS: 'At last: a foundation that's not full of chemicals and doesn't dry out my skin!' • 'balanced my skin tone well, gave enough cover for a fresh, natural look' • 'blemishes weren't noticeable; felt comfortable' • 'very natural finish, smoothed out my complexion and left a nice dewy glow on skin' • 'usual shininess on my skin didn't happen' • 'dewy and healthy finish; good coverage of blemishes'.

INIKA LIQUID MINERAL FOUNDATION
✸✸✸
SCORE: 7.83/10

Yes, mineral make-up does come in liquid form – although obviously other ingredients do feature. Here, that means Aboriginal kaduka plum (the world's richest source of vitamin C), with nourishing rosehip, avocado and coconut oils – in fact, they tag this with an anti-ageing claim. Four shades: we trialled Beige.

COMMENTS: 'Loved the finish – just a bit more coverage than a tinted moisturiser, so perfect for me' • 'I looked very well but not obviously like I was wearing make-up' • 'doesn't shift while exercising' • 'a matte finish that doesn't deaden face' • 'I've been wary around foundation, rarely finding one like this that looked natural and was easy to blend; I'd never have tried it outside of these trials, so thank you'.

ORIGINS PLANTSCRIPTION SPF15 ANTI-AGEING FOUNDATION
✸
SCORE: 7.61/10

Origins' winner promises anti-ageing benefits, too. An extension of the brand's Plantscription age-defying skincare range, this oil-free formula, which comes in a squeezy tube, offers plenty of hydration as well as good coverage and a radiant finish, too. Coming from the Estée Lauder stable, there's a wider range of shades than usual with 11 in total, including for darker skin tones. We trialled Light Neutral.

COMMENTS: 'Looks extremely natural and dewy; I don't normally like foundations as I feel they're too heavy, too obvious, and can't wait to take them off, but I completely forgot I was wearing this one' • 'easy to blend into skin seamlessly; and gave good coverage' • 'very light and natural, didn't feel as if I had make-up on' • 'a little of this goes a long way'.

KORRES WILD ROSE FOUNDATION
✸
SCORE: 7.56/10

On first squeezing out this moisturising base it appears 'radiant' – thanks to the light-diffusing pigments and microspheres – but it then sets to a velvety texture with a soft-focus effect. The wild rose extract adds skin-brightening powers, vitamins A and E also feature, plus silicones and a synthetic chemical SPF15. We tried the shade R2 – a light beige – from a choice of four.

COMMENTS: 'Lovely: great that it contains natural ingredients and is still an excellent foundation' • 'erased dark circles, which pleased me infinitely' • 'covered little thread veins around the nose' • 'a natural finish – I don't think anyone would know I was wearing foundation' • 'a nice, light powdery scent'.

Are you mad for MINERALS?

Whether you love the glowing natural coverage of pure mineral foundation or think that it's a frightful faff, with powder flying everywhere (which it needn't be), this 'alternative' make-up – first popularised in the 1970s – has become mainstream

When you see the phrase 'mineral make-up' today, it often refers to foundation – but many pure mineral make-up ranges now offer everything from eyeshadow and mascara to lippy, bronzer and blusher. However, decoding what mineral really means does need a bit of insider knowledge, because not every product that calls itself mineral is as natural as the label implies.

The truth is that pretty well every make-up range contains minerals – mainly titanium dioxide, zinc oxide, mica and iron oxides – because they are the concentrated pigments that give products colour. When mineral make-up became a buzz, some well-known brands simply relabelled their products to jump on the bandwagon. What makes truly 'pure' mineral brands different is what they leave out: no preservatives, parabens, mineral oil, synthetic colours and fragrance – in other words, no ingredients that can irritate sensitive skin.

Once upon a time, the minerals were mined, pulverised and poured into jars. Nowadays, they are mostly synthesised in the lab – and where natural minerals are used, they undergo an extensive extraction and purification process to remove contaminants such as mercury and lead. Many conventional brands that trumpet the word 'minerals' on the label use plenty of synthetics alongside the actual pigments. (Our daisy rating tells you the two-daisy versions that are purely mineral/botanical.)

For many skin types – including problem complexions – minerals are a huge plus. Many dermatologists agree with mineral make-up

pioneer Jane Iredale that, as well as keeping normal skin happy, pure mineral foundation is a favourite for anyone with skin problems from acne or rosacea to eczema or psoriasis. That's down to the minerals' inherent antibacterial and anti-inflammatory properties. Plus, says Jane, 'it allows skin to breathe and function normally, rather than clogging pores like many conventional products.' The absence of oil may help acne or shiny, oily or combination skin. As a result, women who have found that make-up makes their skin problems worse generally discover that using pure mineral make-up results in a calmer complexion that not only looks better but actually gets better.

Mineral foundations often proclaim an SPF on the label. You can even buy 'brush-on' mineral powder SPFs. While they do offer some sun protection, that's only where the product has been applied. That may be enough for days when you are out briefly – but if you are in the sun for any length of time (or on the water) you should reapply every two hours, and we advise using a proper SPF product underneath, too. (A friend burned with a leading brand of mineral sun defence powder, despite using it according to the directions.)

One concern is the use of nanoparticles in mineral foundation. In general, pure mineral brands seem not to use these teeny particles whereas so-called mineral foundations from mainstream brands may – and in some cases omit to label them, according to research conducted in Australia. (If nanoparticles are Greek to you, read more on page 152.)

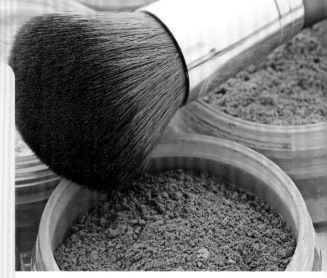

HOW TO APPLY MINERAL POWDER FOUNDATION

We find the biggest concern about using mineral foundation is the perceived mess and fuss. 'I just haven't got the time to do all that,' one woman told us as we researched this. Devotees say it really doesn't take any longer than usual: here's what you do.
NB: If you can, we recommend booking in for a lesson at one of the counters nationwide to see the process demonstrated and also get expert advice on the exact products to suit you.

1 **Assemble your brushes.** A kabuki brush is the traditional applicator but you can use a domed blusher/bronzer brush or invest in those your chosen brand advises.

2 **Apply moisturiser and let it sink in for a few minutes.** If you don't, your skin may look blotchy, warns Jane Iredale.

3 **Apply a primer, if you wish.** Again leave a few moments to absorb. (bareMinerals says you can apply foundation immediately with its oil-free, silica-rich primer.)

4 **Tap a sprinkling of powder into the lid of your foundation pot.** No more than the waft of powdered chocolate on top of a cappuccino.

5 **Dip in your brush and swirl the powder round and round it.** This ensures the powder is evenly dispersed through the bristles.

6 **Start application at the 'edges' of your face and work inwards.** This will make sure it doesn't cake on to your cheeks/ nose. Buff it into the skin in little circles (this is the famous 'swirl' part of the technique). As the powder warms with your body heat, it will subtly change and meld with your skin, so it won't look powdery or dry – just flawless and luminous.

7 **Layer on more where you need extra coverage.** Apply an extra touch if needed.

8 **Top up through the day, as you need.** For advice on which of our award-winning formulations is suitable for carrying in your handbag, see page 20. *Et voilà!*

NB: Several brands now offer mineral make-up in compact cream or liquid form, but still recommend the buffing, swirling approach above.

Mining the history of minerals

The first make-up ever used was based on minerals: when Cleopatra came to power in Egypt in 51 BC, there was a whole rainbow of cosmetics for her to choose from, all made from rocks, minerals and plants. Cleopatra apparently used bright green malachite paste on her lower lids (don't try this at home…).

But mineral make-up made it on to women's beauty radar as a bit of a hippie fad just after the 1960s – bareMinerals, now the market leader, started in the 70s in America with loose powder foundations. Former casting director Jane Iredale launched her eponymous range, also now with a big fan base, in 1994. Australian brand Inika began after the millennium and, in 2010 in the UK, mass-market brand Bourjois diversified with UNE, which includes mineral foundations among its new natural range.

And we love the tag line from Santa Fe-based W3LL People: 'Hippie Tested, Diva Approved'. Add to that 'Make-up Artist Approved' too, as a growing list of fans of this style of make-up will testify.

MINERAL MAKE-UP
our award winners

The beauty world has jumped on the mineral make-up bandwagon in the past few years, but what's on the label isn't always what you get in the formulation. Some brands have relabelled existing products with the word 'mineral', which is technically true as most conventional foundations do contain colour-delivering mineral pigments – but they come alongside not-so-natural ingredients. We are interested in more wholesome credentials. Here are our testers' top choices

LOOSE POWDER FOUNDATIONS
ANTIPODES PERFORMANCE PLUS SPF17 MINERAL FOUNDATION
✹✹
SCORE: 8.6/10

This recently launched, lightweight mineral powder formulation from a New Zealand brand also offers antioxidants (extracts of grapeseeds and kiwi fruit skins). It's good for all skin types, they say, including oily, blemished and rosacea (it's said to actively help reduce facial flushing). If you plan to carry it around in your bag, you can prevent the powder escaping through the teeny holes by swivelling the built-in plastic guard: otherwise it can (like many others) get very messy. From a choice of four shades, our testers had Medium Beige 03.

COMMENTS: 'Lovely to use: lightweight, covered minor imperfections. I use Max Factor Crème Puff normally and this felt much, much lighter, offering a natural, balanced, evened-out skin tone; bye-bye blemishes' • 'easy to apply with a smooth, dewy finish – not shiny, just healthy and natural' • 'helped cover fine thread veins around nose area; felt comfortable on the skin – not tight, and no clogging or breakouts either' • 'fantastic coverage and very buildable to cover any blemishes or marks when you want a night-time look' • 'after a previous bad experience with mineral make-up, I didn't hold out much hope – but how wrong I was: never found a product that makes my skin look glowing but not greasy before' • 'I will never use a liquid base again; I'm converted to mineral foundation – it is much more natural'.

AT A GLANCE

LOOSE POWDER FOUNDATIONS

ANTIPODES PERFORMANCE PLUS SPF17 MINERAL FOUNDATION

INIKA MINERAL FOUNDATION SPF15

BAREMINERALS ORIGINAL SPF15 FOUNDATION

COMPACT FOUNDATIONS

JANE IREDALE PUREPRESSED BASE MINERAL FOUNDATION

GREEN PEOPLE PRESSED MINERAL POWDER SPF15

FINISHING POWDER

BAREMINERALS MINERAL VEIL FINISHING POWDER

INIKA MINERAL FOUNDATION SPF15
✹✹
SCORE: 8.5/10

Inika was started up by New Zealander Miranda Bond, who became a natural beauty enthusiast in a quest to combat endometriosis. Now, her successful skincare brand, which includes a range of mineral make-up, is sold worldwide. Natural titanium and zinc oxides are the key skin-shielding ingredients in this base, with no synthetic or chemical fillers. It's available in seven shades – we dispatched Unity (which is at the fair end of the spectrum). This is best for at-home use with a kabuki brush. Unusually, Inika is one of the few make-up ranges that is halal approved (vegan too).

COMMENTS: 'A fantastic mineral foundation: I've tried a lot but this was far superior and gave my skin a beautiful glow that is generally only associated with youth' • 'natural finish, dewy and non-powdery; covered redness on the cheeks very, very well' • 'really good coverage – as good, or better than, my usual foundation brands, and long lasting, too' • 'fab product: weightless, yet provided evenness, plus perfect colour – and no dry feeling as with some mineral foundations'.

BAREMINERALS ORIGINAL SPF15 FOUNDATION
✹✹
SCORE: 8/10

bareMinerals popularised the buff-and-swirl technique (see page 19), and this is their original (and bestselling) formulation. As

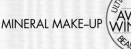

devotees will tell you, this loose powder feels like a cream while you're swirling it on. It comes in a mess-proof, swivel dispenser. Of the extensive shade spectrum (from Fair to Deepest Deep) we tested Fairly Light. NB: To learn the art of minerals, the brand offers in-store make-up lessons nationwide (and internationally).
COMMENTS: 'I love this stuff! Finish very natural; I have slightly oily skin but this stays put very well' • 'I only needed concealer on my darker scars' • 'my skin looks like me but better: like I've been airbrushed' • 'took a little while to learn to apply, but the results were great – skin looks blemish-free and even, as if you're not wearing make-up' • 'good coverage; gave my face a glow – and was easy to reapply in the afternoon to look pretty much perfect again'.

COMPACT FOUNDATIONS
JANE IREDALE PUREPRESSED BASE MINERAL FOUNDATION
✳
SCORE: 8.33/10
Love mineral make-up but hate the fact that the powder often goes everywhere…? Then you'll like this refillable, brushed-gold compact, ideal for applying at home and on-the-go touch ups (using their Handi Brush – like a small kabuki). The soft-focus powder formulation is infused with sea minerals and pine bark extract, offers an SPF20 (with a Skin Cancer Foundation Seal of Recommendation), and comes in an impressive 24 shades – Radiant was ours.
COMMENTS: 'Silky texture, very natural, lasted all day without retouching' • 'this is good for eliminating shine and great in hot weather; love the decadent 1920s-ish compact' • 'buildable coverage from sheer to full finish and balanced my skin tone; a healthy, dewy sheen, not chalky, and doesn't dry skin' • 'looks natural, yet skin appears loads better' • 'loose mineral powders need a perfect technique but this is really easy to build up coverage without looking "made up"' • 'am in love with this and would feel worried if I didn't have it with me!'

GREEN PEOPLE PRESSED MINERAL POWDER SPF15
✳✳✳
SCORE: 7.65/10
This unusual glossy (recyclable) black cardboard compact with a handy mirror gives an impressive level of matte coverage, so you can build it like a liquid 'conventional' base, or dust on lightly as a mattifying setting powder. Our testers' shade (of five) was Caramel.
COMMENTS: 'Very natural finish and managed to balance my skin tone, even around pronounced dark circles; smoothed out redness on my cheeks well' • 'completely perfume free, which I prefer in make-up products' • 'sheer coverage and healthy, lightened effect – I found it very good over tinted moisturiser' • 'nice and light, easy to apply – although more matte than my usual preferred dewy finish' • 'minimised the appearance of enlarged pores'.

FINISHING POWDER
BAREMINERALS MINERAL VEIL FINISHING POWDER
✳✳
SCORE: 8/10
Yet another winner from bareMinerals. A quick whisk of this airy, corn-starch-based translucent powder should keep make-up (including eyeshadow and lip colour, they say) set all day. It's shine absorbing, so particularly good for combination or oily skins, and helps minimise open/large pores, as well as giving a flattering soft-focus finish.
COMMENTS: 'Impressed with this when worn over foundation; helped to reduce look of pores as long as I only used a little' • 'complemented the colour of my foundation, and gave a more balanced complexion – no mess either! It has become a must in my make-up bag' • 'am always recommending this powder for its ability to even out skin tone; and it really helps make-up stay put all day' • 'pores look softer and less noticeable; mattifies and blurs imperfections; lasts all day with no shine breaking through'.

WE LOVE
Sarah is a happy occasional wearer of minerals, admiring the results when she does make the effort (or a kind make-up artist does it for her). But even after years of wanting to – and trying it – Jo still doesn't really love mineral powder make-up. However, we know lots of devotees and might be more motivated ourselves if we had problem skin as it is brilliant for everything from post op/post laser to rosacea, acne and eczema.

Your BEAUTY TOOL KIT

The right kit transforms the art of applying make-up. Maybe it takes a little extra time to acquire the techniques required, but as with any art or craft, the proper tools transform the task

Make-up applied with brushes and sponges lasts longer on the skin, as they press in products (rather than slicking the surface), turbo-charging their staying power.

Having said that, we're also fans of fingertips, particularly for foundation because the product is warmed up as you apply it, so it melds with your skin. But there is no way you can apply, for instance, mineral powder foundation – or powder blusher, bronzer, brow powder and so on – with your fingers.

Interestingly, when we asked brands for 'natural' brushes, some offered us animal bristles such as badger, sable, goat, squirrel, mink or horse, which is logical. But what we really wanted, we discovered, are guaranteed cruelty-free bristles – and this means synthetic (usually a fibre called Taklon). Plus: we like natural sustainable handles, eg, bamboo and recycled ferrules (the metal bit that joins bristles and handles).

Brands such as Ecotools meet all these criteria; we've also been long-term fans of Urban Decay's Good Karma range, Aveda and the Body Shop tools. (You'll find a list of 'Super Synthetics' plus more information on the website of People for the Ethical Treatment of Animals, www.peta.org).

You don't need a huge battery of brushes, so here are the ones we recommend and use ourselves. And remember, says make-up artist Jenny Jordan, an old friend and colleague, the trick to perfect application is blend, blend, blend.

Kabuki brush. The traditional tool to apply mineral powder foundation, this chunky, dense, short-handled brush is brilliant for buffing and swirling.

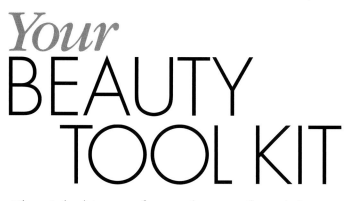

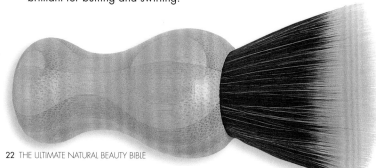

Domed blusher/bronzer brush. Perfect for sweeping colour across your face, you can also use this for buffing on mineral powder foundation.

Foam applicator. Instead of a traditional foundation brush, you might like to experiment with a sponge-on-a-stick.

> TIP:
> You can buy a special brow/lashes brush for separating mascara-ed lashes and grooming brows, but we tend to use an old (washed) mascara brush for both.

Powder brush. A big, fluffy brush – less dense, with longer hairs than a traditional kabuki – that you can use for blusher, bronzer and finishing powder. (You will need this if you choose a kabuki or foundation brush.)

Eyeshadow brush. Essential for applying your base shadow, also shading and highlighting; sweep it over lids and into creases, always blending outwards.

Eyeliner brush. In fact, we find this is fab for applying brow colour; we use it rather like an Italic pen nib, broad side across the thicker part of your eyebrows, then stroked down on end for the more slender outside. For eyeliner, you may prefer a teeny paint brush (as Sarah does), which can also be used to dot on concealer.

Foundation brush. This is optional, as we explain left, but many pros advise it (Sarah sometimes does, sometimes doesn't; for all but her most low-key at-home days, Jo does). Apply foundation to the back of your hand, then dip the brush in that, so as not to overload.

Lip brush. This is a bit of an optional extra, especially if you are using a lip liner pencil, but there's no doubt it gives you a quick, crisp outline.

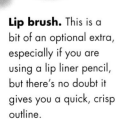

Cosmetic extras

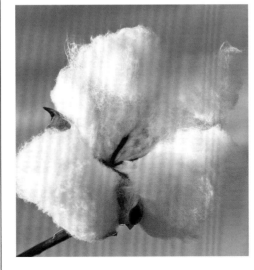

Cotton wool pads, balls and buds. These are now all widely available in organic cotton.

Make-up sponges. We looked for natural versions online but frankly the customer testimonials were generally so dismal we can't recommend you try. You could try cellulose facial sponges designed to remove make-up. (We don't use them, anyway.)

Tweezers. You can find recycled ones but the reviews weren't that great, so you might want to fight your eco-battles elsewhere and stick to Tweezerman.

What have you got TO HIDE?

Many – if not most – women have something they want to conceal, from small flaws, acne, brown spots and dark circles to more significant port-wine stains and scarring. Cosmetics today offer effective camouflage for everyone

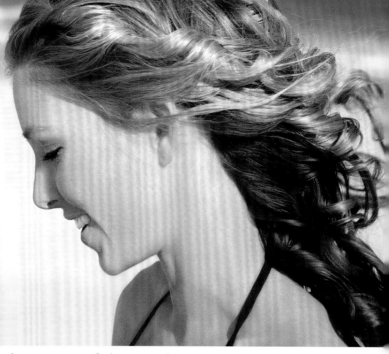

When our very first *Beauty Bible* launched in 1996, we teamed up with a wonderful charity called Changing Faces, which supports people and their families who are living with conditions, marks or scars that affect their appearance. The founder James Partridge, whose patchwork face (similar to Simon Weston's) is the result of a car accident when he was 18, wanted girls and women with disfigured faces to feel as entitled as any of us to buy glam make-up and wander round a beauty hall without feeling they didn't belong.

We're not saying that your (and our) natural desire to soften forehead furrows, correct pigmentation or camouflage dark circles and acne scars is wrong. But it is a reality check to see what some people have to deal with 24/7.

For the one in 111 people in the UK with a significant facial disfigurement, the best route if they wish to conceal it (and not everyone does) is a professional service. In the Directory of this book, you will find a list of resources.

For the rest of us, today's technology is so sophisticated that there is a wide range of effective options to choose from. And to our delight, more natural products are now stepping up to the mark, as you can see from our Award Winners, opposite.

However, one problem that has become clear from questions to our website, www.beautybible.com, is what Liz Earle calls 'concealer confusion'! It's a common complaint that afflicts many would-be consumers and the

symptom is being uncertain of what sort to choose… So here's the low-down: there are two main types of concealer (which are occasionally called 'correctors'). These are:

● Light-reflecting concealers for areas you want to brighten.
● Non-light-reflecting or matte concealers for areas you want to fade.

Light-reflecting concealers brighten dark shadows round the eye. Use them in the inner and outer corners to 'lift' those areas. If the whole eye area is looking shadowy and/or 'tired', apply a thin triangle of light-reflecting concealer (they often come in pen dispensers with a fine brush) under the bottom lash line, going down to a point on the top of your cheekbone, then patting it in – very, very gently – over the area. If you have eye bags, dot and blend a little along the bottom crease line of the bag, above your cheekbone, to soften and blur it. Also try applying under the brow bone to make eyes look brighter and 'lifted'. Sarah also dabs a teeny bit into her frown line, as 'Polyfilla'.

Non-light-reflective (matte) concealers will disguise really dark circles, 'age' spots (aka 'brown', 'liver' or 'sun' spots), scars and small blemishes. For eye bags, use a shade very slightly darker than your skin tone as this will 'knock back' the puffiness more effectively. Then finish with a few dots of light-reflecting concealer, as above.

As you can see from our Award Winners, there is a choice of format: creamy crayons, wand-style dispensers with brushes, and palettes so you can custom-blend your concealer. It is usually best to apply concealer after foundation.

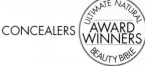

CONCEALERS
our award winners

Concealers disguise a raft of imperfections: light-reflective options work best for shadows and lines, while non-reflective formulas hide blemishes and pigmentation (see opposite for more details). We trialled 25 – here are the top three

WILD ABOUT BEAUTY SMOOTH COVER CONCEALER KIT

✳

SCORE: 8.33/10

This clever 'custom-blend' palette offers a flip-top jar with two shades of concealer in the top, which you can mix (use a finger and the back of your hand) to get your perfect shade. Then unscrew the jar and 'set' with the translucent powder. Being a non-light-reflective option, it's good for spots, red veins and sun spots (though testers also used it under eyes). Wild About Beauty – the brand started by Louise Redknapp – is big on botanicals: here, skin-caring sea whip marine extract, and vitamins C and E. **COMMENTS:** 'Love this: the consistency, the coverage, the packaging, the setting powder – what a great product. It's good for fine lines, evens out pigmentation and hides blemishes beautifully' • 'this product covers redness but still looks natural' • 'the two colours mean you can correct under-eye circles with the lighter shade, while covering up blemishes with the slightly darker tone' • 'very quick and simple to apply; I loved this light concealer with its excellent coverage – fab! A new must-have for me' • 'no cakey-ness, no drying' • 'work colleagues of various ages tried this product too, and loved it'.

LIZ EARLE LIGHT REFLECTING CONCEALER

✴

SCORE: 8.22/10

There are two concealers in the Liz Earle range (Perfect Fix is the alternative) but the wand-style Light Reflecting option is best for dark circles and brushing along furrows and frown-lines, as the light-diffusing pigments deliver a 'blurring' effect. From the four shades, our testers tried Fair 01. This is Sarah's daily choice for under-eye

TIP: When you're covering under-eye shadows, be sure to smooth concealer into the dark corners between the inner eye and nose-bone. It's an effective way to brighten tired eyes.

freshening, brightening and evening out skin tone. It also effectively hides a pigmented spot. **COMMENTS:** 'I'm a long-term YSL Touche Éclat user but this is a different animal – lighter, and seems to have a higher concentration of light-reflective pigments. Blended very well with my natural skin tone without looking patchy' • 'the pen made it easy to apply; it blends well, and lines around my eyes were well concealed' • 'good coverage of veins and not bad on scars' • 'pigmentation was less obvious due to the lightening, brightening effect' • 'a great product which I'd definitely use again'.

GREEN PEOPLE MULTI-ACTIVE PENCIL CONCEALER

✴ ✴

SCORE: 7.45/10

This is a chubby matte pencil that you stroke over redness and blemishes. (Not so effective on dark circles, we'd say, as you really need light-reflective ingredients for that.) They suggest it's applied over foundation or, if your skin's pretty good but just needs a little evening out, over moisturiser. It contains skin-caring botanicals including argan and babassu oils, as well as zinc oxide to soothe touchy skin. It's also said to camouflage spots well, and has antimicrobial ingredients to help heal as it conceals. **COMMENTS:** 'Ridiculously simple to apply and blended easily with a brush, finger or sponge' • 'really good coverage on blemishes' • 'I thought a pencil would be drying and difficult to blend, but oh, how wrong… I've been a Touche Éclat girl for years, but this is genius – it's become my favourite' • 'the easiest concealer I have used; I wore it with BB cream and powder and had compliments on my skin' • 'I'm pale and concealers are usually too dark for me, but the pencil was perfect' • 'this did a great job of concealing thread veins'.

EYES RIGHT

We could make your eyes cross with all the stuff we know about eye make-up but actually there are some basic guidelines that make life simpler. Here's what we have found works on a daily basis – over our many (many) years in the beauty business…

1 **Most women need mascara on top and bottom lashes every day.** Choose black or dark brown. Find one that doesn't clump, shed or end up down your cheeks (that means water-resistant in the case of more natural mascaras). Slender wands are the easiest to use. If you are fluffing powder on your face, leave your mascara 'til last. Don't keep your mascara for longer than three months or it's likely to get gummed-up and bug-ridden.

2 **Apply base on your eyelids.** Sweeping foundation or matte concealer all over your lids makes eyeshadow last longer, look better, and covers any red or discoloration. Or use bone/ivory eyeshadow.

3 **Brighten up the under-eye area with light-reflecting concealer.** Once you get the hang of this, you will do it every day because it makes such a difference. We find wand-style products easiest. Apply after foundation: put a dab in the dark corners either side of your nose, then take it down under your eyes – magic for disguising dark circles and also puffy bags when you stroke it over the creases.

4 **Smoky eyes can be gorgeous but don't suit everyone.** TV make-up artists always applied swathes of cloudy colour to Sarah's peepers until Jo told them not to bother: 'She'll just go to the loo and wipe it all off.' If you do want to try a smoky eye (and it can look fantastic for evening), have a makeover with a pro at a big store (most offer freebies), or see Lisa Eldridge demo-ing her Organic/natural make-up look at www.beautybible.com, which includes a smoky eye. Then decide if it suits you or you prefer a 'clean' look.

5 **'Clean' means neutral and neat.** Mineral eyeshadows come in a dazzling array of colours (we mentioned Cleopatra and her fondness for zingy green malachite on page 19). But we suggest that, unless you are 17 or a woman of colour, you steer clear of rainbow shades and opt for flattering soft browns, taupes, greys, slate blues or dusty purples, accentuated with cream or gold. For a neat, elegant look, keep it on the lids only;

don't be tempted to wing it up in the socket or out towards your temples – then you're straying into the smoky eye zone. The most important thing is to blend the colour in, and then blend it again.

6 **Warm up a high brow line.** If you have a lot of space between the eye socket and your brows, fluff a little blush over. Vice versa, if your brows are crashing down into your eyes, apply a touch of pearlised cream or ivory shadow to highlight that area. NB: We counsel against pink shadow nearer your eyes though, or you risk looking like one of those raspberry-eyed mice.

7 **Crêpey-skinned areas need a light touch with shimmer.** Mineral shadows tend to have an inherent shine, which can draw attention to lines and wrinkles. Keep the colour soft and coverage light on eyelids and avoid anything shiny in the socket.

8 **Eyeliner looks best dotted right into the roots of lashes, then stroked to blend in.** Unless you are a dab hand with liquid eyeliner, use a soft sharpened pencil (see overleaf for our Award Winners). Or wet your eyeshadow and apply it with a small brush. Careful placement can subtly enhance the shape of your eyes: if they are close-set, for instance, start liner in the centre and wing it out. To create a more almond eye, focus on the V-shape at the outer corners.

9 **Well-shaped brows can enhance the architecture of your whole face.** At the very least, tidy up stragglers over your nose and under the arches. (Even Cara Delevingne's fabulous black beetles get a wee bit of grooming.) Visit our website, www.beautybible.com, and search for 'Brow Beat' for lots of details on how to pluck, and the best shape for your face.

10 **Fill in brows with a sharp brow pencil.** Use short hair-like strokes and work in the direction of hair growth. Of the more natural options, we like Liz Earle's Brow Pencil, which comes in two shades, a fair taupe and a dark brown – you don't need more.

EYESHADOWS
our award winners

We trialled cream and powder eyeshadows – over 30 natural options – but the powders were so far ahead that we didn't feel the creams were worth featuring in this book. From flattering neutral shades for everyday to smouldering metallics for perfect smoky eyes, these are your best bets (without a shadow of a doubt)

ORIGINS PEEPER PLEASER POWDER EYE SHADOW
✷

SCORE: 8.11/10

This highly pigmented, silky-smooth shadow 'single' is available in 10 shades: our testers had the classic Copper Penny, a shimmering sheer bronze. (NB: Since it glimmers, keep away from the socket if you have any lines, droops or crêpiness – reserve for the lids.) They come in nifty little round compacts, and if you prefer to put together your own colour combos, rather than go for ready-made combinations (as with the other winners), you'll love these.

COMMENTS: 'Top-quality pressed powder; good colour density: smoothed on and blended well, lasted all day, no irritation with contact lens, no flakiness, no creasing – the perfect eye make-up!' • 'I love shimmery shadow for summer and this was just the right amount without looking OTT for daytime' • 'lovely, silky texture and easy to blend, so I'm going to check out the other shades' • 'equal to the MAC range in quality and high pigment' • 'I loved this eyeshadow; I am so impressed with the results here – not least because it didn't fall onto the face at all, as some do'.

BAREMINERALS READY EYESHADOW 4.0
✷

SCORE: 8/10

bareMinerals clearly listened to their many customers who love the effect of mineral make-up but find it a little, well, messy, at times. They've now pressed the shadow so it delivers the same flattering effect without powder going everywhere. Our testers had The Next Big Thing compact – a mirrored quartet and inside a gleaming gold,

AT A GLANCE

ORIGINS PEEPER PLEASER POWDER EYE SHADOW

BAREMINERALS READY EYESHADOW 4.0

GREEN PEOPLE CITY SKY EYE DUO

TIP:
To get the best out of your eyeshadows, blend into lids with a brush. Don't bother with the fiddly applicators that come with eyeshadows (sorry, they go straight in the bin...). There are now so many great cruelty-free brushes available (see page 22), that we suggest you invest in a set for smooth, long-lasting eyeshadow application.

bright copper, smoky black, and a matte neutral highlighter, plus a double-ended applicator. The shades feature what bareMinerals call their 'SeaNutritive Mineral Complex', which contains cold-pressed borage oil, revitalising caffeine and cucumber to 'power' the product.

COMMENTS: 'Stays on all day even without primer' • 'loved the colours – very wearable – and also the booklet which showed you how to achieve different looks with the shadows' • 'great texture and easy to apply, no fallout, either' • 'nice and soft – the eyeshadow feels creamy, even though it's a powder' • 'good staying power' • 'easy-peasy to use! Lovely silky shadows and they blend like a dream'.

GREEN PEOPLE CITY SKY EYE DUO
✷ ✷

SCORE: 7.75/10

This is a simple black magnetised cardboard and mirrored compact (no plastic waste), which flips open to give you a slate grey with a hazy beige shade. The pressed mineral shadows are finely milled for ultra-smoothness, are talc free, and offer a touch of skin-softening jojoba and sunflower. Ecocert-certified natural, rather than certified completely organic (minerals don't count in their calculations).

COMMENTS: 'I'd never used a mineral shadow but I found this one easy to use and it gave a great smoky-eye look' • 'an almost-creamy texture, even though it's a powder' • 'did not irritate my eyes' • 'love it! One of the best-quality eyeshadows I've used – the only nicer one is by Bobbi Brown' • 'didn't make my hooded eyes too noticeable, unlike others' • 'soft, velvety to the touch and very blendable; smooth, with less dragging than my usual Clinique, Estée Lauder eyeshadows' • 'a handy mirror'.

EYELINERS
our award winners

Do you prefer a fine pencil liner, or a rock-chick smoky eye? Or maybe a liquid for a Marilyn Monroe-esque kitten flick? Whichever eye look is your signature, our panels of testers found great-performing natural eyeliners for each. We tested the eternally classic black, or the nearest shade to it

WILD ABOUT BEAUTY LINE & DEFINE LINER PEN

❋

SCORE: 8.5/10

Despite precious few natural eyeliner pens on the market, this rivals pretty much any liner we've trialled. The felt-pen-style product from Louise Redknapp's range features soothing organic chamomile water. Carbon-black 01 Max is the single shade.

COMMENTS: 'Sooooo easy to use: goes on smoothly and doesn't drag' • 'Fantastic! Had the effect of making eyelashes look instantly thicker; took just seconds to get a brilliant line and, best of all, it stayed put all day yet was easy to remove' • 'my eyes are quite sensitive, but no problems with this' • 'considering I normally look like a clown when I apply liner, this was a miracle product' • 'could also be smudged with a cottonbud for a great smoky look' • 'the best eyeliner I've found – I've used it daily and will replace when it wears out'.

GREEN PEOPLE ANTI-AGE EYELINER

❋ ❋

SCORE: 8/10

With skin-nurturing jojoba, shea butter (to help glide), and vitamins C and E, this will suit even the most sensitive eyes. Testers loved City Grey (the other shade is Forest Brown; no black).

COMMENTS: 'Never thought organic make-up could be this good: it's easy to apply and smudge for a smoky eye, doesn't irritate, and the colour's flattering – looked beautiful in photos, too!' • 'smooth application, didn't drag and was easy to blend' • 'nice and soft, and I felt reassured by its naturalness as I was using it so close to my eyes' • 'goodness me, what an admission, but this is the first time I've used an

---

AT A GLANCE

WILD ABOUT BEAUTY LINE & DEFINE LINER PEN

GREEN PEOPLE ANTI-AGE EYELINER

BELLÁPIERRE EYE LINER

LIZ EARLE EYE PENCIL

TIP:
Invest in a sharpener for your eyeliner pencil, and in warm weather, pop your pencil in the fridge for a while before using it.

---

eyeliner (had to ask a colleague how); it's soft and gentle, makes my eyes look bigger – and I feel naked without it now!' • 'a joy to apply' • 'lovely kohl-like texture which smudges and then stays put' • 'lasted longer than any other pencils I've used and didn't need "topping up"'.

BELLÁPIERRE EYE LINER

❋

SCORE: 8/10

Rich mineral pigments make for the intense colour of these liners. There are five to choose from – we tested Charcoal. Bellápierre adds skin-friendly jojoba and safflower waxes, plus vitamin E, in a hypoallergenic formulation.

COMMENTS: 'Colour stayed true with no smudging. Given that I often heat up (as the menopause takes its toll), this was a star at staying put' • 'a fabulous eyeliner: it has a creamy texture, is blendable, lasts all day without turning greasy – and charcoal is the perfect shade for the over-30s' • 'this didn't smudge or flake, and it's long lasting, too'.

LIZ EARLE EYE PENCIL

❋ ❋

SCORE: 7.67/10

Again, silky waxes make for a smooth finish that doesn't drag, and a texture that can be blended for smoky sultriness. From the choice of three shades, we dispatched 01 Black to our testers.

COMMENTS: 'By far the easiest eye pencil I've used – soft, and with no dragging' • 'butter-soft, glides on like a dream and great for a smoky eye, too' • 'the point kept its shape nicely and hasn't diminished with repeated use' • 'perfect for an eyeliner novice like me' • 'lasted longer between sharpenings than other eyeliners that I've tried'.

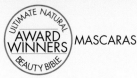

MASCARAS
our award winners

Well, things are really improving on the more-natural-than-most mascara front! Previously for *The Green Beauty Bible* testers were underwhelmed by the performance of the mascaras – but these innovations sweep to victory

ORIGINS GINZING BRIGHTENING MASCARA
✳

SCORE: 8.25/10

By the standards of all our mascara trials, this is a great score. The 'grippy' brush sweeps on a lash-conditioning blend of waxes, plus ginseng and an 'Eye-Brightening Pearl Complex' (with high-contrast black and blue pearl pigments) to make eyes look brighter. Vitamins B complex and E, rosemary extract, hyaluronic acid and glycerine complete the picture. Black only.

COMMENTS: 'No flaking, no clumping, glossy and lustrous – a great product' • 'made my lashes look very long and glamorous, and opened up my eyes' • 'my tiny lashes looked enormous, like false ones – very impressed' • 'an amazing mascara! A colleague stopped me to say what lovely eyes I have (I don't), next day my boss asked what mascara I was using because it really makes my eyes pop' • 'best mascara I've ever used – love it, love it, love it'.

LIZ EARLE LASH DEFINITION SMUDGEPROOF MASCARA
✳

SCORE: 7.88/10

This is Jo's favourite (more) natural mascara: the slimline wand grips her sparse lashes as it's designed to make the most of even the shortest lengths. If it's extra volume you're after, Liz Earle also makes a mascara base. Our panellists tried Black (Brown is the other option).

COMMENTS: 'Couldn't believe how well this performs; will be buying again' • 'didn't flake, crumble or smudge and made lashes look very glossy' • 'lasted all day and didn't run – this survived several bouts of tears (I had quite a traumatic time while trialling it)' • 'found the brush very effective at coating all lashes from root to tip – better than my current mascara'.

AT A GLANCE

ORIGINS GINZING BRIGHTENING MASCARA

LIZ EARLE LASH DEFINITION SMUDGEPROOF MASCARA

WILD ABOUT BEAUTY NUTRILASH MASCARA

NATORIGIN LENGTHENING MASCARA

> **TIP:** Remember to wipe your mascara wand on a tissue before and during use to prevent unwelcome blobs. Truly clump-free options don't exist, in our opinion.

WILD ABOUT BEAUTY NUTRILASH MASCARA
✳

SCORE: 7.88/10

Wild About Beauty claim that the natural, lash-boosting ingredients in this will promote healthy growth (without the use of synthetic pharmaceutical substances, which appear in many lash enhancers). Marine algae extract, 'cotton bloom' and grapeseed feature, together with a moisturising ingredient (new to us) called quackgrass. Black is the only shade.

COMMENTS: 'It separated lashes well, didn't clump or smudge, excellent staying power but removed easily' • 'lashes look more lustrous and healthy' • 'long-lasting even in the rain; wasn't left with panda eyes or clumped mascara at the end of the day; in fact, I could apply a few more coats at night and still look glamorous but not an over-the-top false-lashes look'.

NATORIGIN LENGTHENING MASCARA
✳ ✳ ✳

SCORE: 7.86/10

It's challenging to create mascaras using only natural ingredients (the above three do feature some synthetics), but this is 98.5 per cent natural – quite an achievement. In a choice of four shades (we trialled Black), it conditions with a blend of Arctic raspberry seed oil, essential fatty acids, red algae, jojoba oil and shea butter, and is approved by Allergy UK.

COMMENTS: 'Loved, loved this product: it's excellent at lash-lengthening, with a result almost like natural-looking fine false lashes' • 'glossy and lustrous, very different to most mascaras' • 'didn't irritate my eyes at all; have used every day and will buy again' • 'tested this through a summer of bad hay fever with only minimal smudging, which is fantastic'.

LUSTRE MUST

Give eyelashes a boost with this conditioner. The nourishing blend of sage and olive oil will add length, fullness and shine to both lashes and brows

SAGE LASH CONDITIONER

Fact: we're not at all keen on many proprietary lash-growth-booster products. (Some even contain pharmaceutical substances which may pose risks to eye health.) This lash treatment is as gentle as can be and enhances brow lustre, safely nurturing in the most natural way.

- 20g (1oz) fresh sage (or half the quantity of dried herb)
- 75ml (3fl oz) purified tap, mineral or rain water
- 2 tablespoons olive oil

Place the sage and water in a saucepan, bring to the boil and simmer for 10 minutes. Cool and strain through a muslin cloth or a kitchen towel. Put 1 tablespoon of the tisane into a small-necked bottle with a lid; add the olive oil and give the bottle a good shake.

Before using the lash conditioner, always shake the bottle to mix the oil and water elements. Use a clean mascara wand to apply the mixture to eyelashes. NB: Wash and rinse the wand after use to ensure it's sterile; leave to dry on a radiator or near a heated towel rail.

The oil can also be stroked along brows to add lustre; the sage can have a slightly darkening effect, so you may find you don't need to use so much mascara or brow pencil.

LET'S TALK LIPPY

Or to be precise, the shade you choose and its effect on other people. It turns out your choice of colours influences the judgement they make about your personality – in the first instant they set eyes on you. And it might not be quite the reaction you intended…

We would take a small bet that the first make-up item you ever bought was a lipstick. We'd also gamble on the fact that, for many – perhaps most – girls, that first purchase, and probably many after, veered towards a natural rose or nude rather than full-blown crimson or shocking pink. We've come a long way from the days when lipstick and rouge were associated with 'Scarlet Women' but bold lips do demand a matching confidence in the wearer, new research reveals.

In a recent survey of 1,000 women (commissioned by cosmetic brand Avon) – a real Life, the Universe and Lipsticks exercise – over 80 per cent perceived those wearing a bright lipstick as confident. And over half said they felt more confident themselves when sporting a bright shade. Then it all gets a tiny bit confusing because when it came to going to an interview – for which you'd think you really wanted to feel confident – less than six per cent said they would choose a bright colour.

But don't rely on a bright red lippy to change your whole attitude. 'While it communicates confidence, it doesn't actually build it in the less self-assured,' according to colour psychologist Angela Wright. Red shades also represent a competitive streak and teamed with head-to-toe black 'could be perceived as aggressive', she says.

However, Wright continues, 'when paired correctly, bright colours can portray openness and exude a friendly vibe'. A bit more than friendly, perhaps: women in the survey generally admitted to feeling downright sexier when wearing bright lipstick and over a third said they would choose a brighter shade for a first date.

It might pay to consider your intentions first: red is physically stimulating, raising the pulse rate and physical energy – a reflection of arousal. So make sure you aren't making a statement bolder than your intentions…

While paler shades usually painted the wearer as 'shy', over 60 per cent of the women surveyed said they would wear pale hues for a job interview, the first day of a new job – and meeting their partner's family for the first time. 'Pale or nude lipstick colours are the safe option,' comments Angela Wright. But beware the dark side. Women who wear darker shades were mostly judged as 'unfriendly' – guess that's the Cruella factor. We know the feeling: Sarah chose a dark red matte lipstick for a passport photo years ago – the only one to hand as she dashed out – and it was definitely disturbing whenever she had to show it. (She's never worn the colour since.)

HOW TO FIND YOUR PERFECT LIPSTICK

Red, rose, coral, peach or nude? Pale or bright? Sheer, glossy or matte? Thing is, we can have them all nowadays, in a galaxy of colours. And we are delighted that natural versions now offer such gorgeous shades and textures (see page 36). The only rule is that it should suit you beautifully –so here's how to set about it:

Choose lipstick in a well-lit store, and always try in daylight before you decide.

The colour should complement your skin, eyes and hair: so try lippy when you are not wearing foundation or much other make-up.

The most flattering lip tones are just a shade or two darker, brighter or stronger than your natural colour. To test, apply the product to one lip only (with a cotton bud) and compare. (If you have pale lips, try biting them until they turn pink.)

Try on lots of colours: and notice the tones that really make your eyes or hair pop, advises lipstick guru Poppy King. Keep looking in the mirror until you see the magic happening.

Here are some general guidelines:

● Very pale skins should try nudes and peaches, or soft, natural rose.

● Fair to middling complexions often look best with nude lip liner as a base, and rosy-brown gloss on top.

● Darker complexions can embellish lips with brights of every kind.

● Olive-toned skin looks great in coral, and most shades actually, except for brown (too similar to your skin) and anything with a lot of blue or purple, because they highlight the yellow undertones and make you look sallow.

● Thin-lipped lovelies should stay away from dark shades and opt for creamy textures or tinted glosses to add plumpness and attract the light.

● Pink-toned lipsticks do not suit less-than-white teeth: they accentuate the yellow, so stick to more coral-caramel colours. (NB: Dental hygienists can often brighten and whiten teeth effectively without bleaching.)

● If you are really uncertain, go to a big store and ask several consultants what colour/s they recommend for you. NB: Remove one colour completely before trying another.

● Being a scarlet woman for evening is a great glam look but opt for a sheer red rather than matte lipstick if you like to wear significant eye make-up. If you want to wear bold opaque red, keep eyes more minimal or you risk losing the impact of both.

BERRY SENSATION

Cheap, safe, all-natural and it works instantly: we can't think of anything more we want in a tooth brightener

STRAWBERRY SMILE BRIGHTENER

This makes a delicious and effective brightening paste. Apply as often as you have time – and strawberries.

- 1 ripe strawberry
- ½ teaspoon baking powder

Crush the strawberry to a pulp, and then mix with the baking powder. Paint the mixture onto teeth and allow to set for five minutes. Then use a soft toothbrush to lighten and brighten teeth. To remove the mixture, be sure to brush thoroughly with your normal toothpaste. Rinse with plenty of clear water.

TIP: Eat raspberries: these are reputed to help dissolve plaque... Plus, chew on spearmint leaves and rub a leaf of fresh sage over your teeth: these herbs will brighten teeth, boost the condition of gums and prevent bad breath.

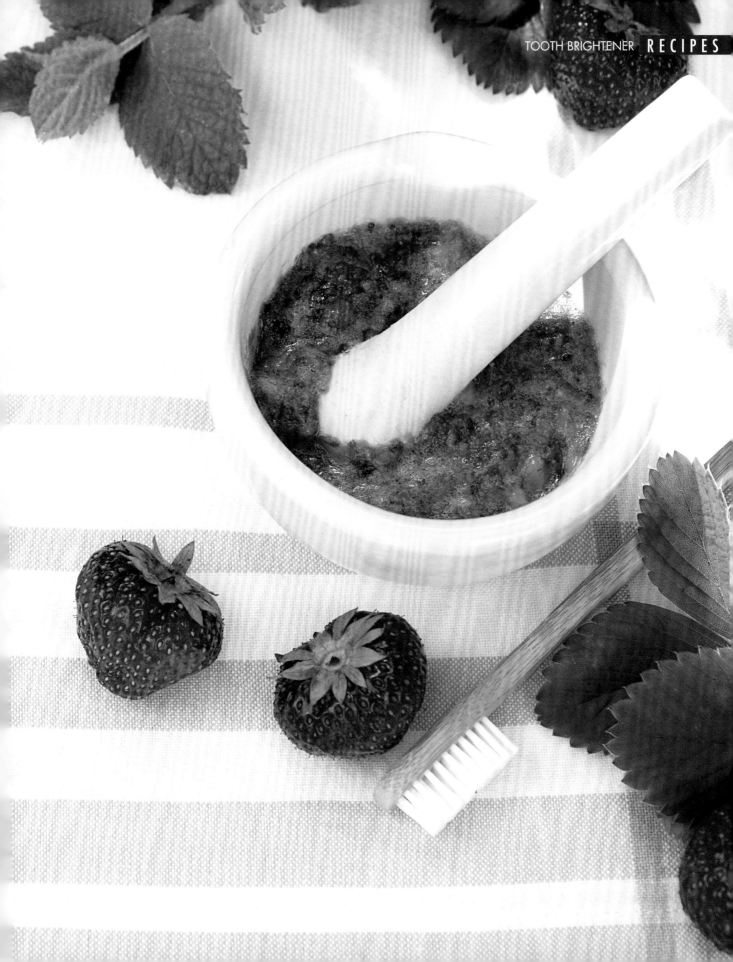

LIPSTICKS
our award winners

These days, there is little difference between 'conventional' and natural lipsticks in terms of staying power, choice of shades and comfort as these winning scores highlight. We've always preferred natural options, and now so do our testers

ANTIPODES HIT ME WITH YOUR BEST SHOT LIPSTICK
✳ ✳

SCORE: 8.14/10

We don't quite get the name, but testers got the point of this creamy mineral lipstick from the New Zealand brand. It has a matte finish with a hint of shine, featuring avocado oil for lip nourishment. Testers had High Pink: a va-va-voom shade; there are neutrals available, too.
COMMENTS: 'Smooth, creamy, comfortable to wear – this lasted well after drinking and eating' • 'velvety with a slight sheen: feels comfy, not dry' • 'a long-lasting lipstick that stays put' • 'I love this lippy: as a redhead, when I opened it I was shocked by the colour – but it looks good on; several people commented' • 'very comfortable; has a suede-like texture that lasted extremely well through drinks.'

NATORIGIN LIPSTICK
✳ ✳ ✳

SCORE: 7.83/10

This lipstick's approved by Allergy UK and the Vegetarian Society: a super-moisturising formula with oils of jojoba seed, sunflower, marula seed, castor seed and sweet almond, plus a trio of soft (and softening) waxes. Testers commented on its lip-hydrating power. There are six shades to choose from: our testers had Lychee.
COMMENTS: 'I have quite dry lips but I found this was very soothing' • 'a soft texture, very creamy' • 'it feels like it's moisturising lips while providing colour' • 'would be fantastic to use in winter to keep lips well hydrated' • 'probably one of the best moisturising lipsticks I've ever used; my sister fell in love with this as soon as she saw it and has bought her own' • 'soft, with a lovely sheen – more of a tint than a full-on colour, but really pleasant to use'.

WE LOVE

We opt for natural lippies as we 'eat' so much lipstick that it probably qualifies as a food group... Jo is a big fan of Dr.Hauschka lip colours which are moisturising and available in great shades, including seasonal limited editions. Sarah is a fan of Essential Care and Neal's Yard Remedies lip formulas which are creamy and come in a spectrum of colours.

NEAL'S YARD REMEDIES LIPSTICK
✳ ✳ ✳

SCORE: 7.81/10

Neal's Yard's relatively new make-up range offers six shades of Soil Association-certified colour combined with care: the softening, moisturising ingredients include organic shea butter and beeswax, their own Organic Beauty Oil, plus sweet orange peel oil for a subtle, refreshing scent and taste. Our testers put the Pomegranate shade through its paces.
COMMENTS: 'Felt very nourishing on the lips, more like a balm; hardly felt like I was wearing a lipstick' • 'a gorgeous silky smooth texture: it was fantastic, delivering a wonderful lustre and no stickiness' • 'I was surprised how long the colour lasted since it feels more like a balm than a lipstick' • 'colour lasts a long time – my 81-year-old mother tried it and she noticed that even though the initial glossiness disappeared, she still had some colour on her lips hours later'.

AVEDA NOURISH-MINT SMOOTHING LIP COLOR
✳ ✳ ✳

SCORE: 7.69/10

We've always enjoyed these Aveda lipsticks for their tingly mintiness. Plant and fruit waxes feature to plump and hydrate. NB: These come as refills (we approve of that); the utilitarian-grey packaging is fine on its own but if you crave extra glamour, spring for the lipstick case, too. Testers trialled Mulberry, out of 20 shades.
COMMENTS: 'Beautiful to apply: felt light and nourishing' • 'left lips feeling smooth and moisturised' • 'I personally liked the simple packaging which made it practical to carry around' • 'gives an attractive, plumped look but not over-glossy' • 'lasted well, though did wear off after eating and drinking'.

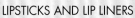

LIP LINERS
our award winners

A pencil helps prevent colour from bleeding, corrects small imperfections in shape, and if used to 'draw' all over the lips, it'll help your lipstick to stay in place for longer. Our one proviso? The lip-liner law is: always choose a neutral shade

KORRES LIPLINER PENCIL
✹✹✹
SCORE: 7.89/10

This Greek brand has come a long way since we first met the founders over a decade ago. The line – which grew out of their popular Athens pharmacy and has now gone global – achieved brilliant results in *The Green Beauty Bible* and testers still love it. Kind-to-skin ingredients in this velvety pencil include shea butter and vitamin E. The liner comes in five shades, though as usual we recommend the one that's closest to natural lips in tone: Neutral Light. That's the shade our testers report back on here; they recommend sharpening this regularly.
COMMENTS: 'Easy to apply and didn't drag; seemed to make lipstick and lip gloss last a little longer and gave a good base' • 'I haven't used a lip liner in years and was a bit frightened of looking very 90s; I remember lip pencil being very dry then and dragging when applied, but this product was soft, smooth and went on very easily' • 'lovely texture; gave subtle definition to my lips' • 'a really great product that is a pleasure to use and looks good on' • 'made my lipstick last longer and I liked the flattering colour a lot; I loved this and think it's a good replacement for my current liner'.

INIKA MINERAL LIP LINER
✹✹✹
SCORE: 7.29/10

From this Australian cosmetics brand (of which we're longstanding fans), a certified-organic creamy pencil featuring a range of cold-pressed plant waxes and oils (including sweet almond, sesame, palm and carnauba wax), blended with natural mineral pigments. Of the four shades Inika offers, the one our testers trialled was Safari – a perfect nude, exactly as we

AT A GLANCE
KORRES
LIPLINER PENCIL

INIKA
MINERAL LIP LINER

LIZ EARLE
LIP PENCIL

WE LOVE
Jo uses the Liz Earle Lip Pencil featured here (in the same Carnation shade), often applying it over rather than under lipstick, to 'seal' the colour in place. Sarah favours the same one but is delighted to find two other good options here (our consumer surveys are useful for us, too...).

recommend. It comes with a sharpener built into the lid, which testers really liked.
COMMENTS: 'This liner lasted from breakfast till after lunch, probably about five hours – pretty impressive' • 'just glides on and didn't dry my lips at all, which is a problem with all the other liners I've tried' • 'my lipstick lasted longer than normal' • 'usually, lip colour lasts until I've had a drink or eaten; by applying this underneath (thanks for the tip!), it stayed put through eating and drinking' • 'the sharpener is brilliant; it's so annoying when a pencil's blunt and you can't find anything to sharpen it with' • 'I found this nice and creamy – a great product that I'd definitely buy again; I don't usually bother with lip liner and this converted me'.

LIZ EARLE LIP PENCIL
✹
SCORE: 7.1/10

Liz's make-up range has done well with our testers – here, with a pigment-rich pencil enriched with vitamin E, cottonseed oil and jojoba. (NB: The first ingredient on the list is paraffin, just for your information; the Liz Earle make-up isn't as natural as the skincare because they didn't want to compromise on performance, and found it hard to achieve with all-natural ingredients, they told us.) The shade Carnation – a great neutral – was dispatched.
COMMENTS: 'Gave a good colour and looked natural; when applied over whole lip area it lasts exceptionally well (up to six hours) and leaves a nice, matte finish' • 'liked this and would buy it again in various different shades' • 'left my lips feeling nourished at the end of the day, and didn't seem to dry them out' • 'my pencil is worn down to an inch-and-a-half tiny stub and I am about to order two more: one for the larder, so I don't run out again'.

LIP GLOSSES
our award winners

Lip glosses are like shoes: you can never have too many. And natural glosses are not only high performers, they're packed with heavenly ingredients that truly are – yes, you know it! – good enough to eat. We'll be adding these winners to our collection

BAREMINERALS MARVELOUS MOXIE LIPGLOSS

✳

SCORE: 8.57/10

bareMinerals launched an entire range with the trademarked Moxie name: it means 'the ability to face difficulty with spirit and courage'. Natural elements of shea, murumuru and avocado butters give the lip-quenching effect, alongside minerals and antioxidant vitamins. It tastes – though not too strongly – of a combo of mint and vanilla, and tingles slightly as it glosses. According to independent trials carried out for bareMinerals, this gloss, delivered by a specially angled wand applicator, enhances lip fullness when used for at least four weeks. Of the 14 shades, our testers slicked on Rebel (pink-mauve).
COMMENTS: 'Absolutely loved this: made my lips look fuller and better' • 'comfortable, and felt more like a light lipstick than a gloss' • 'the applicator makes it easy to avoid "clown mouth" when you're in a hurry' • 'very good coverage, lasts on the lips a couple of hours, and looks luscious' • 'the colour was subtle and the finish (which I loved) very glossy – not shimmery, more of a wet look' • 'a great all-rounder for lips – and a keeper for me'.

AVEDA NOURISH-MINT REHYDRATING LIP GLAZE

✳

SCORE: 8/10

Like bareMinerals' gloss, above, this offering also tastes subtly of vanilla and mint. Plant emollients, including pomegranate oil, plus peptide technology work to smooth fine lines while adding a gorgeous satiny cosmetic slick of non-sticky gloss. Again, there is said to be a lip-plumping effect when used regularly over time. The lipstick in this range has also done well (see page 36), which – considering we trialled nearly 30 natural lippies – is a great

AT A GLANCE

BAREMINERALS MARVELOUS MOXIE LIPGLOSS

AVEDA NOURISH-MINT REHYDRATING LIP GLAZE

ORIGINS DRINK UP HYDRATING LIP BALM

WE LOVE

Jo's fallen for the gorgeous cherry-ish Plum Punch shade of the Origins gloss that's done well here, but also remains devoted to the 'beauty steal' Yes To Carrots C Me Shine Lip Gloss: riffle through her pockets and you'll find a YTC gloss in almost every shade. Sarah's new fave daytime look is Lanolips Lip Ointment in Dark Honey over Liz Earle Lip Pencil in Carnation.

achievement for Aveda. Of the 13 shades, they sent us sheer raspberry-red Cherry Blossom.
COMMENTS: 'Extremely glam – gives you lips like a model!' • 'very comfy, not dry or sticky' • 'I used a similar Aveda product years ago which had an unpleasantly strong mintiness, I'm delighted with this new version' • 'lovely menthol taste which made lips tingle and my breath taste fresh' • 'hard to wear a true red lipstick over 50 years old but this raspberry-red looked youthful, and the gloss stopped any crêpey bleeding' • 'lips felt hydrated and moist' • 'silky and moisturising, like a dry-lips treatment'.

ORIGINS DRINK UP HYDRATING LIP BALM

✳

SCORE: 7.8/10

This has lately made its way into Jo's bag (see *We Love*): a mega-moisturising, glossy gloss incorporating apricot and jojoba oils, barley and wheatgerm extracts, aloe vera, orange peel wax and something new to us called Ximenia Americana seed oil, taken from a drought-resistant tree native to South Africa's savannahs due to its ability to preserve water. This lip 'drink', which is dispensed via an angled applicator, comes in eight shades. Our testers tried Nude Nectarine, almost colourless with a hint of shimmer.
COMMENTS: 'Lovely shimmery look, which suited me as I have three kids and don't have time for a full-on look; it would be fab with a tan and some "bare" make-up' • 'glam, gorgeous and glossy' • 'I eat off any lip product easily, but this seemed to soak in rather well, not just sit on the lips – which was nice' • 'totally different to anything I've used: silky and soft on lips and easy to apply. I'd recommend this' • 'loved the minty fragrance' • 'I have sensitive skin that's also prone to dermatitis and most glosses lead to lips flaking – but this was different, lips were more moisturised than usual'.

LIP BALMS
our award winners

Lip balms are our best friends year round and these days some even offer a pretty hint of colour and gloss, too. We had dozens to trial (they're a cinch to formulate naturally) and the last winner here puts a big Cheshire-cat grin on our (soft, smooth) lips

L'OCCITANE SHEA BUTTER LIP BALM
✳

SCORE: 8.75/10

A swivel-up balm from L'Occitane: one of many of the French brand's shea butter-enriched products that feature in this book. This contains 10 per cent shea, and also features beeswax and carnauba wax for an instantly nourishing, softening and protective action.

COMMENTS: 'Loved this lip balm: extremely rehydrating without being greasy' • 'gave a lovely sheen for a natural no-make-up look; makes a great base for lipstick, too' • 'lips are softer and less dry' • 'I used this during labour with my little baby girl – such a godsend with my awful dry lips – and now it always brings back happy memories and it's kept my lips soft for kissing her' • 'very moisturising, nourishing and long lasting; did not need to be reapplied'.

LANOLIPS 101 OINTMENT
✳ ✳

SCORE: 8.44/10

We're thrilled that two products from our friend, Lanolips founder, Kirsten Carriol have become chart-toppers here. This is the original Lano creation based on 100 per cent pure, medical-grade lanolin, a renowned skin soother and emollient for centuries. The bestselling 101 goes beyond lip soothing and (subtle) glossing: it is great for wound healing, and is suitable for newborn babies, too.

COMMENTS: 'Brilliant at improving softness on my very dry lips, especially over the winter weeks' • 'this is good over lipstick for a more glossy look' • 'felt disappointed and on a losing battle using other lip salves (Carex, Vaseline, etc) – but I'll definitely buy this!' • 'it has absolutely no taste, which I liked: less temptation to lick lips' • 'transforms dryness and cuticles, soothes cat scratches and has softened the horizontal line on the bridge of my nose!'

AT A GLANCE

L'OCCITANE
SHEA BUTTER LIP BALM

LANOLIPS
101 OINTMENT

LANOLIPS
LIP OINTMENT WITH
COLOUR SPF15

BEAUTY
BIBLE LIP BALM

WE LOVE

No surprise here...
we love our very
own vitamin-E
rich Beauty Bible
Lip Balm (right),
of course!

LANOLIPS LIP OINTMENT WITH COLOUR SPF15
✳

SCORE: 8.4/10

With 60 per cent medical-grade lanolin, plus grapeseed, castor seed and coconut oils, shea butter and vitamin E, this is a glossier, tinted version of 101, available in a fab range of five sheer colours. Our testers had Rhubarb, a fruity deep pink and a favourite of ours.

COMMENTS: 'Used this in cold weather and not once did I have chapped lips' • 'a lovely colour that just enhanced my own lip shade; long-lasting: stayed put, even after a cup of tea' • 'lips felt lush' • 'really, really liked this: rich and nourishing, comfortable and the condition of my lips has definitely improved' • 'even when it had seemingly worn off, my lips felt smooth and I didn't feel the need to reapply as I do with other lip balms' • 'lovely tint with an SPF15; perfect for the swimming pool'.

BEAUTY BIBLE LIP BALM
✳ ✳

SCORE: 8.22/10

Some years ago, we launched a single product bearing the *Beauty Bible* name – in truth, to protect our trademark, and because this chunky all-natural balm, with organic shea butter, vitamin E and aloe vera, is actually our favourite-ever lip product (Gill Sinclair at Victoria Health introduced it to us). We're so chuffed that testers truly loved it enough to nudge it onto the award-winners' podium!

COMMENTS: 'Extremely comfortable: moisturising without being too greasy or oily' • 'my husband always suffers from dry lips and he really liked it too' • 'lips were in better condition after just a couple of days' • 'I like the fact this is an un-fragranced lip product' • 'love this balm and will make sure it's within reach at all times' • 'lips look kissable – hell, I'd kiss me!'

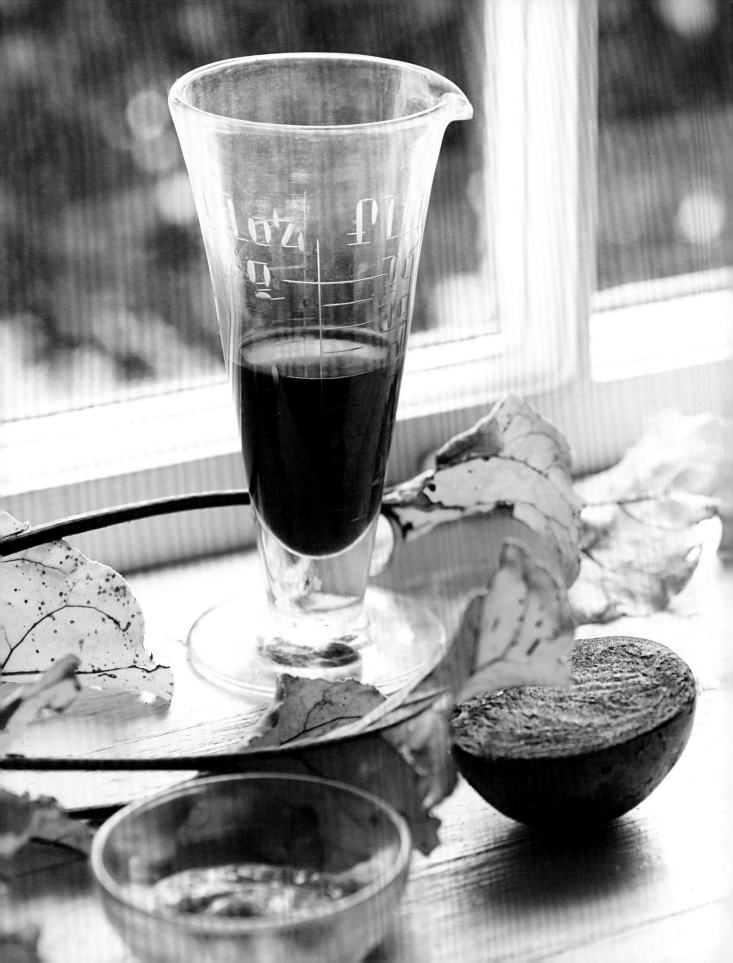

GLOW GETTERS

You don't have to visit the make-up hall to find pretty glosses and stains for lips and cheeks. Have fun creating your own good-enough-to-eat treats

GLOSSY LIP GLOSS

Apply to lips for instant sheen and gloss. Or slick it over lipstick, for shine with a greater depth of colour.

- 1 teaspoon grated cocoa butter
- ½ teaspoon coconut oil
- 1 teaspoon almond oil
- ½ teaspoon beeswax
- 1 teaspoon aloe vera gel

If the cocoa butter is solid, grate it finely (a Microplane is perfect for this).

Melt the cocoa butter, coconut oil, almond oil and beeswax in a double boiler (see page 212); remove from the heat and add the aloe vera gel. Whisk together.

Pour the melted mixture into a small, sterilised container and cool completely.

TINGLY PINK LIP TINT

This produces a fab, strawberry-pink lip tint. You can vary the colour with the amount of beetroot juice you use – just experiment.

- 2 tablespoons sweet almond oil
- 10g (½oz) beeswax
- 3 teaspoons bottled pure beetroot juice (or grate some cooked beetroot)
- 4 drops peppermint essential oil

Grate the cooked beetroot to produce juice, or use a bottled pure beetroot juice (from natural food stores).

Then gently heat the oil and the beeswax in a double boiler (see page 212).

Remove from the heat and add 1 teaspoon of the beetroot juice; whisk well with a fork or small whisk, adding more juice for a deeper colour. Add the peppermint essential oil, whisk again and transfer into a sterilised pot.

BEETROOT AND GLYCERINE CHEEK AND LIP TINT

Benefit Cosmetics popularised the idea of tints for matching cheeks and lips: sheer, liquid colour that delivers the perfect seaside-walk glow. This all-natural version works just as well.

- 45g (1½oz) grated, raw beetroot
- 45ml (1½fl oz) vegetable glycerine

Put the grated beetroot and glycerine in a double boiler (see page 212). Heat gently for 15 minutes, allow to cool, then strain through a tea strainer into a small jug so that you can pour it into a small sealable container.

To use, simply shake before putting a dab on the end of your finger and applying to cheeks, blending well. This amazing stain can also be dotted onto lips: just smoosh them together. (It tastes deliciously sweet.) Finish with the Glossy Lip Gloss (above).

CREAM BLUSHERS AND POWDERS
our award winners

Nothing wakes up a tired face faster than a quick swoosh of complexion-boosting blusher. Whether you choose a powder or cream option is down to personal preference – though we find cream blushers can be more forgiving on older skin. Our testers dusted and slicked on more than 25 mostly natural and organic versions in both textures – reviewed here in separate categories – and found that the following winners were the greatest glow-getters

LIZ EARLE HEALTHY GLOW CREAM BLUSH
✸

SCORE: 8.5/10

Sometimes, due to an admin error, a brand separately sends us two batches of the same product to trial. So 20 of our testers received this and, lo and behold, two separate panels awarded the soft, creamy, vitamin-E-enriched blusher almost identical marks. The Liz Earle team, however, did actually submit two different shades (from the seven available): we tested Nude (a rosy apricot) and Nectar (a deeper, fresh-rose pink) and testers just loved both. (This happens to be our own top 'love' among the more-natural blushers, too.)

COMMENTS: 'Went on easily with a foundation brush and lasted all day and evening' • 'gave a sheer, natural finish like you're not wearing any blusher and look healthy' • 'I was really disappointed when I saw a cream blush to test (I hate them!) and waited till I wasn't working to try this, so no one would see me. But it is now a make-up must have!' • 'a dream: gives a natural, soft, dewy finish; flattering and youthful; non-ageing and doesn't settle into pores – feels like a luxury product; will definitely buy again' • 'it has a skin-like finish; it became part of my facial contours and gave me cheekbones that looked like my own' • 'I'd had this on for seven

CREAM
AT A GLANCE
LIZ EARLE HEALTHY
GLOW CREAM BLUSH

WILD ABOUT BEAUTY
ULTRA DEWY
CRÈME BLUSH

hours when I saw a friend I hadn't seen in a while; he commented on how fab and healthy I was looking. I'm addicted to this blusher' • 'some mornings I can look tired – and that makes me feel tired; this quickly and easily lifts my face without any other make-up'.

WILD ABOUT BEAUTY ULTRA DEWY CRÈME BLUSH
✸✸✸

SCORE: 7.63/10

Louise Redknapp's Wild About Beauty range has done terrifically well in these recent make-up trials. This is a dinky-sized swivel-up blusher stick that can be applied directly onto the cheek and then blended with a finger: the soft-textured colour melds beautifully into skin for seamless results. (No Widow-Twankey blusher, this.) Nourishing ingredients include beeswax and vitamin E. Our testers tried the Fifi shade.

COMMENTS: 'One of the nicest blushers I've ever used – went on really smoothly and felt creamy on the skin' • 'the finish was sheer, the colour perfect and it gave me the most natural "glow" I've ever had from a blusher' • 'a great product: I loved the slight shimmer; it is a face changer that gave me a new look' • 'I totally love it. My only request is: please make a bigger one. This lush blush completely changed my mind about cream blushers'.

BAREMINERALS BLUSH

✹✹

SCORE: 8.63/10

The highest of our blusher scores was for this loose-powder option: one of bareMinerals's earliest products. The brand now has one of the bestselling mineral make-up ranges in the world (Sarah is a fan) using mineral pigments to even out complexions (see pages 20–21), and, as here, to add a pop of colour. To apply the blusher you need to use bareMinerals's signature 'swirl, tap, buff' technique. There's the option of a staggering 30 shades; our testers got glowing with Laughter – a tawny rose hue.

COMMENTS: 'Smooth, natural, velvety finish; blended very easily' • 'I never reapply make-up during the day (I have two young children so it never happens), but this is very long-lasting and gave me a healthy glow' • 'looked scary in the pot but made me appear naturally flushed plus gave a gorgeous, subtle definition to cheeks' • 'lasted well, managing to outlast the daily onslaught of hospital-based ward work' • 'orgasmic! I think this could be a double for Nars blush in Orgasm' • 'I tried it on my teenage daughters, too, and it looks as good on them as me despite the fact they have a different skin tone' • 'my new go-to blusher'.

BELLÁPIERRE COMPACT MINERAL BLUSH

✹✹

SCORE: 8.47/10

This mineral blusher comes as a pressed format in a very generous-sized mirrored compact. Flip up the blusher and you'll find concealed below a generous applicator puff, so generous, in fact, that we'd advise proceeding with caution: it would be quite easy to overdo things and look glowier than you might wish. (We also suggest you ignore these instructions on the box, 'apply to cheekbones and T-zone for a natural-looking glow', we've not met anyone yet who really wants a flushed-pink chin, nose and forehead.) Those caveats notwithstanding, the pretty Desert Rose shade of this silky-smooth powder – which is enriched with jojoba – went down very well with our testers.

COMMENTS: 'Looked natural, gave my skin a pretty glow: I won't use anything else from

POWDER

AT A GLANCE

BAREMINERALS BLUSH

BELLÁPIERRE COMPACT MINERAL BLUSH

WILD ABOUT BEAUTY ULTRA SHEER POWDER BLUSH

GREEN PEOPLE MINERAL POWDER BLUSH

now on' • 'made skin look radiant and healthy in a non-greasy way' • 'very easy to apply; a smooth-texture finish and the colour was long-lasting • 'a wonderful blush that isn't powdery or heavy looking on the skin; fabulous for daytime or evening; would recommend to friends – love it!' • 'very easy to blend'.

WILD ABOUT BEAUTY ULTRA SHEER POWDER BLUSH

✹

SCORE: 8.33/10

Two winners in one category for Wild About Beauty (see opposite page): this powder version comes in a neat little mirrored compact, with a dragonfly embossed on the weightless powder. WAB infuse the powder with vitamins C and E, together with aloe vera to create the soft, buildable texture. Our shade? The peachy-pink Molly, from a range of four colour options.

COMMENTS: 'Sheer finish, not obvious or powdery and looked very natural on the skin: a healthy glow' • 'twelve hours after application the colour and finish were exactly the same as when I first applied it' • 'smooth and natural looking, lovely and stripe-free!' • 'I usually use Chanel blushers but love the smoothness of this one and will consider buying it instead'.

GREEN PEOPLE MINERAL POWDER BLUSH

✹✹✹

SCORE: 7.99/10

Green People really work to ensure that it's not just the contents but the packaging itself which is 'eco', so this certified-organic blusher is packaged in a sturdy, glossy black cardboard palette. As well as containing minerals, the pressed powder is formulated with corn starch, beeswax, sunflower oil and vitamin C. Two shades are available; we dispatched Rose.

COMMENTS: 'A little goes a long way; left a smooth texture on the skin: natural and seamless looking' • 'can't praise this enough: being of the rosy-cheeked brigade, it is difficult to find blusher that masks my rosiness and looks natural – this did both' • 'good to see "green" make-up that's also a pleasure to use' • 'I really, really need blusher to brighten up my face and give it a boost and this did the job pretty well'.

PUFF LOVE

A luxurious face powder to ace your base and blot away shine with an
uplifting fragrance of lavender. Throw it together in just a few shakes

FABULOUS FACE POWDER

Try using this scented face powder to fix foundation or to mattify 'glow'.

- 10g (½oz) rice powder
- 25g (1oz) orris root powder
- 25g (1oz) dried lavender flowers

Put all the ingredients together in a screw-top jar
and then shake, shake, shake. Do not crush the
lavender flowers; you only want them to infuse
the powder with their fragrance.

Do this every day for a week or two, then put the
powder into a sieve and sift into a bowl.

Apply to skin with a velvet puff or a brush.

TIP: You don't always need powder
to keep shine at bay. If your skin
gets oily or starts to gleam, pull
apart the two layers of a tissue, and
lay one over the T-zone (which is
where shine tends to develop). Gently
press onto skin, and you'll find that
the oil is lifted off, without the need
to add another layer of powder.

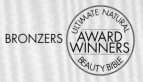

BRONZERS
our award winners

For a sun-kissed boost in summer and beyond, we turn to bronzers. These give a natural glow and offer the right balance between a matte and shimmer finish

DOLL FACE MINERAL MAKEUP BRONZER
✺

SCORE: 8.14/10

This pressed-powder bronzer from a small New Zealand brand looks quite dark in the compact (which has a see-through lid – no mirror), but adds just the right glow, testers felt. There are two shades; they sent us Winter.

COMMENTS: 'A very realistic look: absolutely loved this – it applied well, was silky smooth and gave really good coverage; also makes a good eyeshadow – stayed on for ages and made eyes look more alive' • 'doesn't streak or cake; surprisingly easy to use, blended well and wasn't as dark as it looked in the compact – it is deceptive but the actual product is one of the best bronzers I've tried'.

LIZ EARLE NATURAL GLOW BRONZER
✺

SCORE: 8/10

Formulated to strike a balance between bronzers that are either too shimmery or too matte, this nestles in a chic navy compact. A couple of testers would have liked it to come with an applicator brush, but many already had their own fluffy bronzer brush, which is the ideal tool for this product. One shade only.

COMMENTS: 'Great bronzer: gave me a really natural-looking glow and made skin appear healthy and sun-kissed without a masking effect or looking caked on' • 'comes with a useful application guide' • 'I didn't get the usual "vanishing-make-up-by-lunchtime" scenario; colour lasted throughout the day' • 'this gives a very nice semi-matte finish which didn't clog the skin' • 'fab holiday make-up: just add lip gloss and mascara' • 'liked the compact itself and the mirror was good quality'.

AT A GLANCE

DOLL FACE MINERAL
MAKEUP BRONZER

LIZ EARLE
NATURAL GLOW
BRONZER

AVEDA
URUKU FACE BRONZER

INIKA
MINERAL BRONZER

AVEDA URUKU FACE BRONZER
✺

SCORE: 7.36/10

Aveda's Uruku pigments come from a project between the brand and the Yanawana people of Brazil, who grow annatto (a pigment from the urukum shrub), that gives the red in this bronzer. The low-shimmer product comes in a small plastic sleeve designed to slot into one of Aveda's recycled metal palettes. We trialled 106 Brazilian Sun, one of two.

COMMENTS: 'Very easy to use: just give a swirl of the brush into the buildable colour' • 'gave the coverage I needed; ace at lasting – goes right through from first thing to home time' • 'it was reassuring to use an effective product with green credentials' • 'powders can be worrying, especially if you have wrinkles, but it smoothed on well and gave a good, silky finish' • 'am a big fan of Aveda and I'd definitely buy this'.

INIKA MINERAL BRONZER
✺✺

SCORE: 7.3/10

Sunkissed (one of four) was our shade of this all-natural mineral bronzer (in a little pot – the same format as a loose mineral powder). NB: A couple of testers warned that it was easy to spill the product as there's no 'guard' over the dispensing holes; Inika, please note...?

COMMENTS: 'Skin looked natural, colour more even and it covered up my two small patches of rosacea very well' • 'I always feel that mineral powders are helping to look after my skin while making me look better, too – my skin can "breathe"' • 'the matte bronzer lasted eight hours plus, especially on neck and décolleté where I used it to even out pigmentation' • 'very realistic gentle tan' • 'didn't look like it was "sitting" on my complexion; just blended nicely'.

Super natural
SKINCARE

Clear, radiant skin is one of the biggest confidence-boosters
we know. So here are the products and the insider secrets
that will get you glowing (in the nicest possible way)

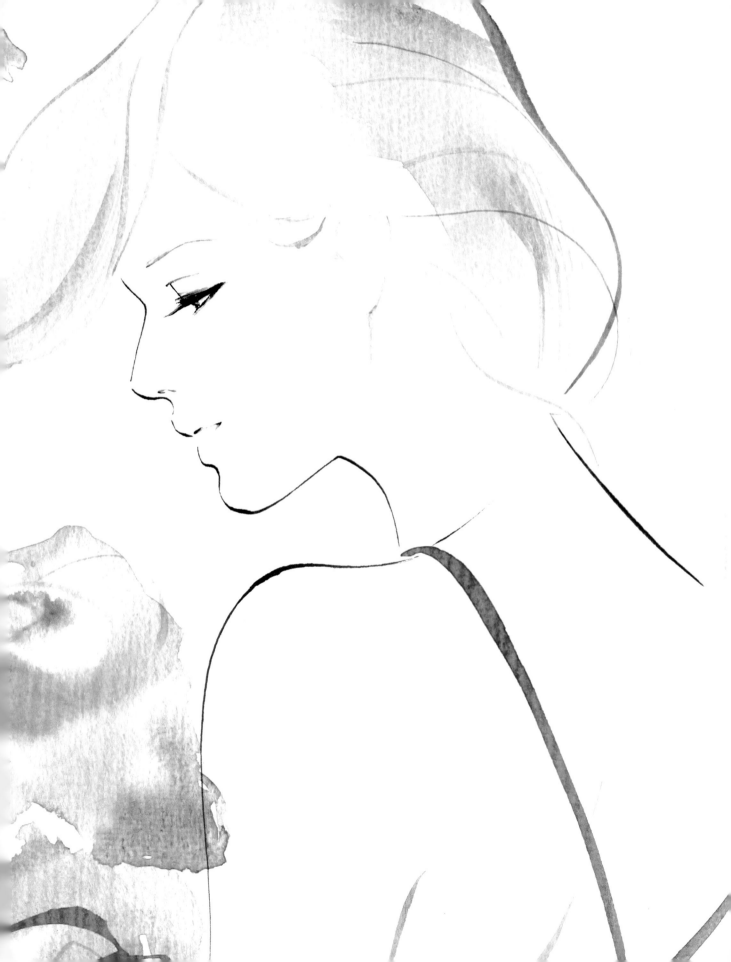

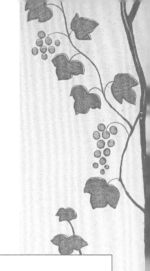

What you REALLY REALLY REALLY NEED

Good skincare isn't rocket science (although some marketing hype makes it sound as if it might be). A few well-chosen products will see your skin right. Here's our shortlist

F act: a groaning shelf of products is not a passport to gorgeous skin. In fact, one of the key pieces of advice we give people is not to use too many items and not to chop and change all the time. Skin cell turnover takes about 28 days – slower as you get older – and you won't see the real benefit of most topicals unless you give them at least that time to work. Some beauty junkies confess to us that they give new products a week then switch, which is a short cut to confusing and possibly upsetting your skin. (NB: Do always stop using a product immediately if you get a sensitivity reaction, though.)

So here are our skincare basics. You will find recipes for many of these throughout the book. But the ones that are pretty impossible to create successfully at home are moisturisers and night creams, serums, and sun preps: so we advise investing in those – ideally after reading our Award Winners.

It might hurt at the time, but de-junking your bathroom shelf (and make-up bag while you're at it) could make your life much simpler and your skin calmer and brighter.

NB: If you are thinking of the old mantra 'cleanse, tone and moisturise', we say: forget the toner, as we do. If you like a fresh sensation, try (organic) rose water.

ESSENTIALS FOR EVERYONE
- Cleanser
- Day cream
- Night cream (younger skins may be fine with their day cream or a light facial oil at night)

OPTIONAL – BUT USEFUL
- Gentle scrub
- Face mask
- Spot zapper for zit-prone skins

FOR MORE MATURE SKINS
- Serum – these deliver lots of nutrients in just a few drops
- Facial oil – layer this with day or night cream, or mix into your moisturiser (or even your foundation) to enrich it if needed
- Neck cream, maybe – if you use a rich night cream, just take that down over neck and bosom (and sweep body products upwards for a double-whammy)
- Eye cream – not essential but can make a difference if you're sprouting crow's feet; also may help with dark circles and/or puffiness

SUNCARE
- Sun preps SPF20–30: if you are going in the sun, don't rely on an SPF moisturiser
- After-sun – good to soothe any sunburn and prolong tan (see our recipe, page 160)
- Self tanners – as with the rest of sun preps, don't try 'cooking' these at home, but you can mix them into face and body moisturisers to custom-blend your own gradual (daily) tanners

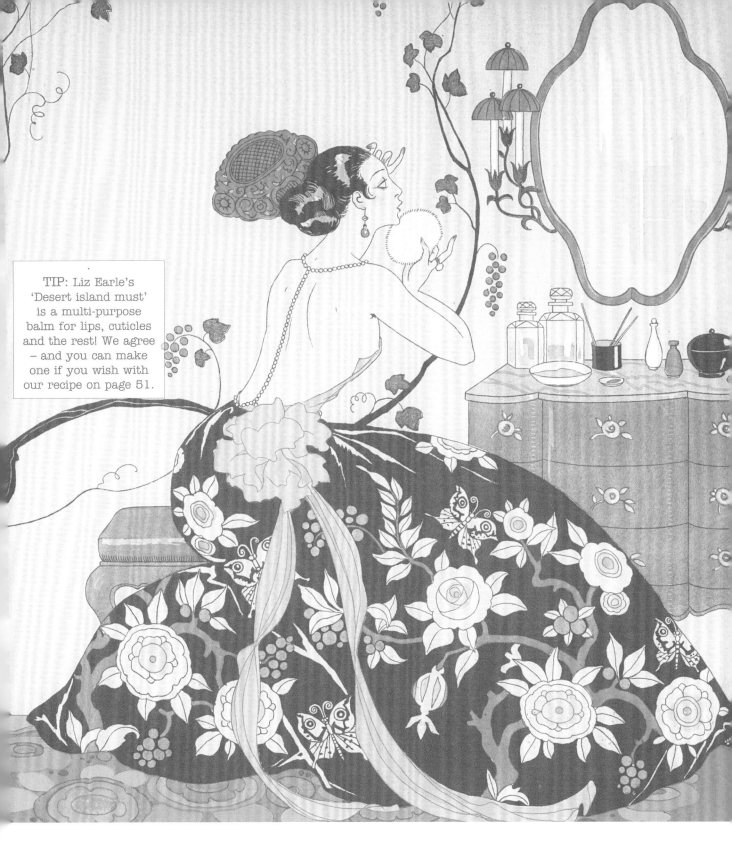

TIP: Liz Earle's 'Desert island must' is a multi-purpose balm for lips, cuticles and the rest! We agree – and you can make one if you wish with our recipe on page 51.

BODY ESSENTIALS: We couldn't do without hand cream, body lotion/butter and foot cream plus a great body scrub. (You'll find recipes for most of these in this book.)

MULTI-PURPOSE BALMS
our award winners

Every woman needs a hard-working balm to tackle dry skin, hard cuticles and even to tame a frizzy mane. But which tick the most boxes for being natural, green and the best at moisturising? Here is the *baume de la baume* of the beauty multitaskers

MARY ELIZABETH SPEARMINT AND TEA TREE NURTURE BALM
✳✳
SCORE: 9/10

The founder of this small skincare company, Cecilia Rathe (an aromatherapist, Reiki master and yoga teacher), created her chemical-free products after being diagnosed with skin cancer. This teeny tin contains a blend of shea butter, oils of hemp, avocado and meadow foam, zingy spearmint, plus antiseptic tea tree.
COMMENTS: 'Love this – great everyday item' • 'it helped a sore armpit to heal quicker after shaving with a blunt razor' • 'better than Elizabeth Arden Eight Hour Cream, in my opinion – a real find' • 'soothed dry patches and rough cuticles' • 'a positive powerhouse in a little tin; smells divine and is reasonably priced' • 'soothed and smoothed some very dry patches on my legs as a result of insect bites'.

WELEDA SKIN FOOD
✳✳
SCORE: 8.62/10

This beauty classic has gone down brilliantly with testers over the years and often sells out. It's a cream in texture rather than the usual balm, blending sunflower seed oil, lanolin, sweet almond oil and beeswax with chamomile, calendula, wild pansy and rosemary extracts – a great barrier against harsh weather and answers many a skin SOS, so it's useful for travel.
COMMENTS: 'A revelation: saw a difference after two days of using this on my feet' • 'lovely lemon, orange, citrus smell' • 'helped my son's dry, chapped skin' • 'soothed patches of dermatitis caused by constant hand-washing looking after my baby' • 'skin has improved by 90 per cent after a month' • 'brilliant for dry patches' • 'compact-size tube for handbag'.

AT A GLANCE

MARY ELIZABETH SPEARMINT AND TEA TREE NURTURE BALM

WELEDA SKIN FOOD

LIZ EARLE SUPERBALM

MELVITA 3 HONEYS NECTAR BALM LIPS AND DRY PATCHES

LIZ EARLE SUPERBALM
✳✳
SCORE: 8.56/10

This has appeared in just about every *Beauty Bible* since we first launched, but we sent it to be tested for this book and, hey presto, another award for this classic balm. It's packed with rosehip, avocado and hazelnut oils, vitamin E, and fragranced with an irresistible blend of neroli, lavender and chamomile essential oils.
COMMENTS: 'Comforting, smoothing; skin around nails has improved, and nails surviving longer' • 'calms itchy burns on hands from cooking and on ears (from straighteners)' • 'my husband – who doesn't believe in products – suffers from very dry skin on his feet and tried this; he was blown away – it has cleared significantly' • 'I'm an air hostess and use this as a do-all beauty item when away on trips' • 'a wonder product for my eczema'.

MELVITA 3 HONEYS NECTAR BALM LIPS AND DRY PATCHES
✳✳✳
SCORE: 8.5/10

Unscrew the lid of this little jar and smell the honey. Then apply it to any thirsty skin zone you choose: the instantly soothing, anti-inflammatory balm is designed to relieve even the most chapped, dry skin. The ingredients include shea butter, coconut and sunflower oils, beeswax – and that generous drizzle of honey.
COMMENTS: 'Totally portable; fantastic results on face and body' • 'definite improvement in dry scaly patches' • 'very soothing and healing on cuts' • 'cuticles so much better after using for a month' • 'a great product I could gush about: I get dry lips and most balms just sit on the top; this tackled the problem from the first application – a real desert-island must-have'.

GOLD REMEDY

Calendula flowers and sunflower oil join forces to
create a skin-soothing natural salve for the first-aid kit

ALL-PURPOSE CALENDULA SKIN SALVE

Keep this balm in the first-aid box to soothe
rashes, itching, sore spots and flaky skin.

- 25g (1oz) dried calendula (marigold) flowers
- 150ml (¼ pint) sunflower oil
- 25g (1oz) beeswax, grated

To make the oil base, place the calendula in
the bottom of a glass jar with a lid. Pour on
the sunflower oil, and leave the mixture to
steep. Shake daily for about three weeks, by
which time you will have a soothing oil base.
Strain the oil through a fine cloth into a bowl,
squeezing and pressing gently with your
fingers until the last drops are filtered.

To make the salve, place a heatproof
measuring jug inside a saucepan containing
about 10cm of water, over a medium heat.
Pour the oil into the jug and add the grated
beeswax. Stir until thoroughly melted.

Take off the heat and test for consistency:
drop a small amount onto a saucer, and put
in the freezer for 1 minute to cool to a thick,
soft ointment. If you want a harder salve,
reheat and add a little more beeswax. For a
softer texture, reheat and add a drop more
oil. (You may need to add more beeswax in
the summer when it's warm outside.)

Then pour the salve into wide-mouthed jars
and allow to cool and solidify.

Store away from heat and light, and apply
whenever skin is inflamed or sore.

CLEANSERS
our award winners

Fantastic skin begins with a great cleanser that will swipe away dead-skin cells along with make-up and any debris left behind by our polluted environment. The result? A fresher, brighter complexion ready for moisturiser. Cleansers are among the easiest products to formulate with natural ingredients and the ones below all scored brilliant marks with our testers

EMMA HARDIE AMAZING FACE MORINGA CLEANSING BALM

✽

SCORE: 9.61/10

Based around moringa seed oil, wild sea fennel and vitamin E, this deliciously fragranced offering from super-facialist Emma Hardie achieved the highest score in 18 years of *Beauty Bible* trials. (We trialled it originally for *The Anti-Ageing Beauty Bible*.) Our testers used it along with Emma's Dual Action Professional Cleansing Cloth (which comes in a pack of three) which we recommend you do, too. See Emma's facial massage technique on page 58. *COMMENTS:* 'This cleansing system – cleanser with exfoliator mixed in, cleanser as mask, plus muslin and facial massage – is easy and left my skin clean, very moisturised and happy' • 'the best cleanser I've ever used; removes all traces of make-up, except waterproof mascara' • 'oily, very rich and feels wonderful going on; an amazing multitasker • 'my skin is much smoother and brighter' • 'stopped breakouts in their tracks and made my skin glow'.

AURELIA PROBIOTIC SKINCARE MIRACLE CLEANSER

✽ ✽

SCORE: 9.43/10

Aromatic: think eucalyptus, chamomile, rosemary and bergamot. Rich and creamy: like an old-fashioned cleansing cream. And high-scoring. This recent British start-up, Aurelia Probiotic Skincare, submitted four products for this book and all have done incredibly well: but this is the second-highest ranking, wowing

testers. It blends ethically sourced bioorganic plant and flower essences with probiotic and peptide technologies, and it is accompanied by an antibacterial bamboo cloth. *COMMENTS:* 'Left my skin soft, smooth and completely moisturised; lovely to the touch (so soft I stroked my face in amazement!)' • 'a perfect texture: non-greasy, light but rich' • 'lovely indulgent product – makes cleansing a pleasure; the eucalyptus smell helps me breathe in the morning' • 'so easy to apply you could use it in the dark' • 'I have loved using this: it made my skin wonderfully soft and I haven't had a single spot (I'm pushing 40 and still get them) – beautiful clear skin for the first time in ages' • 'a little goes a long way'.

ELEMIS PRO-COLLAGEN CLEANSING BALM

✽

SCORE: 9.38/10

A big tub of unctuous balm featuring British-sourced botanical oils – including starflower, elderberry and something called optimega – with fragrant, skin-softening mimosa and rose flower waxes, and Pro-Collagen's signature anti-ager, Padina pavonica, plus a cleansing cloth. Elemis recommend using a separate eye make-up remover. *COMMENTS:* 'Would I buy it again? Yes, yes, yes; I can't live without this, not something I thought I'd say with a cleanser' • 'I use less facial oil as my skin feels like it's already been fed – improved lines and texture of skin on neck and décolleté (I'm paranoid about that)' • 'lovely texture, thick and unctuous – the colour

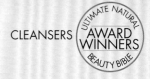

and thickness of honey; melts away make-up leaving a soft, supple complexion' • 'normally I let my sister try products but I won't share this one' • 'I want to give it 11/10! Amazing formulation – dissolves even the toughest make-up. Like a miracle cream: anti-ageing, youthful, invigorating – I feel like a different woman' • 'as someone who suffers breakouts in my 50s, this has really helped to keep skin clear' • 'the cleansing process was so pleasurable I really looked forward to it' • 'the nicest product I've ever tested for *Beauty Bible*!'

ODYLIQUE CREAMY COCONUT CLEANSER
✳ ✳ ✳

SCORE: 9.3/10

This pioneering organic range based in Suffolk was formerly Essential Care. Co-founder Abi Weeds is a member of the Soil Association's Health & Beauty Standards committee. This cleanser comes in a flip-top tube and features a blend of rosemary and French rose extracts, plus clary sage, eucalyptus and olive oils.

COMMENTS: 'Smells subtle, works quickly and removes all traces of make-up, grease and grime – skin felt mega-clean after this, and I'd switch brands in a minute' • 'delicious double cream texture' • 'fab – better than Liz Earle Cleanse & Polish (did I just say that?): worked exceptionally well and even got hair dye off my hairline – no mean feat' • 'does what it says, leaving skin soft, clean and moisturised'.

NEAL'S YARD REMEDIES WILD ROSE BEAUTY BALM
✳ ✳ ✳

SCORE: 9.19/10

This multitasking balm also works as a moisturiser, skin-soother, lip treatment, mask and more, but excels here as a cleanser (with its own muslin cloth). The solid texture emulsifies on skin to melt make-up with a combination of beeswax, jojoba seed and rosehip oils, shea butter and antioxidant palmarosa essential oil.

COMMENTS: 'Can I give this more than 10, like 100? Amazing, beautiful, one-pot wonder: I also used it as a mask and face protector but it takes off make-up easily; I usually double cleanse and still find some residue of make-up

on the cloth with the second cleanse – but not with this' • 'brilliant! Heavenly smell, very luxurious – reminded me of buying frankincense in Far East markets' • 'left my skin feeling super-hydrated with that *ahhhh* feeling'.

JUSTBE CLEANSED CLEANSING BALM
✳ ✳

SCORE: 8.92/10

A new range to us of artisan aromatherapy products made in Scotland. It's 100 per cent natural, but not organically certified. (NB: JustBe's Eye Makeup Remover also did well on page 81.) Coconut oil, coconut butter and beeswax feature, and there's a lovely fragrance from pure geranium and petitgrain essential oils. And yet another muslin cloth…

COMMENTS: 'I loved the smell, texture, result: complete make-up removal without lots of rubbing or scrubbing, even round the eyes' • 'I simply love this – feel like I'm having a nice facial every time I apply the warm cloth to my face; will buy from now on' • 'perfect for my difficult, dry skin, leaving it refreshed, cleansed, clarified but not tight or dry' • 'smelt like walking through an English cottage garden: pleasant to inhale at night'.

DR.HAUSCHKA CLEANSING CREAM
✳ ✳

SCORE: 8.88/10

Devotees are addicted to the gently exfoliating texture of this classic cleanser, based on sweet almond meal, peanut and almond oils, chamomile, witch hazel and more. It comes in a long, thin, easily portable metal tube. Dr.Hauschka recommend applying this cream with a three-minute massage technique.

COMMENTS: 'I sighed as I thought this would be a kerfuffle but the results are so worth it! Skin clean, soft, and dry patches eliminated in a way I've only experienced after a salon facial' • 'love the fact it slightly exfoliates without drying' • 'the orange and lemon scent reminds me of Italy' • 'exceptional: made my face feel so refreshed, but not tight' • 'really surprised by how clean my skin feels, and it's soft, too' • 'loved this product: I used to suffer with dry skin round the nose and that's disappeared now – it's the best cleanser I've ever used'.

WE LOVE

Jo alternates one night on, one night off, between the Elemis Pro-Collagen Cleansing Balm winner here, and that all-time classic Liz Earle Cleanse & Polish which she enrichens with a squirt of facial oil. Sarah's staple cleanser for some 16 years is Cleanse & Polish, which has never caused her touchy skin any problems, removes make-up like a dream, mascara, too (no sore eyes, either) and never leaves her face feeling dry or tight. Occasionally, she feels obliged to test something else but always returns for more of the same.

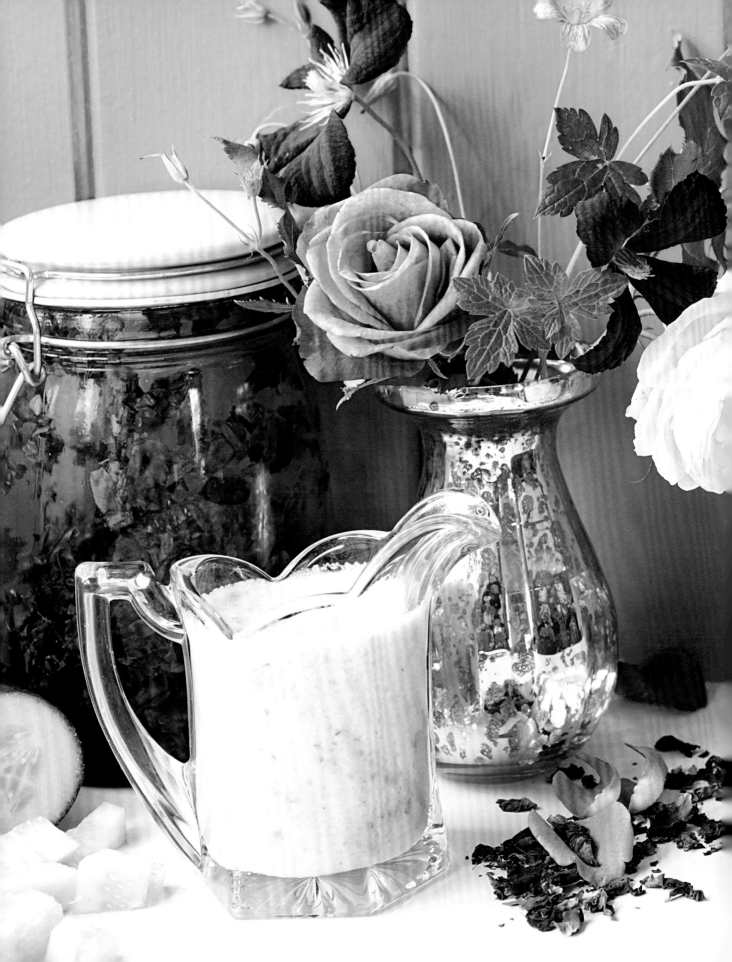

JUST HIT REFRESH

Whether your face is in need of a perk up or you want to wipe away the grime of the day, these fresheners and cleansers are packed with ingredients to pep up, clean and hydrate, leaving your skin ready to start all over again…

TRIPLE ROSE FACIAL FRESHENER

You can either spritz this onto skin as a freshener, or apply with a cotton ball after you've cleansed. It makes a perfect morning cleanser, too.

- 50ml (2fl oz) apple cider vinegar
- 350ml (12fl oz) rose water
- 25g (1oz) dried rose petals
- 2 drops rose essential oil

In a glass jar (with a lid), pour the vinegar and rose water over the dried petals, add the rose essential oil and allow to sit for three weeks. Strain and pour into a sterilised bottle.

GERANIUM CLEANSING BALM

Massage this miraculous, make-up-melting cleanser thoroughly into your face and remove with a muslin washcloth or flannel that has been dunked in hot water; repeat until your face is completely clean.

- 2 tablespoons cold-pressed olive oil
- 10g (½oz) beeswax granules or grated beeswax
- A dozen fresh geranium leaves
- 10 drops geranium essential oil

Heat the olive oil and the beeswax in a double boiler (see page 212).

Place the leaves in the bottom of a sterilised, heatproof glass jar (which has a lid or cork). Pour on the melted oil and beeswax. Put on the lid and leave for three weeks to infuse the mixture with 'geranium-ness'. Then scoop the lot out and reheat in a double boiler.

Strain through kitchen paper or muslin to remove the leaves and when the mixture has cooled slightly, stir in 10 drops of geranium essential oil, before transferring to a sterilised wide-mouthed jar.

MILK, CUCUMBER AND MINT CLEANSER

This is wonderfully cooling on the skin. The milk is lightly hydrating, delivering a veil of moisture that even oily skins need.

- 5cm (2in) piece of cucumber, peeled and roughly chopped
- 50ml (2fl oz) milk, full-fat organic
- 5 mint leaves, chopped (no stalks)
- 2 drops grapefruit seed extract (or 4 drops tincture of benzoin)

Place the cucumber, milk and mint in a blender or food processor and whizz until it is a smooth liquid.

Pour the mixture into a saucepan and gently heat until simmering. Simmer for 2 minutes, then allow to cool. Strain the liquid through muslin (or kitchen paper).

Pour the cleanser into a sterilised bottle and add the grapefruit seed extract (or benzoin). Store in the fridge and use within a week.

DAY CREAMS
our award winners

These creams are packed with botanicals that nurture, plump and smooth all skin types, including combination. They also make a velvety base for make-up. SPF is not included, so remember to layer on sun protection if you're going outside

ORIGINS GINZING ENERGY-BOOSTING MOISTURIZER
✹✹
SCORE: 8.57/10

Lightweight and oil-free, this is a perfect choice for combination or oily skins and 'quenching' enough for drier complexions. It has the Origins signature grapefruit scent (spearmint and lemon oils feature), along with radiance-boosting caffeine and ginseng, plus conditioning wheat, olive and barley extracts.
COMMENTS: 'After first use skin appeared brighter and younger looking' • 'smells fab, makes my dull skin look brighter and feel soft' • 'left skin mattified, and make-up would glide over the top' • 'my partner mentioned I looked less dry and blotchy' • 'this has balanced my complexion, calming sensitivity – skin also less oily, hence fewer pimples – very pleased'.

CIRCAROMA BALANCING FACIAL CREAM
✹✹
SCORE: 8.5/10

Circaroma is a pioneering natural brand we first wrote about aeons ago and we're pleased that a new bunch of testers appreciate its charms. This is designed as balancing, so good for combination skins (we know that a huge number of you categorise yourselves that way), and features lightweight apricot oil, rose geranium, patchouli, French lavender and vitamin E.
COMMENTS: 'Immediately noticed mattifying effect and skin looked more velvety' • 'a lovely, uplifting fragrance, like geranium aromatherapy oil' • 'perfect for day with make-up but also at night as it's hydrating without being heavy' • 'it has reduced the size of my pores – noticed that after five to six days' • 'skin is less prone to becoming oily – noticeably so: I have to touch up my make-up less often, even in the T-zone'.

AT A GLANCE
ORIGINS GINZING ENERGY-BOOSTING MOISTURIZER

CIRCAROMA BALANCING FACIAL CREAM

REN HYDRA-CALM GLOBAL PROTECTION DAY CREAM

AURELIA PROBIOTIC SKINCARE CELL REVITALISE DAY MOISTURISER

TIP: The Aurelia people advise applying their moisturiser using a gentle facial massage technique. That applies to all creams, we'd say – and on page 58 you can read how.

REN HYDRA-CALM GLOBAL PROTECTION DAY CREAM
✹
SCORE: 8.5/10

A pump-action tube of rich moisturiser, ideal for sensitive skins as it features specific skin-calming ingredients such as calendula oil, omega fatty acids (to repair barrier function) and bisabolol (from Roman chamomile) to help with redness.
COMMENTS: 'My skin was dry with fine lines but after first use it appeared smoother, firmer and plumper' • 'a lovely product which has given some great results' • 'the perfect texture: luxurious, smooth and creamy without being gloopy or sticky' • 'a friend commented my skin looked fresh' • 'love this cream: my husband said I looked great, even without make-up!' • 'my complexion looks relaxed and brighter'.

AURELIA PROBIOTIC SKINCARE CELL REVITALISE DAY MOISTURISER
✹✹
SCORE: 8.33/10

The skincare collection from this British brand has notched up some stupendous scores in this book. We'd prescribe this 'whipped' cream as the top choice for thirsty complexions: it delivers baobab, hibiscus, firming kigelia Africana, borage oil and mongongo oil, which is abundant in vitamin E. Jasmine, tuberose and mandarin are responsible for the divine scent.
COMMENTS: 'I'd rate this moisturiser higher than any I've ever used – my skin looks and feels better' • 'excellent product which kept my dry, sensitive skin supple and soft; seemed to fill out lines' • 'face looked healthier, plumped; fine lines seemed to dissolve and larger crevices (on forehead) softened' • 'gorgeous jasmine and orange aroma' • 'wonderful primer for foundation' • 'my other half commented that my skin looks "lovely and fresh"'.

SPF MOISTURISERS
our award winners

To prevent age spots, wrinkles and loss of skin firmness, defending your face against the sun is paramount. Every little SPF helps, so moisturisers that offer extra UVA/B protection are to be applauded. Here are the winning three

L'OCCITANE IMMORTELLE PRECIOUS PROTECTION SPF20
✳
SCORE: 8.36/10

If you've never heard of the immortelle flower – from a wonderful, aromatic plant native to Corsica – you will have done by the time you've read this book, as it pops up all over the place. Immortelle is the foundation of L'Occitane's bestselling skincare range and appears here in an anti-ageing cream designed to firm skin and correct wrinkles, with a useful level of sun protection from chemical sunscreens.
COMMENTS: 'Feels rich, creamy, packed with good ingredients and made me feel like I was feeding my skin – love it' • 'my face is more radiant and healthy looking' • 'made my dull morning skin appear fresh and seemed to have evening-out properties – it almost looked like I'd applied a primer' • 'delivers a lovely dewy glow' • 'a well-designed pot: I could get out just what I wanted, so no wastage' • 'skin feels beautifully hydrated – this is a truly effective moisturiser' • 'sinks in like a dream'.

JOHN MASTERS SPF30 NATURAL MINERAL SUNSCREEN
✳✳
SCORE: 8.29/10

Titanium dioxide and zinc oxide are the entirely natural sunscreens in this pump-action cream. Unlike some formulations it absorbs quickly and any chalkiness rapidly disappears. This is a broad-spectrum sunscreen from the New York organic hairdresser John Masters's suncare range. He asked us to trial it as a moisturiser and make-up base – and it impressed.
COMMENTS: 'Beautifully smoothing and also conditioning' • 'worked well as a moisturiser and left a dewy finish' • 'make-up was easily applied after use and my face didn't become

AT A GLANCE
L'OCCITANE IMMORTELLE PRECIOUS PROTECTION SPF20

JOHN MASTERS SPF30 NATURAL MINERAL SUNSCREEN

APICARE MANUKA NATURAL SUN PROTECT SPF15 FACE CREAM

WE LOVE
Jo is a massive convert to the newish This Works In Transit Skin Defence SPF30 – and is religious about using the lightweight moisturiser on her décolletage as well as her face. Sarah opts for the John Masters sunscreen (left) and always tops up regularly if she is out in the sun.

shiny' • 'comforting and calming; skin felt well protected; it was good as a conditioning cream' • 'most natural sunscreens are thick and clog up your skin, but this doesn't' • 'I shared this with my mum and sister while we were away and we all loved it' • 'this cream is in a convenient handbag-size bottle; I used it on my face and then on exposed areas (shoulders and shins) during my holiday, and it gave brilliant sun protection; my tan lasted longer, too'.

APICARE MANUKA NATURAL SUN PROTECT SPF15 FACE CREAM
✳✳
SCORE: 7.44/10

Apicare gets its name from the bee-derived ingredients – especially nourishing honey – which are a signature of the range. This particular winner features micronised zinc oxide as the sun protectant, alongside natural plant oils (sweet almond, apricot kernel, jojoba and carrot seed), plus a super-strength 'unique manuka factor' (UMF) of 16+. The result is a non-greasy but effective moisturising formula, suitable for all skin types.
COMMENTS: 'Used this on a hot, sunny day, and my skin stayed protected throughout; it also stayed matte for longer (which I didn't expect, due to the oils in the formula)' • 'felt this "firmed" my skin – excellent product which was also very good for my son's sensitive skin' • 'really liked this: it has the creamy, light texture and scent of a good-quality face cream: I'd buy it' • 'skin more dewy and glowing; any tan is enhanced, making you look more healthy' • 'slight lavender scent, not too strong, very pleasant' • 'feels like an expensive moisturiser rather than a sun cream' • 'this compares well with my expensive SPF15 face cream in terms of texture, scent and overall niceness' • 'handy size – convenient for trips to the beach'.

Try the sensational 'new'
FACIAL MASSAGE

Around 20 years ago, we encountered Emma Hardie, a young facialist who had developed her own highly effective method of naturally rejuvenating, lifting and toning faces. Today Emma is known internationally for her golden hands and also for her Amazing Face skincare (which has done so well with our testers, and is a personal favourite of ours). Below, you will find Emma's own how-to guide to achieving a luminous, toned and lifted complexion. Practise it every day as we do – it's worth it

The key to Emma's technique is to stroke *along* the grain of the muscle fibres – that means working in lines, up and down, side to side, and diagonally, rather than in little circles (as often advised by facialists). To maximise the 'lifting' effect, she advises holding the skin taut in the area of the muscles you are working. (We don't always do that if we are in a hurry – but it still feels fantastic.)

Once you get used to the routine, it takes seconds, although minutes are always better when you have more time available.

You can do this with a microfibre cloth while cleansing – as Emma recommends – or after applying facial oil or night cream with your fingertips alone, as we tend to do.

Facial massage can also be a wow on tired mornings and/or when you are suffering from a headache, sore eyes and feel stressed. We all store so much tension in our faces that you will feel soothed and less tense immediately.

This massage has a multi-whammy effect: it is deep cleansing, depuffing (via internal drainage of the tissue), smoothing and toning; plus soothing, brightening and will perkify the many facial muscles. As Emma says, 'it's like yoga for your face'.

NB: 'Don't worry about doing the moves precisely, just follow the general idea,' Emma emphasises. (You can watch her demonstrating it on YouTube if that helps; just Google: 'YouTube Emma Hardie facial massage'.)

If you are doing this while cleansing, use a balm or cleansing oil (for glide). Emma advises using her microfibre Dual Action Professional Cleansing Cloth (see our testers' comments on page 52) but we use the technique with what we have to hand – and quite often, that does mean our fingertips...

TIP: We find scalp massage is fantastic, too: while washing your hair, rub your fingertips and thumbs in little lines and circles from front to back all over your head and right down your neck.

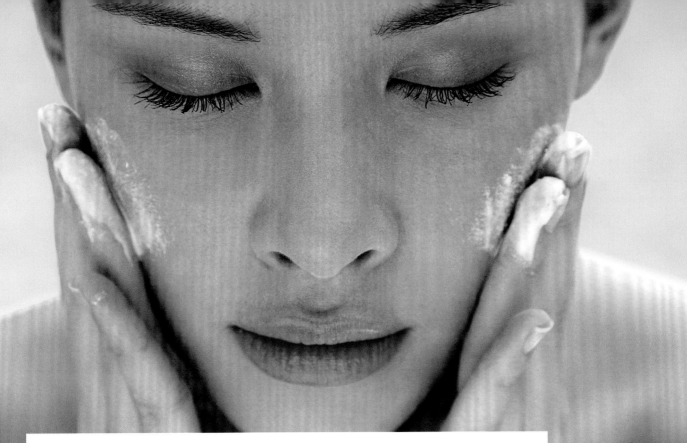

- If you are using a cloth, fold it neatly into a small pad so you can grip it in your hand, and then apply the balm all over.
- Start with your **forehead**: place the fingertips of one hand (the 'holding' hand) in the middle of your hairline to keep your skin taut, then work the pads of the fingertips on your other hand down, in two or three light strokes, towards the gap between your brows.
- Now you are going to do **each side of your forehead**: so move your 'holding' fingers across your hairline out to each temple in turn, and with the fingers of the other hand repeat the strokes downwards to your brows, upwards from brows to hairline, and then diagonally from the middle of your hairline out to each temple.
- Next, stroke the length of your fingers, using each hand alternately, from side to side **across your forehead**, smoothing the skin in the same direction as any wrinkles.
- Hold the skin at each temple, and work your fingers horizontally from side to side under the eyes, moving **down your cheeks**. Repeat diagonally across the cheek and then vertically, stroking over your face each side until you reach your jawline. For each step do one side of the face first, then the other, and move on.
- Move down to your **jawline**: look straight ahead so your chin is lifted. Now stroke down your jawline from temples to chin on each side of your face. Then reverse the process upwards, from chin out to temples (as in the picture above), gently pushing the skin up and out with your fingertips.
- Now place the fingertips of your holding hand just **under your chin**, keeping it firm. Move your fingertips (or cloth) up to your ear, each side in turn, while you push the skin upwards and outwards with the fingertips of your other hand. (You can watch any wrinkles smoothing out as you do this…) Remember to work the area thoroughly under your cheekbones.
- For the **décolleté**, we apply a little oil to our palms then stroke the fingers from side to side and up and down, using the length of our hands flat against the skin.
- And lastly your **neck**: stroke up towards the jawline, using the length of the fingers as well as the palms, cupping your hands alternately – one after the other – round your neck, fingers and thumb upward in a V-shape.

NB: It is literally different strokes for different folks with this massage. Experiment with what perks you up and then incorporate it into your routine. For us it's pinching and lifting along the brow bone, then working horizontally – quite firmly – along the orbital bone under the eyes from nose to temples.

NIGHT TREATMENTS
our award winners

Packed with active botanicals, these overnight sensations work in synergy with the skin's natural cycle to renew and revive complexions

AURELIA PROBIOTIC SKINCARE CELL REVITALISE NIGHT MOISTURISER
✳✳✳

SCORE: 9.5/10

This night treatment has notched up one of the highest product scores in *Beauty Bible*'s history – a fantastic achievement. Rich with firming kigelia Africana, baobab, hibiscus, borage and mongongo oils, plus shea butter, it has a skin-melting texture and a delectable orange blossom, mandarin, rose and lavender scent.

COMMENTS: 'A 5-star rating: skin firmer, fine lines plumper – my husband asked, "have you changed your skincare? Your skin looks amazing"' • 'the smell's so uplifting I sat there hands cupped the first time I tried it – divine' • 'am amazed how quickly I felt a difference in smoothness and softness of skin' • 'the most divine night cream I've ever used (and I've tried a lot)' • 'skin glowing, have recommended to family with sensitive skin' • 'this made a real difference to forehead and laughter lines'.

ORIGINS HIGH POTENCY NIGHT-A-MINS
✳✳✳

SCORE: 8.71/10

This is one of Origins' classics, packed with minerals and antioxidants, plus a time-released resurfacing ingredient to aid cell turnover. And a POMS (Profile of Mood State) study revealed that 87 per cent of panellists experienced a longer, more restful night and tranquil sleep.

AT A GLANCE

AURELIA PROBIOTIC
SKINCARE
CELL REVITALISE
NIGHT MOISTURISER

ORIGINS
HIGH POTENCY
NIGHT-A-MINS

JURLIQUE
HERBAL RECOVERY
NIGHT CREAM

THIS WORKS
NO WRINKLES
NIGHT REPAIR

WE LOVE

Jo double layers product at night: the luscious Emma Hardie Amazing Face AM/PM Treatment Moisturiser, with a facial oil over the top. Sarah puts on oil, or serum (or both on dry days) then night cream.

COMMENTS: 'Skin smoother, more "defined" and brighter' • 'my husband and mother have both commented (she wanted to pinch the pot)' • 'lovely citrus smell to this thick, luxurious cream: in the morning, skin plumped, hydrated, soft and smooth' • 'enhances radiance' • 'lovely to drift off with the scent of orange in my nostrils' • 'skin looked much better on the side I'd been using this on, with open pores slightly reduced too; I'm using it on both sides now to look more "balanced up"'.

JURLIQUE HERBAL RECOVERY NIGHT CREAM
✳

SCORE: 8.29/10

The Herbal Recovery range from this Oz-based biodynamic beauty company has been seducing our testers since our first book. The cream is rich in antioxidant plant extracts, including African birch, 'moth bean' (a first for us), kakadu plum, daisy extract, plus skin-plumping glycerine and hyaluronic acid.

COMMENTS: 'Loved this from the first moment and after three months I can say wholeheartedly that my skin and fine lines have improved in texture and appearance' • 'skin looks more alive and fresher next morning; a luxurious, nourishing product' • 'my friend said I looked really radiant and asked what I was using!' • 'didn't irritate my dry, sensitive, eczema-prone skin and has made a real difference to my complexion – I think I look a little younger'.

THIS WORKS NO WRINKLES NIGHT REPAIR

✳ ✳ ✳

SCORE: 8.29/10

We're such big fans of the No Wrinkles range. This serum-style product (to be worn under a moisturiser) has been formulated to make you 'look like you've had eight hours' sleep, even when you haven't…', with its non-greasy blend of Persian silk tree extract, hyaluronic acid, cactus flower and retinol (vitamin A).

COMMENTS: 'After first use skin looked plumper and more even toned; after a few weeks skin appeared smoother and less lined, make-up went on better and I needed less. This works!' • 'does it make a difference in 24 hours? 24 seconds more like: skin calm, hydrated, rejuvenated and nourished, healthier and brighter' • 'love, love, love this – I've tried most anti-ageing miracle products which don't do what they say and cost the earth, but a definite improvement day after day with this'.

TIP: We recommend Holistic Silk pillowcases (and so do women who've tried them out for us; see directory on page 216). They are definitely worth investing in, if you suffer from night-time 'creases' caused by a regular pillow.

MIRACLE CREAMS
our award winners

Who says there's no such thing as a natural miracle cream? Not our testers, that's for sure, who over a period of months very devotedly put each of these winning all-rounders through their paces on just half their face, for comparison. The following scored high marks – and some with more than one daisy – proving that you don't need to go near a dermatologist's surgery (or a 'derm' brand) to see visible differences. And, say testers, they'll boost your self-esteem

L'OCCITANE DIVINE CREAM
✻
SCORE: 8.61/10

This was the highest-ever-scoring miracle cream in *The Anti-Ageing Beauty Bible*, so we were nervous when we retested after L'Occitane tweaked the recipe for this luscious de-ageing dream formula. It is rich in the Corsican immortelle flower essential oil (used across this entire range by the French brand) which gives it such a wonderful aromatic fragrance. We needn't have worried: out of dozens trialled, Divine once again grabs the top slot here. Nothing we can say about it is more telling than our testers' raves – so here goes.

COMMENTS: 'Skin texture has improved, fine lines less visible, bigger wrinkles slightly blurred – complexion brighter, too; friends commented on how nice my skin is looking lately' • 'the side of my face I've been using the cream on looks more dewy and fresh; lines around my mouth less pronounced on the side I've put it on – I adore it' • 'makes me feel spoiled using it: decadent, like a huge treat with its bottle and thick, luxurious, creamy texture. I will definitely buy again as soon as I've finished this' • 'skin does look better on the side I use the cream on; I am desperate to slather this stuff over both sides of my face!' • 'my dry skin looks brighter and complexion "lifted"; larger wrinkles less prominent; no other moisturiser has had such an anti-ageing and hydrating effect for me before' • 'this cream has boosted my self-esteem: it has improved the look of my skin, plus wrinkles so

AT A GLANCE

L'OCCITANE
DIVINE CREAM

THIS WORKS
NO WRINKLES
EXTREME MOISTURISER

KORRES BLACK PINE
ANTIWRINKLE &
FIRMING DAY CREAM

MANUKA DOCTOR
APINOURISH REPAIRING
SKIN CREAM

GREEN PEOPLE
VITA MIN FIX

SHIFFA TAMANU
MOISTURISING CREAM

much less noticeable; the crêpiness has filled out, and what's important to me personally is the overall reduction in redness and dryness'.

THIS WORKS NO WRINKLES EXTREME MOISTURISER
✻
SCORE: 8.5/10

We just love it when our results are this consistent! This Works also resubmitted their plant-rich vitamin-A-powered cream – an existing winner in *The Anti-Ageing Beauty Bible* – and it did incredibly well with testers all over again, scoring a mere fraction of a percentage point lower. As the name suggests, it's very, very moisturising – thanks in part to lashings of skin-plumping hyaluronic acid.

COMMENTS: 'Quite sceptical to begin with: used it on one side of my face and could see no difference for a while, then, suddenly, I noticed that the line between my nose and mouth on the other side was not as deep – I literally almost look lopsided' • 'loved it! Made me happy to look in the mirror in the morning; melts on and skin looked more youthful, plumper and fresher: people actually said I looked younger' • 'I can't praise this moisturiser highly enough: my wrinkles look reduced, almost no fine lines visible and now a couple of friends have bought it' • 'amazing: after a late night I applied a generous amount and noticed the next morning that my skin didn't have any tell-tale signs: it felt soft, like a silk sheet or a newborn baby' • 'fragrance, feel and texture awesome'.

KORRES BLACK PINE ANTIWRINKLE & FIRMING DAY CREAM

SCORE: 8.43/10

✳

From the Greek pharmacy brand, this is a light-but-powerful cream packed with high levels of pine extract which are said to be rich in antioxidant polyphenols. Quercetin, shea butter, wild yam extract, sunflower seed, sweet almond oils and more also feature. It is recommended for dry to very dry skins.

COMMENTS: 'My face seems plumper, softer, more youthful; little lines definitely improved; I asked my husband to stroke the two sides of my face and he said the Korres side was softer!' • 'I really do think my skin looks younger after using this' • 'creamy texture, smells absolutely divine and lines on forehead reduced' • 'it's the best-smelling face cream I've used; skin looks healthier (which in turn means a bit younger)' • 'I can see a difference in the lines of my face; looking forward to balancing out my creases on the other side now I've finished the trial'.

MANUKA DOCTOR APINOURISH REPAIRING SKIN CREAM

✳

SCORE: 8.33/10

Manuka Doctor scooped 'Best New Brand' two years running in the UK's Cosmetic Executive Women Awards. It features plenty of botanicals, but silicones are also high up the ingredients list – so if you're coming at naturals from more mainstream ranges (the Lauders and the Lancômes, etc.), this is a great 'bridge' brand. It has high levels of skin-softening avocado, super-strength manuka honey, and 'bee venom' extract, which is said to relax wrinkles.

COMMENTS: 'Ironed out crêpiness; skin much smoother and lines softened' • 'my face is much firmer around the eye area, across cheekbones; complexion clearer and brighter' • 'I've softer, smoother skin; fine lines improved' • 'great product, especially for women with oily skin (like me)' • 'love this light gel-cream moisturiser

which sinks in very quickly; lines are much softer and a big reduction in deeper grooves'.

GREEN PEOPLE VITA MIN FIX

✳✳✳

SCORE: 8.25/10

A lightweight, pump-action bottle of organically certified, age-defying moisture, for normal, dry and tired skins. An 'explosion' of vitamins, minerals and antioxidants is how they describe the ingredients, which include vitamins A and E, omega-rich perilla, avocado and evening primrose seed oils, plus rosemary extract.

COMMENTS: 'I was recently away meeting people for the first time and was consistently placed at a younger age than I am – my skin looks really healthy and in good condition' • 'a friend said I looked less tired than I should have considering the amount of sleep I'm getting; I'd definitely buy this again' • 'this is a keeper: a good all-round cream and my skin loves it; I've ordered another bottle already' • 'loved the natural fragrance; I can see the visible difference between this and another organic moisturiser that I use, too'.

SHIFFA TAMANU MOISTURISING CREAM

✳✳✳

SCORE: 8/10

An excellent performance from this all-natural Dubai-based brand, which features rosemary, Chilean rosehip oil (to moisturise and smooth), jojoba, avocado, calendula, and aromatic tamanu oil, which delivers an almost tangy scent and is said to have regenerating powers.

COMMENTS: 'Skin brighter, healthier: I look radiant' • 'love the smell – would buy it for this alone' • 'face is plumped up and "springier"; wrinkles less obvious' • 'skin on treated side smoother and plumper, lines and wrinkles a little softer according to my daughter; after eight weeks I am in no doubt there's a visible difference • 'a really great product; skin much healthier and the texture improved'.

WE LOVE

For Jo, it's L'Occitane Divine all the way. Sarah loves Emma Hardie Amazing Face Age Support Treatment Cream.

How to be NATURALLY CONFIDENT

One of the most rewarding things we do is talking to real women – like you, like us! – at events and book signings (or on the bus…). What we've come to realise is that many women of all ages have, for no apparent reason, a confidence deficit. Here's our take on being happy in your skin – and a few tips we've learnt along the way

The truth is that virtually no one is physically perfect and it is often our imperfections that make us attractive. Supermodels' 'flaws' have often proved their trademark: think of the gap in Lauren Hutton's front teeth, Cindy Crawford's prominent dark mole, and Cara Delevingne's beetling black eyebrows.

Very few of us believe we look fantastic 24/7. We doubt even supermodels wake up, look in the mirror and say: 'Babe, you're gorgeous.' (Not every day, anyway.) The images we see in magazines and ads often bear only partial resemblance to the reality of those so-called 'perfect' women portrayed in them. Not to say they aren't wonderful looking – they just get a lot of help.

We've been on a photo shoot where Linda Evangelista walked in looking puffy cheeked, dark circled and generally un-supermodelish. Then her experience and 'attitude' took over.

Expertly made up and fabulously frocked, she went in front of the camera and 'zipped up' that jawline, contracted her cheeks, posed at the most flattering angle – and transformed into the Linda Evangelista we all recognise. (Afterwards, though, she let it all subside.)

We know for a fact that Jerry Hall hates her ankles and is only ever photographed in a handful of poses. One fresh-faced Russian 'super' is troubled by her eye bags; Kate Moss's skin is said to need a lot of tender loving concealer and Cara Delevingne finds the whole modelling performance so stressful that she has developed psoriasis.

But, ironically, many 'ordinary' women's self-esteem is dented by the flawless images beaming out from the media. Remember: models only look like that from a certain angle, at a particular instant, for the click of a camera – and that's before digital retouching and the rest. (Kate Winslet – famous for being curvy and proud of it – was elongated to Barbie-esque proportions on one *GQ* cover.)

Being flawless is high maintenance – and pretty costly. A lot of famous faces spend a not-so-small fortune on cosmetic dermatology:

having lines filled, cheeks plumped, jawlines tightened and/or the top layers of their skin peeled away. And many of the slender women you see in movies, ads, on TV and the ballet stage, too, are on permanent semi-starvation diets. You may be able to squeeze into those skinny jeans or figure-hugging LBD after dieting but weight loss also affects your skin, brain and hormones (cutting out fat is a sure-fire way to age prematurely as we have seen). Is that really worth it? The short answer is no. We are all for being fit and shapely but please do it safely – by eating well and exercising. (Read more on this hobby horse on page 112.)

We also try to point out that, often, the so-called 'flaws' women fret and angst about are nigh on invisible to other people. They point out a sun spot or wrinkle we can hardly see, or fret about open pores that we have to get a magnifying glass to register. And – perversely, sadly – they miss all the good bits.

SO, PLEASE: HAVE A SECOND GLANCE IN THE MIRROR. We are conditioned to see the things we don't like and end up putting too much emphasis (and often too much make-up) on them. Put on your rose-tinted specs, take another look, and appreciate just one feature you do like. Clue: it's usually something other people notice: that infectious smile; wow-factor hair; peachy skin; hourglass figure; shapely legs; even pretty ear lobes, or luscious lips. And please don't reject compliments: treat them like presents and respond nicely with a 'thank you'.

And, now, accentuate the positive! We encourage you to dress and make up to maximise your assets. (There are plenty of ways to disguise the negative if you choose.) If you're curvy, make the most of those curves. If you have fabulous hair, prioritise spending on a good cut (and maybe colour) that shows it off. Gloss up a pretty mouth, buy sparkly earrings, flaunt your legs in (faux or real) Louboutin heels…

It's not just about focusing on the external. Yes, this book is about beauty. (And wellbeing, too.) But does that mean we're only interested in the outer layer? Not at all: we look at the bigger picture. Your feelings of self-worth should extend beyond the physical. Research has shown that individuals who have the healthiest levels of self-esteem acknowledge other qualities in their lives: the fact they are great at being a friend or family member, have a specific talent, a rewarding job – or are just lovely to be around. In the grand scheme of things, these all far outweigh the importance of having legs that go on forever, or a waist as trim as a starlet's.

Truly, your soul is reflected in your outer appearance: a heartfelt smile, the light in your eyes, the way you behave to others – even your voice. And that's what people remember, not your imperfections.

Aim for a balance between inner and outer confidence. This book is full of tips and products that we know can make a difference to your appearance. But we are encouraging every woman to get a sense of the big picture, the image of you that others see. It's natural that self-esteem has peaks and troughs: sometimes it's down to sheer lack of sleep, or an unavoidable blow like a loved one becoming sick, or losing a job. (Or being unable to find one in the first place, for that matter.) But there is so much each of us can do to feel better about ourselves, most of the time.

When you take care of yourself it shines out. The very best recipe for beauty, health and self-esteem begins with looking after ourselves – face, body and soul. Exercise doesn't just shape you up and keep you fit: it releases a plethora of feel-good endorphins that surge through the body. Eating a well-balanced diet will improve mind as well as body. Cutting out excess caffeine can reduce a sense of panic and stress, and – together with a hug, a funny film and a good night's sleep – has unfurrowed many a fretful frown line that was troubling its owner and denting her confidence.

We can all find achievable ways to boost our self-esteem. As the song says, 'latch on to the affirmative… spread joy up to the maximum'. When confidence shines out, that is the essence of true, natural beauty…

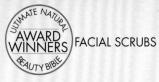

FACIAL SCRUBS
our award winners

Scrubs are fantastic at ditching the dirt! But the exfoliator should be gentle and packed with botanicals to nourish newly revealed skin. Our testers loved these

LIZ EARLE GENTLE FACE EXFOLIATOR
✳

SCORE: 8.67/10

One of our favourite facial scrubs, which decongests and softly buffs dull-looking skin with fine jojoba beads in a skin-softening cocoa butter base, infused with the uplifting scent of purifying eucalyptus. It's good for clearing blocked pores and blackheads, they suggest.

COMMENTS: 'Not too scratchy; didn't irritate my sensitive skin but left it glowing' • 'loved using this: the skin on the treated side of my face is soft and much brighter' • 'does a great job without the harshness' • 'lovely, fresh, zingy scent – you can really smell the eucalyptus' • 'someone at work commented: "you look different – oh, you're not wearing any make-up"; I did have make-up on, but much lighter than I'd normally wear' • 'skin felt moisturised afterwards which isn't something I expected'.

JURLIQUE PURELY AGE-DEFYING REFINING TREATMENT
✳✳

SCORE: 8.55/10

Apricot seed powder powers the exfoliating action of this slim-tubed scrub, which also features willow bark extract, a natural source of salicylic acid (a 'beta-hydroxy' acid). To counter that, they add soothing bisabolol and calendula, plus the 'Jurlique Biodynamic Blend' – a skin-boosting infusion of organic and biodynamic herbs and plants from their Adelaide farm.

COMMENTS: 'Expected skin to be red and rough but it wasn't – it looked glowing' • 'immediately liked this skin-polisher: face felt and appeared refreshed' • 'my uneven skin tone has been reduced and looks smoothed and plumped – I'd consider other Jurlique products after using this polisher' • 'my daughters think my skin looks lovely and even my husband has noticed!' • 'love the lemony smell' • 'this has

AT A GLANCE

LIZ EARLE
GENTLE FACE
EXFOLIATOR

JURLIQUE
PURELY AGE-DEFYING
REFINING TREATMENT

LAVERA
PURIFYING SCRUB

ÉMINENCE
STRAWBERRY RHUBARB
DERMAFOLIANT

reduced the appearance of pores, smoothed out skin texture and lessened the patches of discolouration – I cannot praise it enough'.

LAVERA PURIFYING SCRUB
✳✳

SCORE: 8.5/10

A fresh-scented gel option from a German brand that's been at the forefront of natural skincare for decades. The exfoliating action is down to jojoba beads, alongside plant extracts including witch hazel and safflower. They recommend avoiding the eye zone – but that holds true for all facial scrubs, please note.

COMMENTS: 'This is now a must for me before a big occasion' • 'skin felt lovely and smooth, fresh and clean after use' • 'gentle not scratchy – usually my skin feels tight and dry after a scrub, but not with this' • 'loved it: I sometimes get dry patches but this really helped – and left my skin with a glow and very well-hydrated'.

ÉMINENCE STRAWBERRY RHUBARB DERMAFOLIANT
✳✳✳

SCORE: 8.5/10

Here's something a little different from this certified-organic Hungarian brand: you turn the nozzle and pour a little of the fruit-scented, lactic-acid-boosted powder – which also incorporates rice powder, thermal mud, oatmeal and pore-tightening chickpea flour – into the palm of your hands. Then add a few drops of water to create a paste, and apply using a circular motion to the face.

COMMENTS: 'This is gorgeous: the dry powder scent changes to a lovely rice smell when water is added, and it's an amazing texture on the skin – leaving a soft complexion' • 'liked the fruity, light smell' • 'lots of comments about how nice my skin looked' • 'skin felt very clean and "alive" afterwards'.

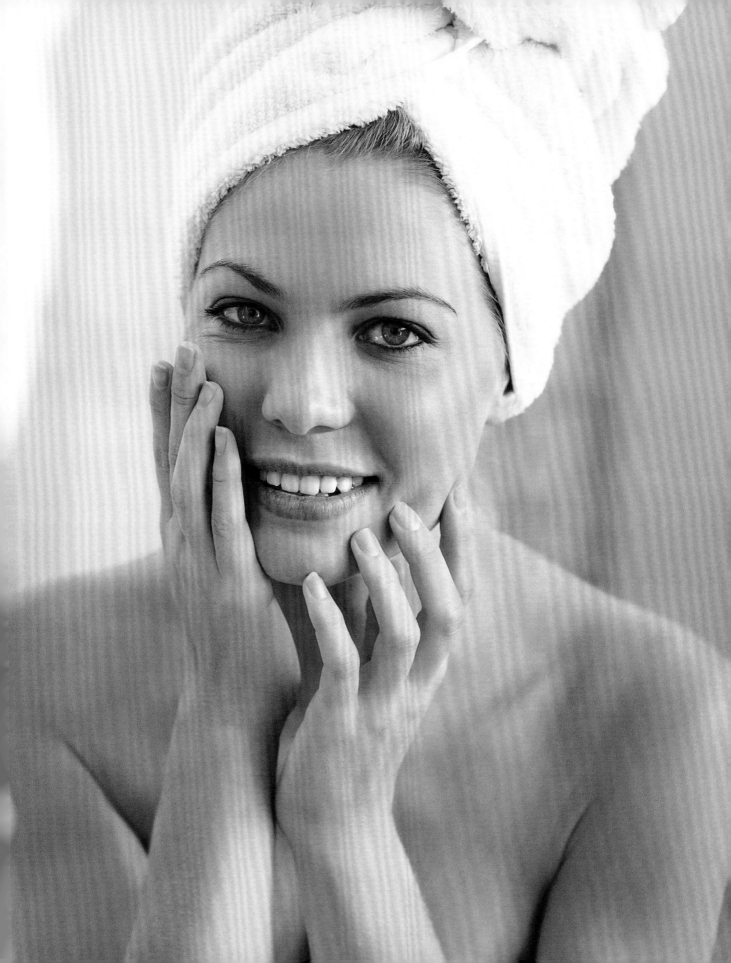

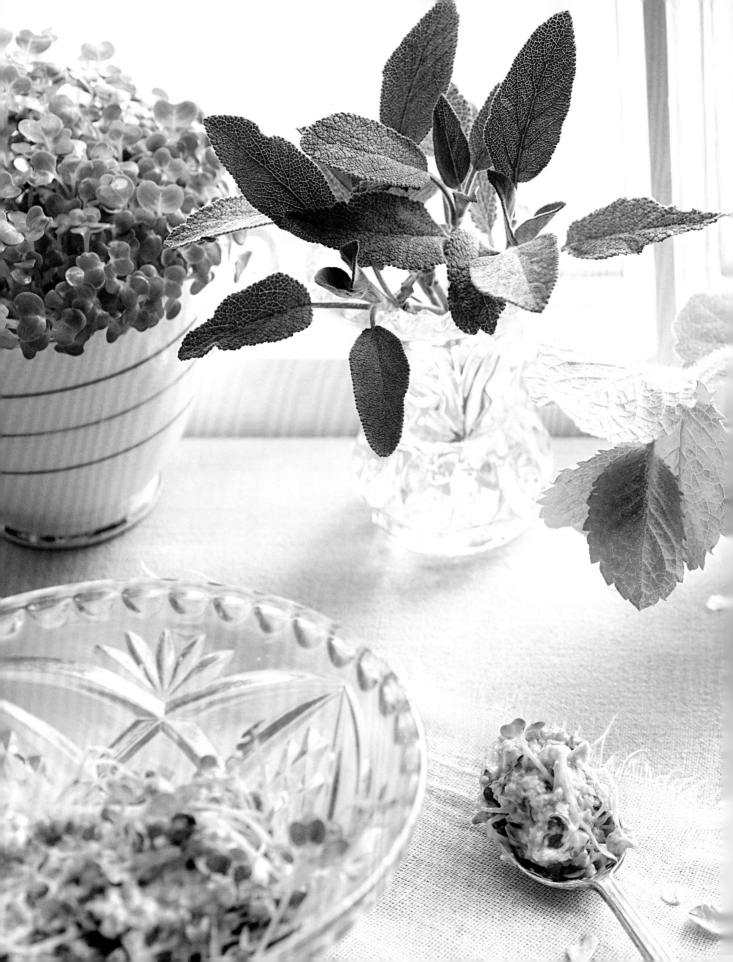

GENTLY DOES IT

Do you have problem skin that is prone to break out at the slightest 'insult'?
If so, the last thing you want to do is pile on aggressive chemicals. Opt for
a kind approach, instead, with this deep-cleansing facial steam and buffer

PEPPERMINT AND THYME FACIAL STEAM

Lots of problem-skin sufferers like to steam their skin (actually so does Sarah). Mint and thyme are the perfect herbs for this because they are effective antibacterials, helping to purify the complexion. The mint also has an antiseptic effect. Facial steaming is the best way to clean your skin pore-deep to get rid of city grime or dirt, encouraging pores to expel toxins. However, it should be avoided if you have a tendency for broken veins (like Jo).

- 2 handfuls of fresh mint leaves
  (or 1 tablespoon dried mint)
- 1 teaspoon fresh thyme leaves
  (or ½ teaspoon dried thyme leaves)
- 600ml (1 pint) water (preferably purified tap or mineral water; or allow tap water to sit in an open bottle for 24 hours until the chlorine dissipates)
- 2 drops peppermint essential oil (optional)

Place the mint and thyme leaves with the water in a pan, and bring to the boil. Remove from the heat and add the peppermint essential oil.

Allow to cool slightly, and then pour the mixture into a heatproof bowl.

Sit down with the bowl on a table in front of you, hover your face over the bowl, covering your head with a thick towel and making sure the sides are closed. As you lean over the bowl, the steam will open the pores and cause you to perspire, helping to release toxins and debris.

Repeat the facial steam once or twice a week. It's good to do it before using a face mask, to increase its effectiveness.

CRESS AND OATMEAL SKIN BUFFER
for oily skin

The cress in this recipe is packed with antioxidant vitamins A and C, plus it is highly antiseptic and antibacterial. The oatmeal has a skin-soothing effect, and together they are great news for oily skins.

- 1 small bunch cress, with leaves and stalks
- 2 tablespoons plain yogurt
- 60g (2½oz) coarsely ground oatmeal
- 4 pieces of 30cm (11in) square muslin

Purée the cress and yogurt in a blender. Pour the oatmeal into a bowl, add the purée and mix well.

Pile 2 tablespoons of the mixture in the centre of each cloth, gather the fabric and secure with a piece of string, ribbon or raffia. The bags will last for several days if you keep them in a plastic bag in the fridge

After cleansing at night, moisten your face with water and dampen one cress bag. Massage oily or blemished zones with the bag, squeezing it gently to release the extracts. Leave the skin to dry naturally.

FACE MASKS
our award winners

We heart face masks, possibly something to do with the on-box commandment to 'relax for 5/10/15 minutes', while the formula works its softening, brightening, hydrating, glow-restoring magic. Because how often in life do you get told to lie back and do nothing? We sent over 40 different masks to *Beauty Bible* panellists. And from their horizontal positions, they report on the real winners...

LIZ EARLE INTENSIVE NOURISHING TREATMENT MASK
✳

SCORE: 8.94/10

A regular winner just about every time we run our trials, and dry- and sensitive-skinned testers fell for this richly hydrating mask all over again. (This is not one for oilier complexions.) The intensive skin drink calms complexions with comfrey, while shea butter and borage seed oil hydrate and help the skin's barrier function. (NB: This is one of the few Liz Earle products that features a combo of parabens; if that bothers you, find out more on page 153.)
COMMENTS: 'Skin felt really soft and glowing – shiny, clear and fresh' • 'this was easy to relax in, didn't feel like my face was cracking, as with some masks I've experienced in the past' • 'very indulgent and nourishing – a treatment to make you feel pampered' • 'what a fantastic product! My skin feels so soft and revitalised; it has made a major difference' • 'by far one of the best face masks I've ever used – just fabulous!' • 'my skin drinks this up – even as a quick fix; one of the best for injecting moisture into parched skin' • 'like a spa at home'.

OSKIA RENAISSANCE MASK
✳ ✳

SCORE: 8.69/10

Although this British product features fruit acids (from passion fruit, lemon and pineapple), it's never bothered our touchy skins. They just love the luscious gel-like texture of this rose-tinted mask which targets all skin types and is great on mature complexions. It's wonderfully aromatic

AT A GLANCE

LIZ EARLE
INTENSIVE
NOURISHING
TREATMENT MASK

OSKIA
RENAISSANCE MASK

MV ORGANIC
SKINCARE SIGNATURE
MINERAL MASK SET

ESPA LIFT & FIRM MASK

DR.HAUSCHKA
REJUVENATING MASK

L'OCCITANE
IMMORTELLE
BRIGHTENING
MOISTURE MASK

with rose, chamomile – and a pleasant tanginess from the combination of passion fruit and papaya enzymes, which also work to brighten skin. A previous winner, re-tested for this book, and it wins a fresh award from us.
COMMENTS: 'Amazing: very brightening straight away; skin felt so soft for a couple of days after use' • 'unbelievable product; I was going out and didn't want to, which showed in my face, but this was a great pick-me-up' • 'a complete feeling of relaxation as you inhale the product (gosh, I sound like a complete moron!)' • 'first time I used this I was blown away, and couldn't believe the results: a healthy glow and freshness were so immediate' • 'this is brilliant at plumping and refreshing the skin, plus calming redness' • 'you look in the mirror afterwards and think "wow this works"'.

MV ORGANIC SKINCARE SIGNATURE MINERAL MASK SET
✳ ✳

SCORE: 8.57/10

There's a DIY vibe to this Aussie skin brightener, from a brand that Sarah loves. The kit features a dry powder that is based on skin-friendly powdered minerals, plus a mixing bowl and a fan-shaped applicator brush. Just add water. (The pack should last for 20 applications, they say.) It's good for normal to combination/oily skins, we'd say, though drier complexions could add a few drops of oil – or perhaps some MV Rose Skin Plus Booster (see page 75).
COMMENTS: 'Looked a bit of a faff when I opened the box, but it's easy to mix and apply; skin looked calmer and pores appeared smaller

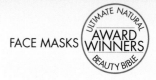

afterwards' • 'skin was left more nourished and even toned' • 'liked the texture: cooling but not drying at all' • 'the very first thing I noticed was clean pores: almost a "where did they go?" moment' • 'skin felt soft, revived and smoothed, and next day, refreshed with a lovely tone'.

ESPA LIFT & FIRM MASK
❋
SCORE: 8.57/10
Though the second ingredient is kaolin clay, the addition of argan and grapeseed oils make this appropriate even for 'maturing, stressed or dehydrated skin types'. Antioxidants and something that glories in the name of 'Pelan silt' (another mud) also feature, and we reckon any skin type would suit this.
COMMENTS: 'Smelt lovely and felt great on the skin' • 'looked like it would set "hard", but never did – very comfortable' • 'loved this: pleasant to use and benefits really noticeable; skin looked soft, smooth, clear and "evened out"' • 'afterwards I felt more perky and had a glow about me' • 'in the short term it left my skin looking tauter (good effect!)' • 'I'd buy this again, as I've found few masks that don't irritate my sensitive skin'.

DR.HAUSCHKA REJUVENATING MASK
❋ ❋
SCORE: 8.53/10
There are several masks in Dr.H's range, but this one's designed to 'bring life and vitality to pale, dry skin' (but would also suit deeper skin tones, we think: it isn't just for English roses…). Botanicals include apricot, borage, jojoba, peanut and wheat germ oils, with glycerine and extracts of carrot and chamomile. A lot of the Dr.Hauschka range has been repackaged in plastic but this still comes in one of the squeezy metal toothpaste-style tubes.
COMMENTS: 'Face felt smoother and softer without being left feeling dried out at all' • 'skin

looked plumped immediately, and felt better for a couple of days after use' • 'enjoyed this particularly when I was feeling tired or poorly – a good "rescue" mask' • 'absolutely loved this: skin looks soft and plump' • 'as soon as I started applying this mask, my skin was going "hey, this is great – give me more"' • 'face velvety smooth and feels "caressed"'.

L'OCCITANE IMMORTELLE BRIGHTENING MOISTURE MASK
❋
SCORE: 8.39/10
This is absolutely one of Jo's favourite masks. It's another product from the age-defying Immortelle range: it has a rich, crème-fraîche texture and lashings of that aromatic Corsican essential oil (immortelle), together with moisturising fig extracts and daisy-derived brighteners. Don't throw the box out till you've first read the instructions advising you to apply in a way that boosts micro-circulation, for even more glow.
COMMENTS: 'Complexion more even and felt youthful; love the thickness of the sumptuous cream, like it was full of goodness and luxurious, too' • 'skin looks healthy, toned and my complexion is amazing' • 'I could still feel the effects over 24 hours later; face feels thoroughly and deeply moisturised' • 'have also tried this as a night cream and it works wonderfully – going to bed with a lovely fresh fragrance on your skin and waking up to a plumped-up, soft, dewy face' • 'not only did make-up go on more smoothly, but I noticed my now-radiant skin peeking through my foundation; looked younger and refreshed'.

> TIP: Anything that is moisturising for faces is good for slathering on hands, too; so, while you lie relaxing with your mask on, do treat the backs of your hands as well.

POWER PACKS

You can nourish your skin with simple mixtures of ingredients, most of which you will already have in your kitchen. These home-made masks are super-quick to put together, and will make your face feel and look delicious

CUCUMBER MASK
for sensitive skin

Ultra-sensitive skins like gentle, soothing cucumber. Any leftover mask will keep for a day or two if stored in the fridge.

- 10g (½oz) brewer's yeast (if you can't find this, pulverise brewer's yeast tablets in a herb grinder)
- 10g (½oz) finely powdered oats
- 7.5cm (3in) chunk of cucumber, peeled
- 2 tablespoons plain yogurt
- 1 teaspoon honey
- 1 drop rose essential oil

Mix the yeast and oats in a small bowl and set aside. Liquidise the cucumber in a food processor or herb grinder until it's literally liquid, with no seeds or chunky bits.

Add the yogurt and honey and whizz again for a few seconds. Add the yeast and oats to the cucumber mixture, followed by the rose essential oil; whizz until smooth.

Apply to a cleansed face and leave for about 20–30 minutes.

Remove with a wet muslin cloth, or splash with water. Follow with toner and moisturiser.

VITA-CARROT MASK
for mature skin

This is good for even the most sensitive skins. Carrot is incredibly rich in vitamin A, which has an anti-ageing activity when applied to the skin topically.

- 1 large carrot
- 1 tablespoon sweet almond oil
- 5 drops jasmine essential oil (optional)

Peel and liquidise the carrot, then sieve and strain off the juice (you can drink this), reserving the pulp.

Next, blend the pulp with the sweet almond oil and add the jasmine essential oil, if you are using it.

Cleanse your face, then lie down with your head on a towel. Apply the pulp to your face and relax for 10–15 minutes.

Remove with a wet muslin cloth, or splash with water. Follow with toner and moisturiser.

TOMATO FACIAL MASK
for oily skin

The fruit acids in tomato are great for getting rid of blackheads, to which oily skins are prone. They also brighten dull skin by gently loosening surface cells.

- 1 ripe tomato

Slice the tomato thickly, then lie down and apply the slices directly onto your face.

To mould the slices round your nose, cut the tomato into shape.

Leave the tomato slices for a few minutes, then rinse and pat dry.

STARFLOWER MASK
for dry skin

This is Jo's all-time favourite mask, created by her husband Craig Sams: 'I love the way it softens and "plumps" my dry skin,' she says.

- 50g (2oz) aloe vera flesh
- 2 tablespoons plain yogurt
- 2 capsules of starflower (borage flower) oil
- 10 fresh borage flowers (in season)

Aloe vera flesh is quite hard to blend, so it is easiest to whizz all the ingredients in an electric herb chopper. (You'll need to snip the starflower oil capsules, and squeeze out the oil.)

Massage the mixture into the skin of the face and neck, and leave for about 15 minutes whereupon the most extraordinary thing happens – your complexion will have soaked up almost all the mask, and will be left looking plumped-up and younger.

FACIAL OILS
our award winners

Testers who have never tried facial oils before are often blown away by their plumping, smoothing, general age-defying effects – they are also surprised by how (in many products) the formulas sink in so fast that skin is not left greasy. They are a cinch to formulate naturally so we were able to put dozens through their paces – and these award winners combined a high pleasure factor with serious skin benefits. PS: We are huge fans, too

ESPA REPLENISHING FACE TREATMENT OIL
❈❈
SCORE: 9.38/10

A divine, aromatic experience with this super-high scorer. Coconut, sweet almond, avocado, macadamia nut, carrot and evening primrose create the rich base in which essential oils of neroli, sandalwood and patchouli work their cell-renewing magic. Suitable for all skin types but especially dry, dehydrated or ageing complexions. NB: Several testers commented they'd love the tall, screw-top bottle to be repackaged in a more 'squat' flask.

COMMENTS: 'One of the best things I've ever applied to my face – smells divine, my skin felt like it was drinking up this oil: it was left nourished, but not greasy at all' • 'gives a lovely warm feeling to skin as you apply it: very soothing and a great treat before you go to sleep' • 'so effective, it's worth paying the slightly higher price: my husband said my skin looked great... and he never usually notices! Thinking of buying a tanker load' • 'lovely, woody, warm scent' • 'will I buy again? Yes, yes, yes; I'm 42 and have had several clients who've never met me before tell me I look 30; has really improved my skin and far exceeded my expectations' • 'the best product I have ever used: gave an instant glow, and lines around my eyes and on forehead less visible'.

AT A GLANCE

ESPA
REPLENISHING FACE
TREATMENT OIL

AURELIA PROBIOTIC
SKINCARE CELL REPAIR
NIGHT OIL

AD SKIN SYNERGY
FACE OIL NOURISHING
NIGHT TREATMENT

MV ORGANIC
SKINCARE ROSE
SKIN PLUS BOOSTER

SUTI
NOURISH ORGANIC
FACE OIL FOR NIGHT

SUTI
REJUVENATE ORGANIC
FACE OIL

AURELIA PROBIOTIC SKINCARE CELL REPAIR NIGHT OIL
❈❈
SCORE: 9.15/10

Every product this newish British brand submitted for our trials rocketed up the charts and won an award. This oil in a dropper bottle bursts with the fresh but intoxicating scent of orange blossom, alongside lavender, rose and mandarin, plus exotic mongongo and Kalahari plant oils, baobab (a new buzz ingredient) which delivers omega 3, 6 and 9 fatty acids, and firming, toning kigelia.

COMMENTS: 'My skin looked fresh and plump after just the first application; on the odd night I didn't use it, I noticed my face wasn't feeling as good' • 'love this product: it smells absolutely divine (floral, sensual), sinks into skin with little effort and a little goes a long way' • 'oh my word, how much do I love this...? I could smother myself in this oil – the smell is amazing' • 'enhanced radiance and made me look younger' • 'everyone has commented on how good my skin looks and how my complexion has evened out (after three children I had pigmentation) – I now don't have a single blemish' • 'my mother and husband have both commented on my glowier softer skin' • 'really rate this due to the noticeable effects; also it's fragrance, lightness, non-greasiness, and quick absorption – it's a great product'.

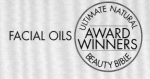

AD SKIN SYNERGY FACE OIL NOURISHING NIGHT TREATMENT

✻✻

SCORE: 9.12/10

A winner in previous books, this was retrialled – and received a very similar score. It has a nourishing base of sweet almond, coconut, evening primrose, jojoba, grapeseed, rosehip and coconut, along with frankincense, jasmine, lavender, ylang-ylang, rose geranium and Roman chamomile essential oils. (Mostly organic, though the end product isn't certified.) Dispensed via a small metal spray — the oil appears in drops, not as a mist. It was put through its paces by combination-skinned testers. *COMMENTS:* 'My skin had a plumpness I've never experienced before, with a lovely, dewy appearance' • 'face smoother and wrinkles on forehead less visible' • 'I now have the soft peachy skin of a newborn's bottom' • 'soothing fragrance: I felt I slept better after applying it' • 'my boyfriend said it makes my skin look "glowy"' • 'seems to last about nine months, so very good value for money' • 'a lovely foot treat, too, if you have a willing slave (sorry, partner) to rub it in' • 'loved this: easy to apply; sinks into my oily/combination skin really fast'.

MV ORGANIC SKINCARE ROSE SKIN PLUS BOOSTER

✻✻

SCORE: 9.07/10

Fragranced with Bulgarian rose oil, geranium and rosemary, this is from a cult Aussie brand. It targets dry, delicate and hormonal skins and is also formulated to act on redness and rosacea, soothing the complexion. *COMMENTS:* 'Has enhanced the tone and brightness of my skin' • 'texture of my face is like the Sahara, but this has made a massive difference – my skin just adores it and feels very smooth' • 'loved, loved, loved the delicate rose scent – in fact, there was nothing I didn't love about this' • 'received comments that my skin looks nice and I never usually get compliments of this nature' • 'a hero product: the tiniest amount of this magic yellow oil has made an amazing improvement to my dry, sensitive skin: less sore, patchy, flaky – and with a glow all of its own'.

SUTI NOURISH ORGANIC FACE OIL FOR NIGHT

✻✻

SCORE: 8.93/10

This is a spectacular result for the small, Sussex-based aromatherapy brand: two of their oils are award winners here. Most ingredients for both are certified organic (though these final products haven't been through the certification process). This version is the slightly richer night oil, with avocado, macadamia, apricot kernel, sesame and argan oils, plus aromatherapeutic jasmine, patchouli, bergamot and geranium. Suti infuse their oils with crystals, which they believe energises the ingredients. *COMMENTS:* 'The best oil I've ever used; I've recommended it to my friends – complexion much healthier' • 'fine lines seem diminished and skin looks plumper in the morning; I've been getting great comments about my skin since I started' • 'Suti – what a cutie! This smells heavenly; look forward to using it every evening and inhaling the aroma' • 'absolutely fab! Compared to my usual facial oil, this doesn't "creep" into eyes' • 'loved this from day one: didn't cause any spots – a great product'.

SUTI REJUVENATE ORGANIC FACE OIL

✻✻

SCORE: 8.86/10

Rosehip, evening primrose, jojoba and argan oils are the key skin-nurturers here, endowed with a lovely soft fruity scent by lashings of tangerine and orange oil, plus frankincense and rosemary. They recommend this for morning use after cleansing: just a drop should do. (We prefer oils for night – and this can be used then, although they recommend the previous winner specifically as a pre-sleep treatment.) *COMMENTS:* 'Skin plumper, firmer and dewy: radiant immediately' • 'the smell is divine: a rose and tangerine aroma' • 'face looked smoother and lines seemed to fade' • 'have had comments from several friends' • 'I felt like I was "feeding" my skin with fantastic ingredients that could only do it good' • 'sinks in beautifully; skin feels firmer and brighter – I am a major fan!' • 'a friend commented my skin is looking good which is always nice to hear!'

WE LOVE

Jo goes to bed with facial oil over her face, neck and décolletage: either Liz Earle Superskin Concentrate, or a wonderful product from Face Matters called Evening Elixir, which has an addictive blend of geranium, mandarin, jasmine and lemon essential oils. Sarah is a fan of the AD Skin Synergy and MV Organic products reviewed here and, for day, is fond of a (very expensive) drop of By Terry Huile de Rose Nutri-Regenerating Firming-Lift Oil. (PS: We like droppers please.)

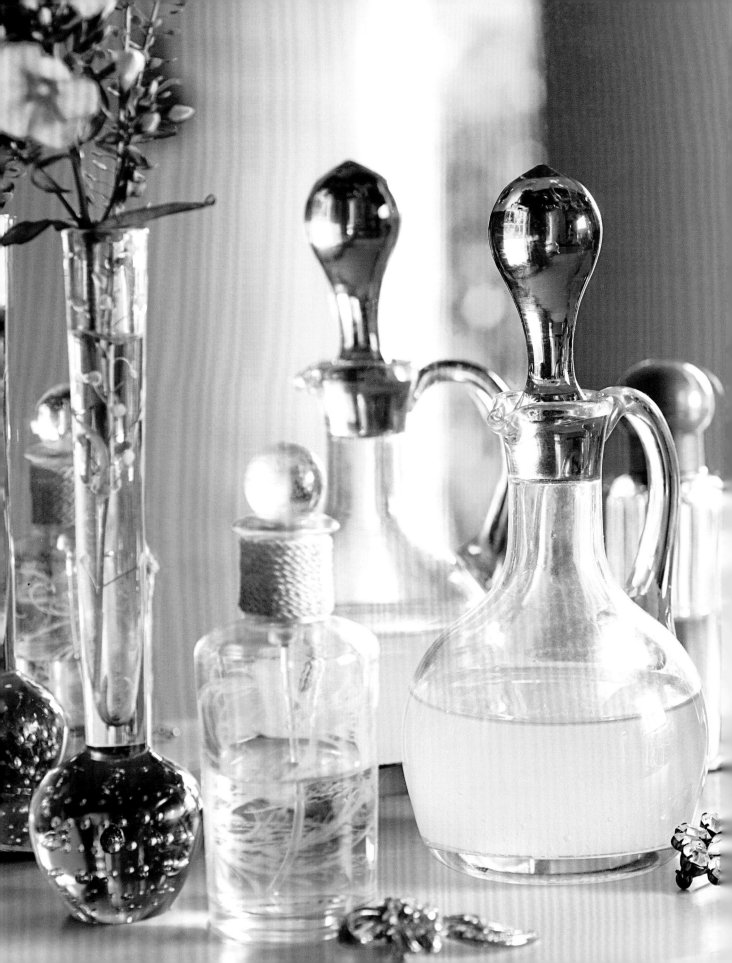

PRETTY SLICKERS

Facial oils are a cinch to make: simply pop in a small screw-top jar or bottle and shake vigorously to blend. Shake again before using

OILY TO NORMAL SKIN

Mention 'facial oil' to those with a shiny complexion, and they may run a mile. Yet botanical oils can work to rebalance and normalise greasy or oily skins. Many people need to overcome their prejudice against oils – we suggest you give this formula a go, at night, for two weeks, and you may well be very surprised (and delighted) by the results.

- 2 tablespoons grapeseed oil (this is the best oil for oily skin, although jojoba is also brilliantly rebalancing)
- 10 drops juniper essential oil ● 15 drops petitgrain essential oil ● 5 drops frankincense essential oil
- 5 drops marjoram essential oil ● 10 drops lemon essential oil

NORMAL SKIN

Normal skin? Lucky you! This blissful scented oil can be used instead of a night-time moisturiser. We always advise a real-time assessment of skin's needs on a daily (or, in this case, nightly) basis: an oil is great when your normal skin is feeling in need of a little extra nourishment. That might mean every night – or it might mean twice a week. Try to tune into your own skin's condition and use accordingly; if it feels dry or rough to your fingertips, it would love some well-oiled TLC.

- 2 tablespoons avocado oil ● 15 drops rose essential oil ● 10 drops geranium essential oil
- 5 drops neroli essential oil ● 5 drops palmarosa essential oil ● 10 drops calendula essential oil

DRY OR MATURE SKIN

These oils are all excellent for ageing and sagging skin – and this is the blend we make for ourselves. Our favourite essential oil is probably neroli (orange blossom oil), which has a natural cell-rejuvenating action as well as a divine, sweet fragrance. If you don't want to use a blend like this (but please do try it, you might be converted!), simply add a drop or two of neroli to your usual night-time moisturiser as a booster: blend in the palm of your hand, and massage into skin.

- 1 tablespoon sweet almond oil ● 1 tablespoon argan oil ● the contents of 2 capsules wheatgerm oil
- 10 drops frankincense essential oil ● 10 drops sandalwood essential oil ● 10 drops patchouli essential oil
- 15 drops neroli essential oil ● 5 drops clary sage essential oil

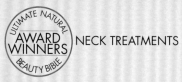
NECK TREATMENTS
our award winners

There was little between these top creams and serums, score-wise – but plenty of the 30 or so tested languished down in the sixes. These are the neck's best (natural) things

DR.HAUSCHKA REGENERATING NECK AND DÉCOLLETÉ CREAM
✹✹
SCORE: 8.06/10

There are some stonking results in challenging categories for the renowned biodynamic brand. They take top prize here for a tube of rich cream boosted by strengthening horsetail, oils of jojoba, sesame, sunflower and macadamia, shea butter, and fragrant Rosa Damascena.
COMMENTS: 'Fabulous, yummy, gorgeous; smells quite exotic' • 'definite reduction in fine lines and crêpiness has improved' • 'a smoother neck and décolletage' • 'wrinkles softened, skin less dry and neck lines dramatically reduced, leaving a fresh and younger complexion' • 'this is a lovely product with a fresh, clean scent' • 'great – to anyone over 40, I'd say: "go for it!"' • 'wow, a massive difference in 10 days; I've bought this so I can keep my fab new neck'.

LOVE YOUR SKIN CENTELLA & WILLOW BARK FACIAL SERUM
✹
SCORE: 8/10

Tiny brand, big score: Love Your Skin is a British brand created by a skincare expert with 40 years' experience. It punches above its weight with this light facial serum (which they submitted for this category); it incorporates beta-hydroxy acid, willow bark, firming Centella Asiatica, meadowsweet and senna.
COMMENTS: 'The skin on my neck looks firmer and healthier after using this light, clear gel, which sinks in fast' • 'my chest area feels hydrated, younger and smoother: a lovely cream' • 'my neck was smoother, fine lines and crêpiness reduced – much more toned' • 'my neck has never looked so good and I'm now addicted to this product!' • 'yes, yes I would buy this and have put it on my birthday list'.

AT A GLANCE

DR.HAUSCHKA REGENERATING NECK AND DÉCOLLETÉ CREAM

LOVE YOUR SKIN CENTELLA & WILLOW BARK FACIAL SERUM

LIZ EARLE SUPERSKIN MOISTURISER

LIZ EARLE SUPERSKIN BUST & NECK TREATMENT

WE LOVE

Jo remains devoted to Liz Earle Superskin (right), while Sarah religiously takes all face products down to her chest, which has worked so far. As with any treatment, it is regular – and we mean daily – use that maintains any improvements.

LIZ EARLE SUPERSKIN MOISTURISER
✹
SCORE: 7.63/10

Here's the legendary Superskin, yet again, voted in by a new crop of neck slatherers. Lusciously textured, it's crammed with rich fatty acids and antioxidants: oils of cranberry seed, rosehip and borage, plus shea butter and pomegranate – these all contribute to its nourishing power.
COMMENTS: 'My neck is smoother, lines seem reduced and not so deep; décolletage seems less crêpey' • 'after two weeks of use, the skin on my neck and chest felt and appeared smoother, and crêpiness caused by sun damage was vastly improved – I wouldn't have believed the difference if I hadn't seen it happening myself' • 'neck more toned, less lined' • 'I usually use Crème de la Mer and thought this wouldn't be as good – but it was fab!'

LIZ EARLE SUPERSKIN BUST & NECK TREATMENT
✹
SCORE: 7.42/10

Just behind the Superskin moisturiser comes this treatment targeted at necks (and bust). You may have read of it in our previous books, but we did send it out all over again – and here it is on the winners' podium. Botanicals include kigelia extract, mangosteen, quince, green algae and white lupin, to 'plump' this fragile zone.
COMMENTS: 'My necklace lines are less noticeable and my décolleté smoother with fewer wrinkles, too' • 'this product is amazing! I can't sing its praises highly enough: it's easy to apply, I even worked it down to the cleavage and the little crêpey lines vanished!' • 'what can I say except I loved this product: texture, scent, even the dispenser; more importantly I liked the velvety-smooth skin; recommended for anyone who feels bad about their neck area'.

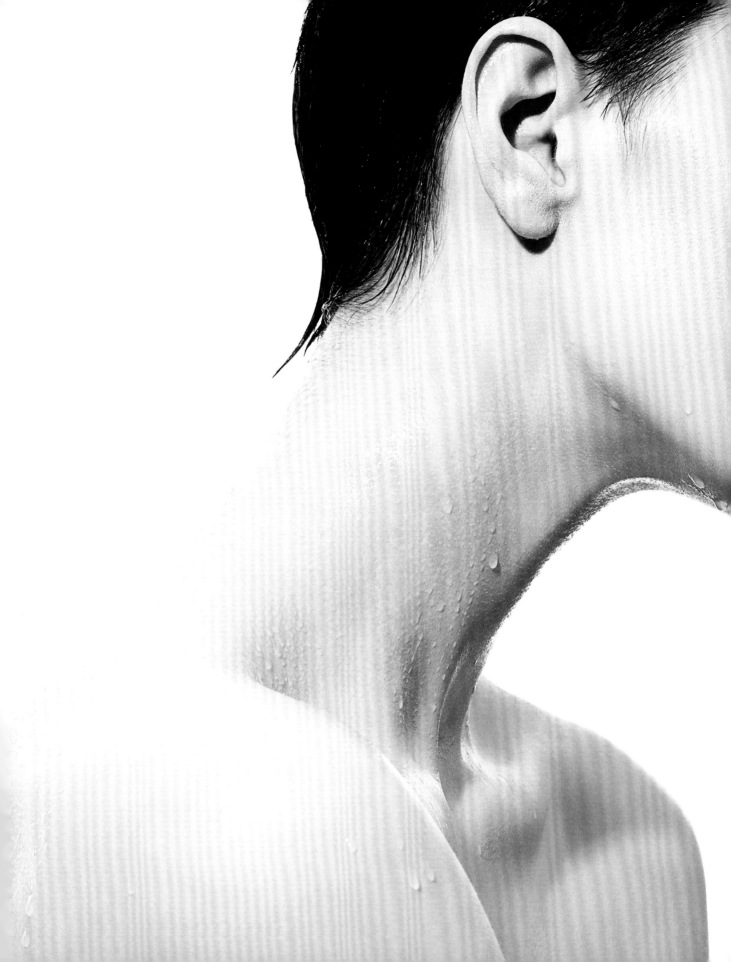

SWIPE AND GO

The fragile eye zone requires a super-gentle cleanser. This moisturising oil-and-herbs formula is as effective as any conventional remover

GENTLE EYE MAKE-UP REMOVER OIL

In our (wide) experience, the most effective conventional eye make-up removers blend oil and water in a shake-before-use product. Recreate their cleansing power by applying this oil on a damp cotton pad – and your skin will benefit from the nurturing blend, too.

- 5g (approximately 1 teaspoon) dried eyebright
- 10g (½oz) dried calendula (marigold) flowers
- 2 tablespoons olive oil
- 2 tablespoons avocado oil
- 2 tablespoons sunflower oil

In a screw-top jar cover the dried herbs with the oils and leave for about four weeks on a windowsill to infuse the gentle, soothing plant goodness. Check the oil from time to time to make sure the herbs remain submerged.

After the required time, strain and strain again, either through kitchen towel or muslin, and pour into a dry, sterilised bottle with a screw top or a cork – or even better, a bottle with a drop dispenser.

You can speed the process by 'cooking' the herbs in the oil in a double boiler (see page 212) for 15 minutes.

Cool thoroughly and strain as before, then transfer to a sterilised bottle.

To use the infused oil, put 3–4 drops onto a damp cotton pad that you've squeezed to get rid of excess moisture. (Use a dropper if your bottle doesn't have one.) Swipe the cotton pad across the eye area, but avoid getting the formula into your eyes. Be sure to use a clean pad for each eye.

EYE MAKE-UP REMOVERS
our award winners

On our wish list: a product that is tough on make-up (even waterproof mascara) but gentle on eyes. Our panel tested 20 and these mostly natural options delivered

ESPA BIO-ACTIVE EYE CLEANSER
✹✹
SCORE: 8.14/10
The pale-blue liquid in this shake-before-use glass bottle of luxury eye make-up remover is enriched with hyaluronic acid (one of our top skincare ingredients, known for its visibly 'plumping' effect). It features a non-greasy coconut oil derivative, lash-conditioning moringa extract and a dash of antioxidant malachite. It's 99 per cent natural – so teensy quantities of synthetics in here – but we thought it's so darned close it deserves two daisies.
COMMENTS: 'Needed just one thorough wipe to remove all make-up' • 'I love this make-up remover: it's the best one I've ever used (and I'm 52 so I've used a lot). It removed waterproof mascara with one or two light wipes' • 'this product has changed my thoughts on eye cleansers; previously, I would not have used one but this takes off everything with a swift wipe' • 'really refreshes your eyes' • 'no sensitivity (hurrah!), very gentle but also effective (a Holy Grail)' • 'safe for contact lenses, so I'm happy'.

JUSTBE CLEANSED EYE MAKEUP REMOVER
✹✹
SCORE: 7.85/10
From an artisan aromatherapy brand that's new to us, created by a Scottish aromatherapist (Gail Bryden), this soft balm-like remover is designed to be squeezed onto a damp cotton pad before gliding over eyes. The make-up-melting elements are coconut oil, coconut 'solid', and coco glucoside, with jojoba, vitamin E, beeswax and a subtle fragrance from geranium and petitgrain essential oils. They say: the remover can also be used for all-over facial cleansing with a muslin cloth. We say: the small bottle

AT A GLANCE
ESPA BIO-ACTIVE EYE CLEANSER
JUSTBE CLEANSED EYE MAKEUP REMOVER
NATORIGIN EYE MAKE-UP REMOVER EMULSION

WE LOVE
Jo finds that the reformulated Eye Make-Up Remover by Melvita – a soothing, cornflower-rich lotion – is the best way to take off her eye make-up at night. Sarah relies on her long-term favourite Cleanse & Polish by Liz Earle, which swipes off eye make-up without stinging.

would be very convenient for travelling – but it won't last long for regular all-over use.
COMMENTS: 'No traces of make-up on pillow, and no smudging the next day' • 'very effective' • 'the balm texture makes all the difference: very efficient at removing make-up, and it almost felt like I was pampering my eyes; luxurious indeed' • 'incredibly gentle, didn't trigger any soreness or sensitivity – in fact, soothed the area' • 'this remover, in its hygienic pump, has become a favourite of mine: it's almost like an eye treatment in itself'.

NATORIGIN EYE MAKE-UP REMOVER EMULSION
✹✹
SCORE: 7.83/10
The award-winning NATorigin range is certified by Ecocert and this offering has featured in a previous book of ours. It was retested this time, receiving more good scores and comments. The lotion-style remover contains soothing raspberry seed oil and red algae extract. Sensitive-skinned readers may like to know that the hypoallergenic NATorigin brand is the only one approved by Allergy UK.
COMMENTS: 'This removed my waterproof mascara without any effort' • 'found this very gentle (even on my eyes which are sensitive after laser surgery)' • 'performs magnificently: two swipes on each eye and all make-up was completely removed, including mascara' • 'skin felt moisturised and softer after use' • 'I loved the "baby lotion" smell and the gentleness of this product; I have sensitive eyes, but they felt moisturised and conditioned: I'd buy this' • 'I was pleasantly surprised by this lotion (which is easy to squeeze onto cotton wool), as I normally use liquid removers, but this was very beneficial to my sensitive eyes'.

CLEAR IDEAS

Acne can cause emotional distress at all ages but there are plenty of natural ways to prevent outbreaks

From the occasional breakout to angry red blotches, acne is a pain, physically and psychologically. As well as teenagers – where raging hormones are the principle cause of outbreaks in 90 per cent – acne is increasingly affecting older adults, due in the main to a combination of stress, which causes hormonal imbalances, and environmental pollutants. Drug treatments (to regulate hormones, and/or control bacteria) can be effective but they may have side effects. However, there are many lifestyle remedies that can help.

- **Don't let skin dry out:** even oily complexions need moisturiser or the sebum glands go into overdrive; for the same reason avoid using harsh moisture-stripping cleansers such as those containing benzoyl peroxide and/or pore-blocking petrochemicals, usually labelled paraffinum liquidum. Look out for products labelled non-comedogenic (which won't cause blocked pores) or non-acnegenic.

- **Don't scrub your face or squeeze spots:** your skin may respond better to a weekly clay-based mask (containing antibacterial manuka honey if possible).

- **Keep face cloths scrupulously clean:** wash at a high temperature and use a fresh one each time. Never leave lids off pots and bottles – bacteria gets in like a flash.

- **Try pure mineral make-up:** it camouflages, protects and heals while letting skin breathe. Try bareMinerals, Ineka or Jane Iredale ranges.

- **Get out in the sunlight:** it helps skin heal by enhancing the body's production of vitamins A and D.

- **Try avoiding cows' milk products:** the hormones that are fed to cows (or produced during lactation) and pass into milk can aggravate acne. If you love chocolate, opt for very dark versions, which are full of good-for-the-skin antioxidants.

- **Cut down on all sugar.** Foods that are high in sugar – that's anything ending with 'ose' if you're scanning the label on packets – cause increased insulin production that in turn signals the body to release extra androgens (male hormones), which are involved in pimple formation. Eating whole fruit, particularly antioxidant-rich blueberries, kiwi fruit and watermelon, will do your skin good but juice and smoothies contain high concentrations of sugar and no fibre. Follow a low GI (glycaemic index) diet. A useful book is Antony Worrall Thompson's *GI Diet*, which explains the principles of GI and gives lovely recipes.

- **Learn to relax:** if you suffer from stress, try yoga, meditation or exercise (whatever you enjoy); and practise simple deep slow breaths whenever you start to feel stressy.

- **Try supplements:** clinical pharmacist Shabir Daya, who specialises in natural remedies, advises the herb burdock root, or Clarify Blemish Formula (by LifeTime Vitamins), which contains a range of acne-fighting ingredients including vitamin A, zinc and alpha-lipoic acid.

GENTLE SKINCARE
Dr Rabia Malik, who specialises in treating skin holistically, recommends these simple, natural skincare products.

'Over-the-counter skincare products often contain too many ingredients, plus synthetic chemicals, which may aggravate problem skin. I often recommend MV Organic Skincare Gentle Cream Cleanser, followed by their Pure Jojoba oil. One Love Organics Skin Savior Waterless Beauty Balm and Easy Does It Foaming Cleanser are also good for calming irritated skin.'

SPOT ZAPPERS
our award winners

Botanicals have a long tradition of zapping spots effectively – and healing the scars. Our panellists – all blemish sufferers – voted these four the business

ELEMENTAL HERBOLOGY PERFECT CLARITY BLEMISH MINIMISER

✻

SCORE: 8.83/10

This is an exceptional score for a blemish-buster from a range founded by qualified acupuncturist Kristy Cimesa. The treatment contains a blend of anti-inflammatory lavender, rosemary and tea tree oils, with salicylic and lactic acids to clear pores and exfoliate, plus antibacterial sulphur, renowned for preventing blocked pores.
COMMENTS: 'Very easy to apply from a small tube with a concealer-style brush; love this product and the cooling feel when applied to skin' • 'didn't dry spots or make them flake like more astringent products; good on hormonal red lumps' • 'nice herbal, tea tree-ish, clean smell' • 'made a red lump disappear altogether – I absolutely would buy this again' • 'really does work! Noticed an immediate cooling effect and redness reduced by end of day' • 'my stepdaughter uses this on her teenage acne with amazing results and is a total convert – though the price means she'll keep pinching mine'.

TISSERAND TEA TREE+ ANTI-BLEMISH STICK

✻

SCORE: 7.56/10

Perfect for on-the-go zapping, you apply the light antibacterial gel (with tea tree and kanuka oils, plus witch hazel) via a slim wand with a sponge applicator (do wash this frequently). This is very affordable as well as portable.
COMMENTS: 'Easy to apply, helped to clear spots quickly; also worked well on insect bites and cuts' • 'spot came to a head quickly, dried up and started to heal – good product' • 'usual scar site was much clearer and I didn't have a red mark where the spot had been' • 'banished red lumps, and easy to carry round'.

AT A GLANCE

ELEMENTAL HERBOLOGY
PERFECT CLARITY
BLEMISH MINIMISER

TISSERAND TEA TREE+
ANTI-BLEMISH STICK

BAREMINERALS
BLEMISH REMEDY

INLIGHT
SKIN-EASY BALM

BAREMINERALS BLEMISH REMEDY

✻

SCORE: 7.5/10

This award-winning spot treatment comes in the form of a nude-tinted powder (yes, a powder) which conceals while treating breakouts with natural sulphur, plus the bareMinerals ActiveSoil Complex, common to all their skincare. It comes with a little brush for precise application.
COMMENTS: 'Did a good job of camouflaging redness; cover lasted for a long time' • 'helped stop further breakouts: used the powder on a wider area of my face as a preventative at night, and it reduced the number of blemishes' • 'calming effect, spots less inflamed' • 'where has this been all my life? This sealed the spots and then healed from the inside out – love it'.

INLIGHT SKIN-EASY BALM

✻✻✻

SCORE: 7.39/10

This powerful healing balm comes from a natural and organic range created by a homeopathic Italian doctor who moved to Cornwall. Active ingredients include neem oil, propolis, tea tree oil and plantain extracts, with lavender, lemon peel and frankincense essential oils. The beeswax and oil base makes it best for night-time use.
COMMENTS: 'After a few hours, this calmed the redness of a hideous zit; by day three it had completely gone – I'd buy this' • 'prevented the spot getting too red and angry, though you need to leave 10 minutes before applying concealer; certainly worth trying' • 'over 12 hours, spots became less inflamed and skin texture improved; good for giving the complexion more clarity' • 'helps to reduce pain and redness on the many spots on my face and back – effective and worked fast' • 'my husband used it on inflamed ingrowing hairs in his beard and rated it very highly'.

IT'S CRUNCH TIME

With acne affecting all ages now, some experts believe a key cause is the skincare products. These treatments use natural actives from apple and

APPLE ZIT-BLASTER

If you feel a pimple coming on, pour boiling water over a thin slice of apple in a bowl and wait a few minutes till the apple's soft. Remove from the water, let it cool till warm, then place on the pimple as a poultice. Leave in place for 20 minutes, then peel off and swipe skin lightly with a moistened cotton wool pad.

TIP: Being scrupulously clean is vital with skin that's prone to spots. Wash and soap your hands thoroughly before you touch your face. Wash flannels, face cloths and towels on a hot setting, and use a fresh one daily. Also, be sure to put lids back on all pots, jars and bottles to stop the bugs getting in.

APPLE SKIN-CLEARING TREATMENT

Apples are packed with enzymes that help the skin shed dead cells, as well as being powerfully antibacterial. The fruit acids in apples have a rebalancing action on the skin's pH level, helping prevent infection. Use this treatment regularly – at least once a week – and you should see an improvement in acne, breakouts and even boils.

● 1 apple, chopped

This couldn't be simpler: put the apple in a blender and whizz into a pulpy juice. Put a towelling band over your hairline, lie down with your head on a towel and smooth the apple pulp over your face.

Leave for 15–20 minutes, then rinse thoroughly and apply a light moisturiser everywhere except the T-zone.

FOR SPOTS

synthetic chemicals found in mainstream
willow to target spots and blemishes

WILLOW BLEMISH-BUSTER

The salicylic acid in the willow leaves will dry
out spots effectively.

- 10g (½oz) fresh willow leaves, chopped
- 50ml (2fl oz) apple cider vinegar

Put the willow leaves in a jug and pour the
vinegar over them, then put in a screw-top
bottle and shake well.

Keep in the refrigerator and shake the
bottle every day for a week.

Apply with a cotton wool ball to pimples.

TIP: Most commercial toners for oily complexions work by stripping
the skin. What happens then? Oil production revs up to compensate,
so these products actually make the problem worse. (What's more,
the common ingredient benzoyl peroxide is a potential allergen.) Our
advice is to go gently, so that skin can rebalance itself. If you like the
freshness that a toner delivers, just make a tea of 2 tablespoons of
dried chamomile and 1 tablespoon of dried rosemary. Strain out the
herbs and keep the bottle in the fridge. Used on cotton wool, it gently
cleanses and soothes, and often your skin soon settles down.

REDNESS RELIEF
solutions for rosacea

Such a pretty name for a chronic skin condition that causes such distress

About one in 10 people suffer from rosacea, which mainly affects the face, neck and chest areas. Symptoms invariably begin with episodes of flushing (like blushing), which can start in early teens or childhood; these bouts usually last up to five minutes and may continue occurring for years without any other skin problems arising.

The underlying cause is that the blood vessels in the faces of rosacea sufferers are hypersensitive to a number of triggers, so the vessels dilate and flood with blood more than non-sufferers. The repeated dilation and constriction creates constant blushing and flushing.

Over time this repeated pattern results in long-term facial inflammation, causing redness that looks rather like permanent sunburn. It can be blotchy and tends to affect cheeks, nose and chin but can spread to the forehead, neck and chest. The skin usually looks dry, scaly and/or swollen.

Small blood vessels may become inflamed and show through the skin. Eventually these can become permanently dilated and visible (thread veins). Some rosacea sufferers develop papules – round, red lumpy bumps – or pustules, which are pus-filled swellings. (They look similar to teenage acne but are actually quite different; there are no blackheads and skin is dry and flaky rather than greasy.) There is one comfort in that rosacea, unlike acne, rarely causes any scarring.

Other symptoms include a feeling of burning or stinging, dry rough skin, raised red patches (plaques), and sensitivity to cosmetics. Half of rosacea sufferers also have problems, usually mild, with their eyes, such as sensitivity to light, dry/sore irritation, eyelid problems such as cysts, plus styes or inflammation (blepharitis).

OK, so it's not good, as we know all too well from our friends who suffer this condition daily. But there are many things you can do to help reduce skin inflammation.

BEAT THE BLUSH
Naturopathic doctor Nigma Talib, based in London and New York, recommends the following strategies to calm down the chronic inflammation that underlies this condition.

First, treat your gut...
Healthy gut equals healthy skin. Digestive problems are reflected in the skin and an imbalance of gut flora, the 'good' and 'bad' bugs, can cause rosacea to flare up. Treating this can help: to find out how, see supplements, opposite. Antibiotics can knock out good gut flora: conventional doctors tend to prescribe them for skin problems and in the short term they may help, but used long term (especially without probiotics) they may cause more problems.

Check your stomach acid levels. A lack of acid can prevent proper absorption of trace minerals and may provoke the growth of skin-aggravating bacteria. (See supplements.)

Do you have food intolerances? Hidden food sensitivities can cause reactions from four minutes to four days after eating a meal. Dr Talib believes that over 70 per cent of people are intolerant to various foods and know nothing about it – although many have a 'gut' feeling that they are eating something that triggers the flushing. She suggests having a blood test for food intolerances. (See Directory on page 216 for resource.)

Avoid common food triggers, including:
- Caffeinated drinks (tea, coffee and chocolate, also cola, energy drinks and sodas) and foods (chocolate, some ice cream, frozen coffee-flavoured yogurt).
- Foods high in histamines (fermented alcoholic drinks and vinegar, canned fish, processed meats, yeast and yeast extract, soy products, mushrooms, citrus fruit and tomatoes) and some vegetables (including aubergines). For a complete list, see www.allergyuk.org.
- Spicy foods (except anti-inflammatory turmeric and ginger, see below) and additives – principally nitrates (used in fertilisers), sulphates (found in tap water) and MSG (monosodium glutamate).

Do eat an anti-inflammatory diet based on simple fresh food, organic if possible. Avoid overloading with big meals, choose small portions high in protein, vegetables, some fruit and lots of fibre:
- Organic meats and wild fish (such as salmon), which have more anti-inflammatory omega-3 fatty acids than other sources.
- Bright-coloured organic fruit and veggies, particularly orange, red, and purple (papaya, blueberries, oranges, strawberries, kiwi, broccoli, cauliflower, red cabbage, peppers and Brussels sprouts).
- Olive oil, turmeric and ginger.
- Drink digestion-boosting aloe vera juice and use filtered water where possible.

Consider taking these supplements – discuss with your healthcare practitioner first.
- *Probiotics* (friendly flora or 'good' bugs), also known as biotherapeutics, can help slow an overgrowth of 'bad' bacteria and/or yeast in the gut.
- *Vitamin D3*: this is essential for skin repair and support; ask your healthcare practitioner to test your vitamin D levels and to prescribe the appropriate dose.
- *L-arginine*: this amino acid helps strengthen the blood vessels that rosacea weakens over time.
- *Vitamin B12* and *folic acid*: the B vitamins, especially B12, tend to be deficient in rosacea sufferers because low stomach acid levels prevent them from being absorbed effectively from food.
- *Digestive enzymes*: supplements can help redress the lack of stomach acid.
- *L-glutamine*, a key amino acid: helps to prevent excessive inflammation, and restores balance to the gut after damage has occurred.
- Also talk to your health practitioner about taking supplements with *Betaine HCL* (HCL is hydrochloric acid, the type found in your gut and can help people who have a deficiency in stomach acid).

- Have a test for *Helicobacter pylori*, a treatable infection which is often found in people with rosacea.

Use gentle skincare and mineral make-up.
In a survey of over 1,000 patients, the National Rosacea Society (www.rosacea.org) found these common cosmetic irritants: alcohol (66 per cent), witch hazel (30 per cent), fragrance (30 per cent), menthol (21 per cent), peppermint (14 per cent) and eucalyptus oil (13 per cent). Plus, astringents and exfoliators were deemed too harsh for sensitive skin.

It is wise to test products first (on your neck rather than face). If you do have a reaction, note down the ingredients. (For example, a synthetic preservative known as MI, methylisothiazolinone, is causing what dermatologists are calling 'an epidemic' of redness and swelling, and we think rosacea sufferers would be wise to avoid it. More on page 153.)

We have heard anecdotally that aloe vera suits some people with rosacea; choose topical skincare based on the succulent plant as well as drinking its juice. And we have read reports that full-fat organic milk swiped on as a cleanser is successful (it's high in another essential fatty acid, CLA or conjugated linoleic acid). Natural facial oils have also helped friends we know with rosacea.

Make-upwise, Jane Iredale, one of the pioneers of pure mineral make-up, says 'minerals allow skin to breathe and function normally, rather than clogging pores like many conventional products. The principal minerals we use – titanium dioxide and zinc oxide – calm inflammation and do not harbour bacteria, so they help clear and prevent skin problems.' Jane advises Liquid Minerals Light Reflecting A Foundation to camouflage redness, then PurePressed Base (powder foundation) or Amazing Base Loose Mineral Powder. (For more about mineral make-up, see page 18, and for our Award Winners, see page 20.)

And finally, try not to get het up. Fretting and stressing produces cortisol, the fight-or-flight hormone, which is a villain for touchy skin. Breathing techniques, such as those used in yoga, are wonderful for 'bringing you down' rapidly. Simply centring yourself – taking your mind to your heart or tummy, rather than your brain – and letting your shoulder blades drop down as you inhale gently and exhale very slowly helps enormously. Also, find pastimes that you love to distract your brain from worry: from painting to knitting, pets to building drystone walls, it doesn't matter. But give yourself somewhere to go in your mind that frees it from fretting.

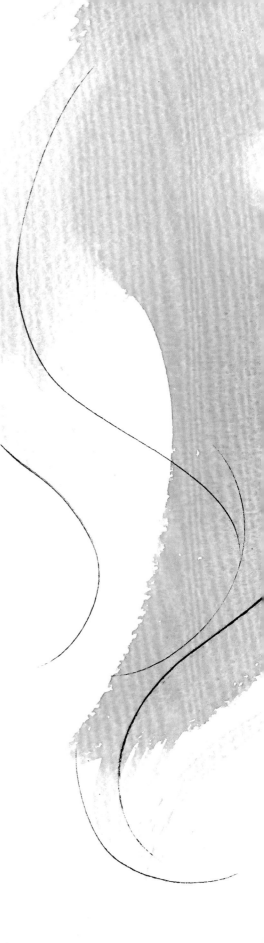

Bright Shining EYES

Your eyes can be your biggest asset – or a big beauty angst. So we offer effective natural strategies to keep them luminous – plus the products that fix bags, shadows, lines and more

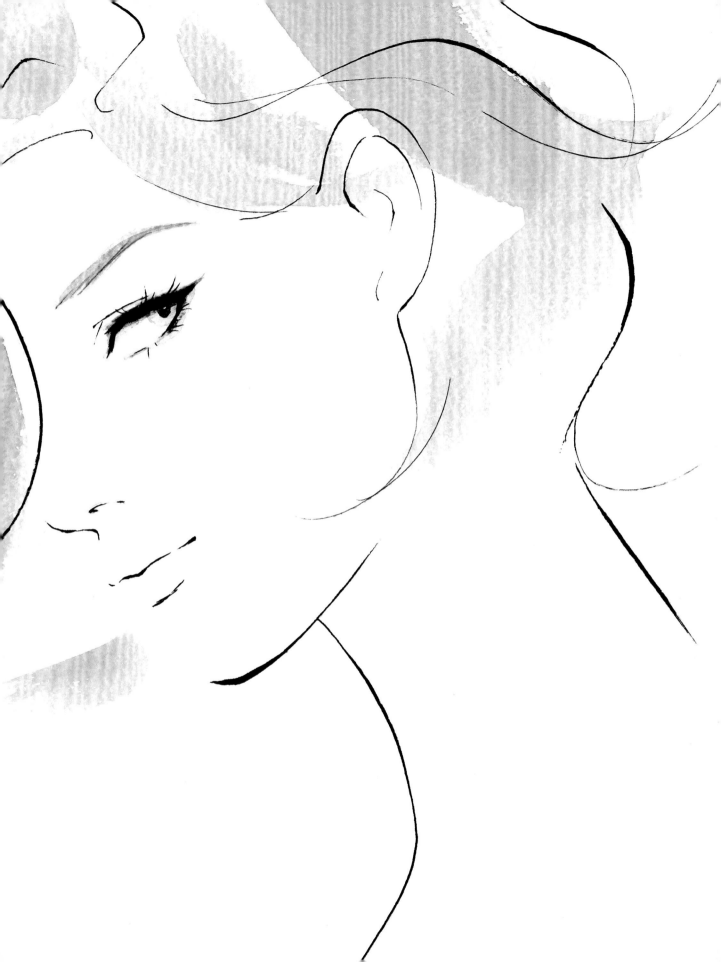

REJUVENATING EYE TREATMENTS
our award winners

Saggy, baggy, crêpey: gravity plays horrible tricks on eyes as we age. But thanks to some extremely effective botanical ingredients, we've always found the more natural age-defying eye creams perform well against higher-tech options. That proved true yet again with this selection, used on just one eye by our testers for the period of the trial – unless they wrote and literally begged us to be able to use the product on the other, because their eyes were becoming 'lopsided'. (It happens in our trials more often than you might think!)

DR.HAUSCHKA REGENERATING EYE CREAM
❋❋

SCORE: 8.43/10

A truly fabulous score for this biodynamic brand – one of the earliest natural ranges – which really wowed our testers. This cooling, soothing, super-lightweight cream sinks in fast, nourishing the fragile eye zone with active botanicals including oils of jojoba, sesame and sunflower seed, shea butter, plus birch and daisy extracts. Rosa damascena gives a light, rose scent.

COMMENTS: 'Instantly brightening, lines smoother – and I can see a difference in the eye I used it on' • 'fine lines seemed to disappear – this product is a keeper' • 'the wrinkly bits look less so' • 'loved the luxurious creaminess' • 'a very nice eye cream for day and night use' • 'fine lines and crêpiness reduced, dark circles less noticeable' • 'slight matte effect which I liked, and made make-up application easier' • 'my sister noticed reduction in my dark circles and wanted to try it herself, too'.

BAREMINERALS RENEW & HYDRATE EYE CREAM
❋

SCORE: 8.19/10

bareMinerals has become world-famous as a make-up brand but they're less well known for

AT A GLANCE

DR.HAUSCHKA
REGENERATING
EYE CREAM

BAREMINERALS RENEW
& HYDRATE EYE CREAM

ESPA LIFT & FIRM
INTENSIVE EYE SERUM

L'OCCITANE IMMORTELLE
DIVINE EYES

BALANCE ME WONDER
EYE CREAM

JURLIQUE HERBAL
RECOVERY EYE CREAM

their skincare. At the heart of this formulation is the 'ActiveSoil Complex', but there's nothing grubby about the Renew & Hydrate Eye Cream, which also features Alpine skullcap and elder-flower extract.

COMMENTS: 'Really impressive: from first use the treated eye was wider open, smoother and generally looking better. I thought it was just me who noticed this but a friend asked if I had a sore eye as the untreated one looked closed' • 'didn't upset my sensitive eyes at all – definitely the best eye cream I've used, and I will continue' • 'nice, expensive feel; very pleased with the results' • 'crêpiness 100 times better' • 'lovely, light, floral smell with a hint of aromatherapy products – liked it' • 'my parents thought I looked less tired!' • 'have finally found a worthy alternative to my Gatineau Paris cream (and it's natural and cheaper!)'.

ESPA LIFT & FIRM INTENSIVE EYE SERUM
❋

SCORE: 8/10

The advantage of serums over creams is they can be applied directly to the eyelid. (Put a rich cream that close to the eye, and there's a risk it will travel into the eye itself, triggering irritation and puffiness.) So, if crêpey eyelids are your beauty woe, this golden-toned serum in a little pump bottle is probably your top choice. It is packed with micro algae and a fern tree extract to lift, firm and boost cell renewal; plus de-puffing golden root, and nourishing omega-rich Inca Inchi oil.

COMMENTS: 'A bit of a miracle product; my skin has aged pretty well so far, apart from the eye area, which is covered in crow's feet and starting to get bags – but this appears to have rolled away about five years' worth of ageing in about six weeks – *love it!*' • 'loved the creamy feel and cooling effect of this serum' • 'have had a few people comment that my eyes looked more lifted and less lined – will buy again'.

L'OCCITANE IMMORTELLE DIVINE EYES

✸

SCORE: 7.95/10

Our book *The Anti-Ageing Beauty Bible* helped put L'Occitane's Divine range – whose signature ingredient is immortelle oil from the Corsican 'everlasting flower' – firmly on the skincare map. And not only has the newly revamped Divine Cream done incredibly well in this new trial (see page 62), but the accompanying eye product – with 'a patented complex of seven active ingredients' – is an award winner, too. Immortelle oil has proven rejuvenating benefits, and gives a beautiful aromatic scent to the range.

COMMENTS: 'Very effective at reducing puffiness, dark circles and refreshing the eye area but – miracle of miracles – it seems to soften crêpiness and made skin around my eyes smoother' • 'the first eye cream I've used that hasn't irritated my eyes' • 'I had sore, red, dry areas at the side of my eyes which diminished after using this; my eye area is brighter, hydrated and feels much more comfortable' • 'shift work entails me getting up at 4am and I've had several comments as to how wide-awake I look at that time in the morning – it's got to be the cream!' • 'smoothed out fine lines: the whole area looks more open'.

BALANCE ME WONDER EYE CREAM

✸ ✸

SCORE: 7.94/10

We're longstanding fans of Balance Me – voted Best British Brand at 2013's Cosmetic Executive Women (UK) awards. And our testers gave a good score to this soothing, brightening, 'lifting' cream. Dispensed through a small pump, Wonder Eye Cream blends virgin coconut, rosehip and carrot oils with plumping hyaluronic acid, lemon, cucumber oil and witch hazel.

COMMENTS: 'Wrinkles appeared less prominent' • 'I used my normal (Clarins) cream on one eye and this on the other; my daughter (aged 26) said she could see a difference in favour of the new cream' • 'love this product and would recommend to all my friends; it improved the look and quality of skin around my eyes' • 'a natural product that works really well'.

JURLIQUE HERBAL RECOVERY EYE CREAM

✸

SCORE: 7.94/10

There were more Jurlique winners in this book, then Jurlique informed us (as we were going to press) that they were reformulating – so we had to drop most of them. Happily, this classic keeps the same formula, and our testers still approve, so it remains. The small tube of cream is infused with cucumber extract, safflower, marshmallow, aloe vera, antioxidants – plus ingredients to combat dark circles and puffiness, including arnica, eyebright and rice bran protein.

COMMENTS: 'Skin looked plumper after use and the laughter lines round my eyes were less prominent after six weeks' • 'nice creamy consistency, absorbed quickly and felt "light" on the eye area; eyes appeared more wide awake' • 'lines and wrinkles looked improved after using for three weeks; I would buy this and recommend to my friends' • 'a pleasant floral, lavender smell' • 'the side I tested it on looks "lifted" compared to the other side'.

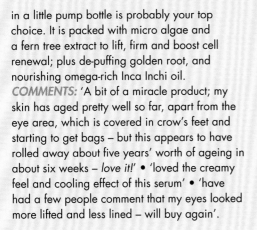

WE LOVE

Liz Earle Superskin Lip & Eye Treatment, with its lightweight texture, is a long-term favourite of Jo's (and doesn't irritate her sensitive eyes). Sarah has had problems with products on her sensitive – sore, red, puffy – peepers for so many years that she avoids them, but is tempted to try the winners here.

TIP: Flaming obvious, this. But it bears repeating because we hear from women so often that eye creams don't work – only to discover that they use the products occasionally. The reason we consistently get high scores for eye creams from our testers is: they use them according to manufacturers' instructions, which generally means twice daily.

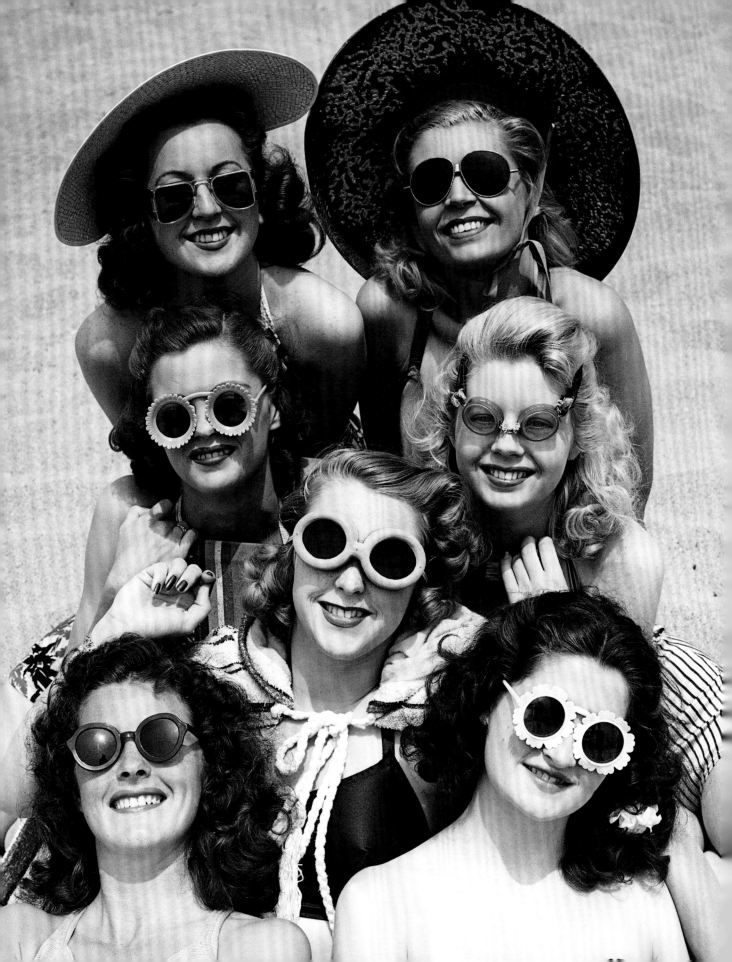

How to keep your EYES SMILING

We get lots of questions about eye problems – from dark circles and puffy bags to tired, sore peepers. Here we focus on helping them stay happy and, above all, healthy

PROBLEM: Dark circles and/or puffy eyes and eye bags

SOLUTION: If you're short of sleep, get more and better (see page 196 for help on this). That might be obvious but it should help. Dark circles and eye bags are often linked to food allergies or intolerance, so if more sleep makes no difference, cut out wheat entirely for a week and see if that helps. (Sarah's eyes can be practically invisible under the bags in the morning if she's had pasta or sandwiches the day before.) If that doesn't work, try avoiding all cow's milk products. There could well be other foodie culprits, so for details of an elimination diet, read *Solve Your Food Intolerance* by Dr John Hunter. In general, stick to fresh food, preferably organic; processed and/or conventionally grown foods may contain additives that you are sensitive to. Cut down on alcohol, sugar and sugary foods, and salt (often hidden in processed foods) and drink lots of still, pure water between meals to flush out toxins.

For an immediate rescue strategy, stroke ice cubes (wrapped in clingfilm or a hankie) over your eyes. If you have longer and can lie down briefly, brew a pot of chamomile tea with two teabags (you're looking for German chamomile, *Chamomilla recutita*) and lay the slightly cooled, slightly squeezed bags on your eyes – you need to lie down for obvious reasons. Slices of cucumber are also very soothing, and raw potato contains an enzyme which helps de-puff

TIP: Remember, the biggest favour you can do your eyes is to invest in wraparound sunglasses – big ones with thick side bars – that will shield the eyes themselves from sun damage and environmental pollutants, and also the fragile skin around them.

skin – lay slices straight on your eyes, or grate some potato and pop in a clean cotton hankie.

Then camouflage dark circles with a little concealer (see page 25 for our Award Winners), patted on thinly with your ring fingers: don't rub, pull or drag the skin. If you use cream around your eyes, be sure not to get it too near: products should be applied on the orbital bone, the bone of the eye socket, and from there they travel to the skin nearer the eye all on their own. Another cause of problems can be eye products and cosmetics: if you suspect a culprit, bin it immediately – or the problems may continue and be much harder to solve. Remember: even natural ingredients can cause problems – Sarah's eyes flare up if the herb eyebright gets near them (apparently that happens quite commonly, despite its eye-friendly name…).

Puffy eyes also respond brilliantly to an instant 'bag-draining' detox in the shape of a run or a vigorous session on the treadmill, followed by a sauna or Turkish bath – or the low-tech solution: steam your face over a bowl of very hot water, with some essential oil such as rosemary to perk you up. (It works wonders for your skin, too.)

PROBLEM: Tired itchy dry eyes

SOLUTION: First, the mucous membrane round eyes needs to be lubricated, like every other part of your body – so drink more water. Aim for eight large glasses of pure, still water between meals (more appealing if you flavour it with lemon, lime, ginger or mint). Also make sure you eat plenty of omega 3 essential fatty acids (see next page) and follow the suggestions for an anti-inflammatory diet on page 86.

Second, dry environments will dry your eyes, so if you work in an office put a bowl of water and/or an ioniser on your desk; if you have a centrally-heated house, put a bowl by all the radiators. For instant help, try the chamomile teabag trick (see previous page), or treat your poor sore eyes to a squirt of Eye Logic Spray Relief for Dry Eyes (formerly Clarymist), a gentle product that you spray on your eyelids (and it doesn't make your make-up run). It contains a phospholipid found in soy lecithin, which is also the most common one in natural tears, and is said to help 80 per cent of cases of dry eye where the cause is tear evaporation, compared to other gels and drops, which are only effective in 20 per cent.

Eye Logic is fine for contact lens wearers too but do check in with your optometrist, as there are now lenses that may help dry eyes.

PROBLEM: Red bloodshot eyes
SOLUTION: Sleeeeep! And clean up your diet. If you've excluded conjunctivitis (visit your doctor to make sure) and the veins in your eyes are always on show, the likeliest villain is lack of sleep. Pollution doesn't help, so if you spend a lot of time walking around in a polluted town (as we do), always wear your big shades.

We have also noticed a big difference in terms of brighter whites of our eyes with a bit of light detoxing and green food supplements such as Sun Chlorella A (our old favourite).

You could also try the detoxing foot pads (brands include Bodytox and Patch-it by NutriWorks), which work for us and other people we have talked to. After five to seven days, we have noticed brighter eyes, with whiter whites (and better skin, too).

PROBLEM: Computer Vision Syndrome
SOLUTION: Long hours at the screen can lead to all sorts of problems, as many of us know too well. The symptoms of CVS include sore, tired, burning, itchy, watery or dry eyes, blurred or double vision, headaches and a sore neck. You may have trouble when you try to move your focus between the monitor and papers on your desk. Some people notice increased sensitivity to light or see colour fringes or afterimages when looking away from the monitor.

The first thing to do, according to integrated health expert Dr Andrew Weil (www.drweil.com), is to ensure that your computer is in the best position:
● Make sure you are sitting straight in front of it, about an arm's length away.
● The top of the screen should be at your eye level or just below, so you are looking down slightly. You can get a sore neck if the screen is too high or too low.
● Your keyboard should be directly in front of the monitor.
● If you are working on a wide screen, position the document you are working on straight in front of your eyes.
● Put your reference books and papers in front of you at the same distance and angle from your eyes, and on the same level.
● Minimise glare from bright lights by putting your light source at a right angle to the screen.
● To reduce eye strain, take periodic breaks and focus on more distant objects. Schedule a five-minute break every hour. Stand up and move around or simply lean back and close your eyes for a few minutes.
● Blink frequently. If you have dry eyes, it may be due to blinking less than usual when you look at the screen. If that doesn't help, try artificial tears (available over the counter from any chemist, or Eye Logic, mentioned above left).
● Have an eye check every two years, annually if you have glaucoma in your family.

SMILE WITH YOUR EYES

According to the late Dr David Servan-Schreiber, a psychiatrist and writer, watching the way people smile – with their eyes or not – is a simple test of whether they are really happy to see us. A forced smile – the sort we 'put on' in social situations where we really aren't feeling warm and at ease – mobilises only the muscles round the mouth, showing our teeth. A 'real' smile, however, also uses the muscles round our eyes.

The order for smiling with your eyes comes from the deepest and most ancient region of your brain, known as the limbic system, which we can't control with our cognitive brain. As Dr Servan-Schreiber explained: 'A warm smile, a real one, lets us know intuitively that the person we are talking to is, at that exact moment, in a state of harmony with what he or she thinks and feels.' In other words, they are happy to be there with us.

Of course, it works the other way too. People are getting the same intuitive messages from us. As Dr Servan-Schreiber wrote in his life-changing book *Healing Without Freud or Prozac*, the key way to help ourselves communicate better with the outside world is to be loving and kind. Then, no matter what else is going on, people who look into your eyes will see 'the sweet soul shining through', as one poet put it – and that's real beauty in our book.

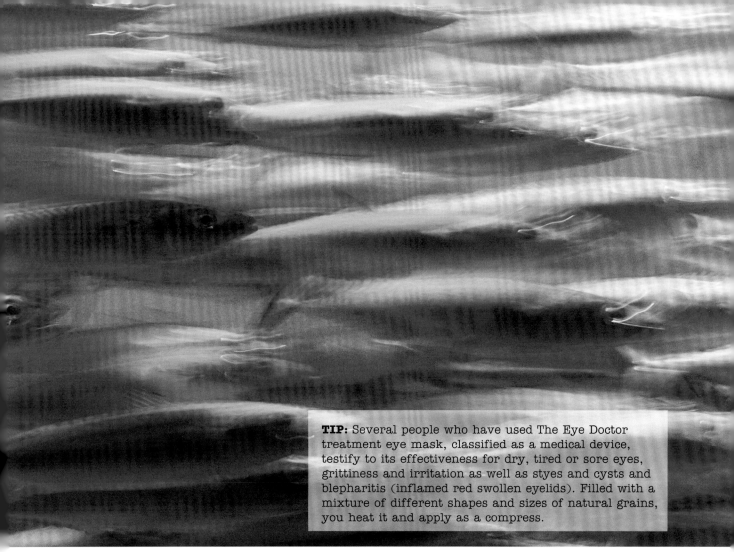

TIP: Several people who have used The Eye Doctor treatment eye mask, classified as a medical device, testify to its effectiveness for dry, tired or sore eyes, grittiness and irritation as well as styes and cysts and blepharitis (inflamed red swollen eyelids). Filled with a mixture of different shapes and sizes of natural grains, you heat it and apply as a compress.

FEED YOUR EYES WITH FISHES

There is some evidence that specific nutrients can help some vision problems. A large ongoing study called AREDS (Age-Related Eye Disease Study) found that taking a supplement containing a high-dose combination of vitamins C and E, with zinc and copper, nutrients called lutein (found in green veg) and zeaxanthin (in orange and yellow ones) and beta-carotene, significantly reduces the risk of developing advanced age-related macular degeneration (AMD), a very common cause of blindness in older people. (Antioxidant supplements did not, however, help prevent cataracts.)

Omega 3 fish oils are vital for the development of vision in pregnancy and after. While they have not been shown to help in preventing advanced AMD, people who had the highest level of omega 3 fatty acids in their diet were much less likely to develop macular degeneration. They are also important to keep eyes lubricated and avoid dry eye syndrome.

The best food sources of these 'good' fats (which help your health generally, including your heart, mood and fertility – and your skin, hair and nails), include the following:

● Eat cold-water fish at least twice a week: salmon, mackerel, tuna, sardines and herring. Look for wild-caught varieties rather than farmed fish, which often have higher levels of chemicals.

● If you don't like eating fish, consider a supplement: pharmacist Shabir Daya recommends 'Power of Krill', which offers omega 3s as phospholipids that go directly to your cells so you need much less. Unlike fish, krill are teeny-tiny shellfish found at the bottom of the ocean, so some experts believe that they are less polluted and there is less risk of over-harvesting.

● Also eat lots of dark green leafy veg, walnuts and flaxseeds.

● Avoid foods fried or processed with sunflower and corn oils, the omega 6 fatty acids that, in excess, can damage our health.

EYE REFRESHERS
our award winners

Revitalising tired eyes, helping to banish puffiness and dark circles, all make for the toughest beauty challenges out there. And what the respectable results below reflect is that some testers for each product got fantastic results, while others were less impressed, which brought the average down a little. You may still have to deploy trial and error to find what works for you, but we think these six are the very best place to start – as scores for some products we dispatched languished in the doldrums (as low as 4.33/10). A bit of an eye-opener, that…

A'KIN WHITE TEA & CORNFLOWER EYE DAY GEL

✳

SCORE: 8.08/10

This is good news for anyone on a budget: the least expensive of the six award winners comes out top. The lightweight, antioxidant-powered gel sinks in swiftly, soothing and de-puffing with a cooling combo of (as the name suggests) white tea, cornflower, sambucus (elderberry), vitamin C, plus pro-vitamin B5, dispensed through the fine nozzle at the end of the tube.

COMMENTS: 'Cooling and definitely makes eyes feel less weary' • 'eyes felt alert, bright, more wide-awake; very refreshed and revitalised' • 'a great eye treatment with multiple results: uplifting, calming, soothing and a pleasure to use' • 'reduced puffiness and also helped with the appearance of wrinkles around eyes; I really liked it' • 'this actually makes it easier to apply make-up over the top' • 'I'm hoping with continued use this will help soften fine lines, but the initial soothing effect alone makes it a keeper – this product was amazing and performed much better than some of my expensive eye creams' • 'within a couple of days I noticed an improvement in the fine lines around my eyes – and then after two

AT A GLANCE

A'KIN WHITE TEA
& CORNFLOWER
EYE DAY GEL

LIZ EARLE
EYEBRIGHT SOOTHING
EYE LOTION

ORIGINS
NO PUFFERY COOLING
MASK FOR PUFFY EYES

DARPHIN
ANTI-FATIGUE
SMOOTHING EYE GEL

GREEN PEOPLE
FIRMING EYE GEL

REN
ACTIVE 7 EYE GEL

weeks, a definite transformation, which means I'm looking less tired'.

LIZ EARLE EYEBRIGHT SOOTHING EYE LOTION

✳

SCORE: 7.88/10

This does double duty: as long as you're not wearing waterproof mascara, it effectively cleanses the eye zone – but in this case, our testers tried it as a treatment for their weary eyes. (The how-to: soak a couple of cotton pads in the liquid – which you can pre-chill – and place over peepers, allowing the organic aloe vera, witch hazel and cornflower to cool and refresh.) This is one of the Liz Earle products that still contains a couple of parabens: if it worries you, find out more on page 153.

COMMENTS: 'A simple product which does exactly what it says on the bottle: my eyes feel so revitalised after use' • 'working with computers all day, every day in a badly air-conditioned office with artificial lighting all contribute to my tired, puffy, old-before-my-time peepers, but this sorts that out so simply that I now take it to work to give my eyes a bit of a pick-me-up at lunchtime – and it does wonders' • 'I adore this stuff: it refreshes your eyes if

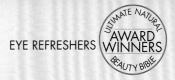

they're feeling tired; and it's great for soothing and refreshing the skin, plus reducing redness after brow-plucking' • 'yet another of my new Holy Grail products' • 'this made a real difference to my tired, saggy, baggy eyes – both appearance and comfort'.

ORIGINS NO PUFFERY COOLING MASK FOR PUFFY EYES
✳
SCORE: 7.63/10
The No Puffery range is growing all the time at Origins (see We Love, right), and our testers loved this small flip-top tube of skin-chilling green gel. Use it for 5–10 minutes as a mask, or apply sparingly in the morning and let it work its de-puffing, brightening magic all day. Key ingredients are bag-banishing yeast extract and calming hoelen mushroom, aloe vera and cucumber extracts; it also has a pretty scent from damask rose essential oil.
COMMENTS: 'I don't believe in miracle creams but this has changed my mind: immediately after application puffiness and dark circles are diminished – a fabulous product' • 'this is definitely a must-buy: makes the skin under my eyes much less puffy after use; I'm now a big fan' • 'reduced the dark circles under my eyes: I used it on one eye the first time for comparison and could see the difference straight away' • 'excellent the morning after a late night'.

DARPHIN ANTI-FATIGUE SMOOTHING EYE GEL
✳
SCORE: 7.57/10
Gels really were the top de-bagging choice for our panellists in this category: this option from Darphin features circulation-stimulating caffeine, vitamin C, and an age-defying walnut extract, to work on fine lines at the same time. They recommend application with an outwards tapping movement, to help lymph drainage.
COMMENTS: 'This is a fantastic product; definitely brighter eyes with no dark circles; less tired and hydrated' • 'used this on tired eyes at work and it really refreshed; a great pick-me-up' • 'I put this in the fridge if my eyes are feeling particularly sore, and then it's doubly refreshing' • 'my daughter commented that my eyes had no bags after using it in the morning; a lovely, reinvigorating eye gel' • 'this really is a fantastic product'.

GREEN PEOPLE FIRMING EYE GEL
✳✳✳
SCORE: 7.56/10
Again, a patting, tapping action is suggested (as in the Darphin entry) with this pale white gel, which uses chicory and something called Tara bush to firm and tighten instantly. This bush extract, together with chicory, are also included to promote collagen production and therefore help fight the signs of ageing. It's alcohol free, so suitable for sensitive and fragile skins – and the all-natural product is certified 86 per cent organic. It works well under make-up, they say, and can be used any time of day – or night!
COMMENTS: 'Really liked using this after a hard day at work, or the morning after partying, as it has an instant cooling and refreshing effect on the eye area – am also now going to check out other Green People products' • 'a total eye treat: helped me to feel awake in the mornings' • 'a light gel that sinks in faster than I can tell you (so make-up goes on really well afterwards); I am prone to puffiness and this helped so much – the most effective cream or gel I've used for that' • 'a great product: it has a non-greasy texture and feels cooling and tightening (in a good way)'.

REN ACTIVE 7 EYE GEL
✳
SCORE: 7.5/10
This is also seriously cooling, and can be used under or over make-up. (In fact, the slender pump-action bottle would fit brilliantly inside a make-up bag – and that's probably the best place for it, as we found it knocked over easily.) Extracts of fig, rumex (a slightly sexier name for sorrel!), arnica and ginseng, vitamin P from rose damask water, plus hyaluronic acid are the REN revivers here.
COMMENTS: 'When applied in the evening this had a refreshing lifting effect' • 'great mixed with foundation in the under-eye area; peepers definitely feel brighter' • 'cooling and refreshing and bagginess reduced' • 'there was immediate improvement in puffiness which continued for a long time into the day, yet the area around the eyes remained very well hydrated'.

WE LOVE
We're both fans of the rollerball action of Origins No Puffery Cooling Roll-On for Puffy Eyes: the cold of the metal ball really does work to smooth away the puffiness that's finally, finally catching up with Jo – and has been well known to Sarah for too many years! Sarah also rates Bright Eyes by Goldfaden MD, an American botanical brand developed by a doctor; plus a recent arrival, the effective Aurelia Probiotic Skincare Eye Revitalising Duo, with a rollerball brightener plus a de-puffing eye cream.

NOW AND ZEN

Sit back and relax while these treatments reinstate calm to over-tired eyes

LAVENDER EYE PILLOWS

These eye bags are wonderfully relaxing: helpful for getting to sleep, for an at-home spa treatment or whenever you have some quiet time. The weight of the grains seems to calm the eyes – and, in turn, the mind. They make wonderful gifts, too. Your herb pillow should last for about a year. Renew it when the next lavender harvest is in.

- 23cm x 26cm piece of natural fabric (cotton, linen or silk)
- 150g (5oz) dried lavender flowers (or a mix of half and half lavender and flaxseeds)
- 6 drops lavender essential oil (optional)

Cut two rectangles of fabric, measuring approx 23cm x 13cm. With right sides together stitch a 1.4cm (½in) seam around the two long sides and one end of the pillow, either by hand or using a sewing machine. Turn right side out.

Put the lavender flowers (and flaxseeds if using) in a bowl, add the lavender essential oil drop by drop and swirl to mix.

Using a funnel, pour the mixture into the bag. Hand-sew the remaining side to close.

TIP: You can also put slices of cucumber over and under the eyes to help combat puffiness.

CHAMOMILE EYE BAG BANISHER

Chamomile has a near-miraculous effect on tired and puffy eyes. If you know you're heading for a morning-after-the-night-before, make this chamomile infusion before you go out and it'll be ice-cold and ready for bag-blitzing the next day. (It will keep for just a few days in the fridge.)

- 10g (½oz) dried chamomile flowers
- Mineral, purified tap or rain water

Place the flowers in the bottom of a mug and fill with boiling water.

Allow to cool and strain into a sterilised jar, which you should pop into the fridge. Soak cotton wool pads in the cold tea and place over the eyes. (Pads are better than cotton wool balls because they cover more of the eye zone.) Relax for 15–20 minutes. During this time, use the pads of your fingers to tap outwards along the orbital bone above and below the eye, to help de-puff.

CUCUMBER REFRESHING GEL

This jelly-like recipe is very cooling when dabbed lightly onto the orbital bone around the eye (essentially, the socket area).

- 2.5cm (1in) slice aloe vera leaf, or 1 tablespoon aloe vera gel, from a natural food store
- 2.5cm (1in) slice cucumber
- ¼ teaspoon corn starch
- 1 tablespoon witch hazel
- 1 drop grapefruit seed extract

Place the peeled aloe vera leaf or the aloe vera gel with the cucumber in a pestle and mortar and pound (or whizz in a herb grinder) until they are smoothly blended.

Then put in a double boiler (see page 212) with the corn starch and heat until almost boiling.

Allow to cool slightly. Add the witch hazel and grapefruit seed extract, then pour into a small, sterilised glass jar and put into the fridge to cool thoroughly.

TIP: If eyes are puffy in the morning, take a leaf out of supermodel Linda Evangelista's book and reach for a cube of ice. Wrap it in clingfilm and stroke away eye bags, working in an outward direction. The cold will help to reduce the swelling.

POTATO DE-BAGGER

Try this simple de-puffer: the decongesting action of the potato acts to reduce swelling.

- ¼ large potato

Slice the potato in 5–10 very thin slices, or grate it on a coarse grater, so that it can easily be moulded to the skin.

Simply spritz the eye area with plain water and arrange the potato around the eyes. Leave in place for 10–15 minutes – and the puffiness will soon start to disappear.

ROSE PETAL EYE REVIVER

Your eyes will feel calmer and more soothed, and what more romantic way to do it?

- Large handful rose petal leaves (unsprayed and organic, dried or fresh)
- A few drops of rose water

Pound the rose petals in a pestle and mortar, adding the rose water drop by drop until the mixture becomes a mask-like, not-too-runny consistency.

Lie down somewhere peaceful and scoop a small handful of the mashed roses onto each closed eye; pat into place.

Relax for 15–20 minutes, then swish the roses away. For an effective, de-puffing variation, use a few drops of cucumber juice in place of the rose water.

Blissful BODYCARE

Looking after your body with good food, drink and exercise isn't just vanity – it's at the heart of wellbeing. And here's everything you need to be softer, smoother and more sensual, from neck to toe

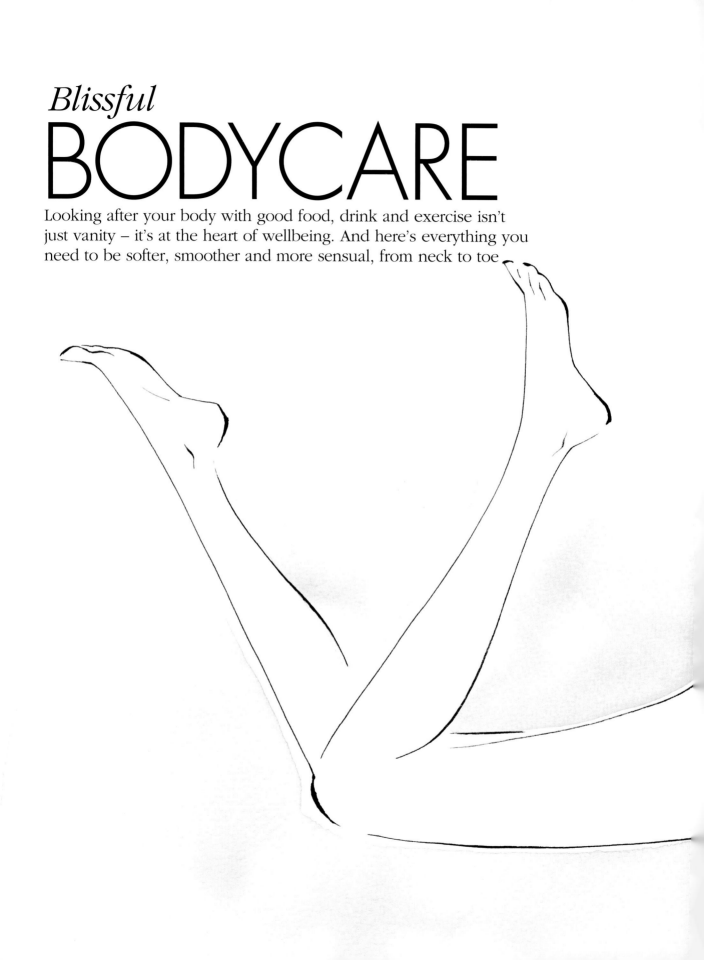

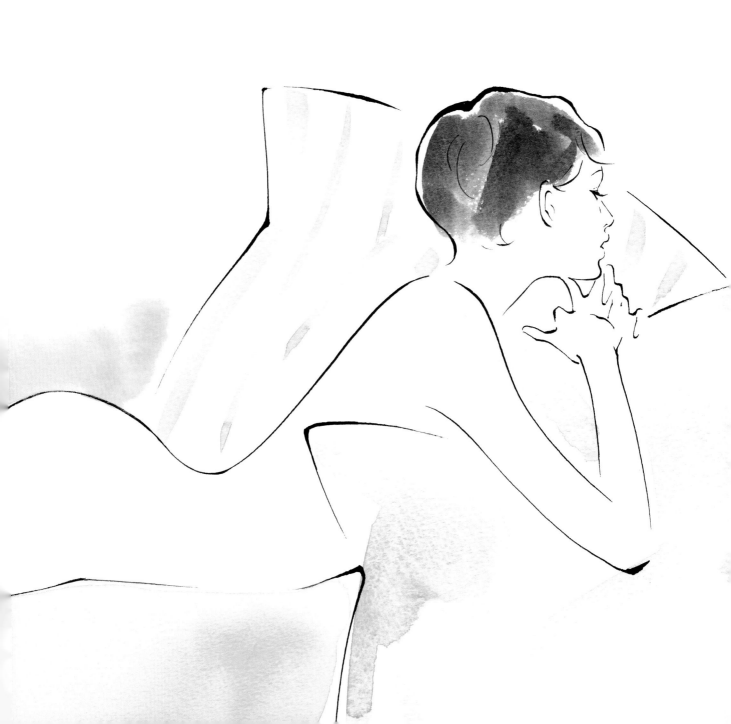

Doing what comes
NATURALLY

The fact you're reading this book indicates that something draws you to natural beauty products. Alongside that often comes a delight in living more naturally in general and we find that keeps us – and our bodies – happy

We grew up in the days before cook-chill foods, with vegetables from our family gardens and allotments. Weekends meant being dragged out on long walks (now we go voluntarily, daily...). Beauty technology was in its infancy – we still used granny's glycerine and rose water as a face tonic and the only body product was probably talcum powder. As the years went by, all that changed: we moved to London, often ate convenience foods and slapped on increasingly more high-tech products from top to toe.

Then came a revolution in our thinking – and doing. We both started writing (on different magazines and newspapers) about the environment. We became involved with issues around organic food (Jo is married to Craig Sams, an early campaigner for organic food and past Chair of the Soil Association). And we addressed other concerns such as Fairtrade ingredients – largely through the late and very much missed Anita Roddick, founder of The Body Shop and a dyed-in-the-heart green goddess whom we both knew.

Jo's light-bulb moment came a couple of decades ago when she put on some body lotion. Watching it sink into her skin, she thought: 'Where is that going?' Eating organic food and opting for a more natural lifestyle generally, it suddenly didn't make sense to be slathering on a cocktail of synthetic chemicals. And compared to the small amount of product we put on our faces and necks, the amount

we slather over our bodies, chest to toe, is so much greater.

Sarah's concern was also 'what's it doing?'. Although our skin has an effective barrier to keep invaders of all kinds from getting in the bloodstream, some substances undoubtedly penetrate those defences. In some cases, that's on purpose – for instance, patches carrying pharmaceutical drugs (including HRT) or nicotine – but sometimes not. Skin problems such as eczema impair the skin barrier, so it doesn't work as effectively and many experts say that at least a small percentage of what we put on our skin is likely to penetrate anyway. And unlike the food we eat, cosmetics will not go through the liver's detoxifying process.

Today, without being obsessive, we generally opt for natural cosmetics. We prefer skincare with as few synthetics as possible, partly because, like Dr Rabia Malik (see page 82), we find that a short list of mainly natural ingredients is less likely to irritate sensitive skin. We also like the fact that many natural ingredients have been used safely for centuries to soften, smooth and protect skin – and you can carry on that tradition, if you wish, with the

There are simple (and low-cost) ways to incorporate natural wellbeing into your life

- **Grow your own herbs and salad leaves: it's addictive, soothing and delicious.**
- **Use cotton hankies rather than paper tissues.** ● **Hang washing outside on a line or drying rack: it smells fresher and saves energy – and money.** ● **Air rooms: open windows in the morning but remember to turn down the heating first. (Jo swears she can only sleep if she has fresh air at night too, so hotels with hermetically sealed windows are out...)** ● **Get outside every day for exercise and light: you need both (see page 146 for more on sunlight and vitamin D).** ● **Explore your neighbourhood green spaces both at home and work: a stroll round a park at lunchtime can dissipate work stress.** ● **Use natural wax candles instead of electric light for evening meals: saves energy, may help you sleep better and boosts romance.** ● **Buy or make natural household cleaning products: lemon, baking soda and borax work as well as commercial cleaners in many cases – and smell nicer. See www.thedailygreen.com for ideas; also www.supergreenme.com by green campaigner Diana Carney (married to Bank of England governor Mark Carney).**

recipes in this book. (Though, of course, not all natural ingredients are irritation-free: just think of nettles – ouch!)

Sustainable provenance is a key factor for us. Given the choice of, say, a body butter using Fairtrade ingredients from a women's cooperative in a developing country or one pullulating with molecules invented by a white-coated chemist in an industrial laboratory, we'll take the Fairtrade option, please. And we actively dislike – and voice our opposition to – over-packaging. Hacking our way through layers of petrochemical-derived plastic packaging frays our tempers (and our nails...), so we applaud recycled/recyclable and refillable containers.

But it's not just about cosmetics. True wellbeing is about loving and appreciating and making the most of the world we live in. Think for a moment of the exhilaration you feel with a good walk by the sea, with the wind in your hair and the sun on your face. And if you're in a town, just making your way to the nearest park and watching dogs bounding around can turn a blue-mood day into a happier one. For Sarah, it's the joy of being with her horses in the

West country – even on a winter's night... As GP Dr William Bird (who pioneered the concept of 'green gyms' – exercising outside whenever possible) says, 'We're programmed as humans to be with the natural environment. When we see trees, the sea, fields and woods we overwhelmingly feel at peace. It's to do with evolution: nature has a strong effect on a deep part of the brain. It gives us a sense of belonging and of wellbeing.'

It always amuses us when scientific research 'discovers' that activities which are entirely natural for human beings are – gosh! – actually good for us. Two recent headlines revealed that 'exercise can be as good as drugs' and 'gardening can prolong life'. These related to specific groups but we'd say they are almost a necessity for all ages.

Both of us love gardening; even when Jo was based in a crowded part of West London, her roof terrace provided salad leaves year round, and even new potatoes. Now we are both lucky enough to have gardens in the country, which give us great joy, some foodstuffs – and lots of flowers for the house, another source of pleasure.

BODY WASHES
our award winners

Although relative newcomers to our bathrooms, body washes have become an integral part of most women's beauty ritual, whether you prefer baths or showers. Fragrance certainly plays a huge part in the pleasure factor, and our testers – who washed their way through a total of 50 products – agreed: these are all chock-full of aromatic botanicals and smell divine. More importantly, we wanted to identify body washes with kind-to-skin, non-stripping detergents and foaming agents (natural obviously) – and these all fit the bill…

L'OCCITANE LAVENDER SHOWER GEL
✳ ✳ ✳
SCORE: 8.86/10

One of L'Occitane's organically certified products (by Ecocert) – and the first of two of the brand's winners in this indulgent category. Flip open the top of the bottle, breathe in deeply, and you can smell wafts from their PDO (Protected Designation of Origin) lavender, harvested in Haute-Provence. Known as 'blue gold', lavender was one of the first flowers distilled by Olivier Baussan, the founder of L'Occitane.

COMMENTS: 'Refreshing, calming, foamed perfectly (not too much, but just right); great for morning showers' • 'I often find it hard to drop off to sleep and this acted as a calming aid' • 'I loved this product. Skin didn't feel tight or dry after I'd showered with this gel' • 'the most heavenly lavender scent; this is the body wash you want to shower with in the morning to ease you into the day in the most gorgeous, pampering way' • 'I'm an aromatherapist and very sensitive to "synthetic" lavender, but this conveys the most natural, fresh, earthy, fragrant aroma of the lavender plant that I have ever experienced in a bodycare product'.

AT A GLANCE

L'OCCITANE
LAVENDER SHOWER GEL

JOHN MASTERS
BLOOD ORANGE &
VANILLA BODY WASH

DR.HAUSCHKA
LAVENDER
SANDALWOOD
CALMING BODY WASH

REN MOROCCAN
ROSE OTTO
BODY WASH

L'OCCITANE
ALMOND
SHOWER OIL

BURT'S BEES
FABULOUSLY FRESH
PEPPERMINT &
ROSEMARY
BODY WASH

JOHN MASTERS BLOOD ORANGE & VANILLA BODY WASH
✳ ✳
SCORE: 8.57/10

John Masters is a wonderful 'natural' hairdresser from New York whose products have always gone down well with our testers. His offering here blends refreshing pink grapefruit with blood orange, but to our noses it's the rich, cocooning smell of vanilla that wins through in this silky wash. (It features high levels of organic ingredients but the final product isn't certified, hence just two daisies.)

COMMENTS: 'This has a lovely fragrance that makes me think of orange sweeties – a real pleasure to use, smells gorgeous, plus no nasties – this is a keeper' • 'I spend a lot of time outside playing sport and sometimes shower two or three times a day, especially during hot weather – but even after extensive washing, this didn't dry out my skin and has such a lovely scent' • 'a little goes a long way' • 'skin felt fab and smooth – definitely more silky than after using a normal wash' • 'probably the nicest shower gel I've used: it feels like it's good for my skin, rather than stripping it' • 'the fragrance smells warm and real, not synthetic; my

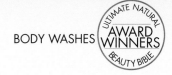

nine-year-old daughter has eczema and swims a lot, and enjoys using this because it leaves her skin comfortable and not itchy'.

DR.HAUSCHKA LAVENDER SANDALWOOD CALMING BODY WASH
✹ ✹

SCORE: 8.5/10

With a creamy texture, this smells lavishly lavender-y, blending that aromatic note with the amber-like warmth of sandalwood. (The aroma of sandalwood is pretty subtle compared to the lavender.) Like much of Dr.Hauschka's updated packaging, this product now comes in a lightweight, travel-friendly plastic flip-top bottle. Some testers felt it could have lathered more – but, in fact, a rich foam tends to dry out skin. *COMMENTS:* 'I loved this; my skin felt lovely afterwards and it was a real "spa" experience' • 'this did not leave my skin dry' • 'when the lid is closed on this, it's firmly closed; I like being able to take luxury products away from home, and I could travel with this knowing it wouldn't leak' • 'lovely, calming lavender fragrance, perfect before bed' • 'gorgeous smell, goes on well, leaving skin clean, refreshed and calm' • 'felt gentle and mild on skin' • 'the aroma filled the shower cubicle and bathroom when I used this: an authentic lavender fragrance as if you'd crushed the flower in your hand'.

REN MOROCCAN ROSE OTTO BODY WASH
✹ ✹ ✹

SCORE: 8.5/10

Ever since they launched the Moroccan Rose Otto range, REN have been wowing *Beauty Bible* testers with their gloriously scented bath and body treats based around one of the perfume world's most expensive fragrance ingredients. This is equally rosy-rich, packing a scented punch while it gently cleanses. One of Sarah's favourites, see We Love (right). *COMMENTS:* 'Left a fresh scent afterwards – very pleasant' • 'lovely fragrance – a gentle, old-fashioned rose kind' • 'I've seen benefits to my skin since I gave up soap – fewer breakouts – and this must have contributed to the

improvement' • 'really love it!' • 'heavenly fragrance' • 'I have very sensitive skin which is irritated by a lot of products but I was able to use this with ease' • 'truly gorgeous and pampering – definitely one of my star products' • 'one squirt does my whole body'.

L'OCCITANE ALMOND SHOWER OIL
✹

SCORE: 8.31/10

The second L'Occitane winner in this category is something a little different (and is a favourite of Jo's): it is a marzipan-ish oil that emulsifies on contact with water, but really does leave a veil of satin-softness on the skin, eliminating the need for additional moisturisation. *COMMENTS:* 'I've never come across a body wash that acts like a rich, nourishing moisturiser – it's everything that dry, dehydrated skin needs' • 'the nicest-smelling body wash I've ever used; the almond scent was still on my skin hours later' • 'using this while shaving my legs left them looking super-smooth and smelling great' • 'I have had to hide this shower oil from family members!' • 'how can an oily product be so cleansing, light, refreshing, and smell pleasantly fragrant, too? It's utterly wonderful'.

BURT'S BEES FABULOUSLY FRESH PEPPERMINT & ROSEMARY BODY WASH
✹ ✹

SCORE: 8.3/10

What a peppy product this is! Described as 'an energising boost for body, mind and spirit', the gentle plant-based body cleanser, which comes in a generous bottle, is packed with awakening, aromatics and would be brilliant, we think, for a morning shower. You won't need a Java jolt after washing with this... *COMMENTS:* 'Smells minty and zingy: an instant wake-up for the skin and senses' • 'it smelt like I'd fallen face-down into a mint bush – heavenly; put me in a really positive mood' • 'skin left soft and looked dewy' • 'felt energised all morning' • 'skin was moisturised without the need for extra body lotion' • 'after using I felt refreshed and alive' • 'full marks from me and I'm usually a mean marker!'

WE LOVE

Jo's not big on body washes – 'what's wrong with soap?' – but if pressed, likes the tangy Pomegranate Creamy Body Wash by Weleda. And (when she's in too much of a hurry to apply body lotion or is shaving her legs), she uses the award-winning L'Occitane Almond Shower Oil featured left. Sarah has always loved body washes; yes, it's the fragrance but also the ease of a quick squidge rather than losing a bar of soap in the shower. Her current favourites are Melvita Gentle Shower Gel and absolutely the REN Moroccan Rose Otto Body Wash that our testers also loved. PS: the only soap by Sarah's bath side – brought back from Syria (in more peaceful days) – has lasted for years and is the best she has ever used.

BODY SCRUBS
our award winners

We're all for beauty shortcuts and the fast-track to smooth, gleaming skin? A brightening, deep-cleaning body-scrub session to see off any rough patches and reveal the soft, healthy skin beneath. Our teams buffed their way through dozens of natural scrubs out there – and there are plenty as they're so easy to formulate – and awarded some incredibly high scores to these six winners. For more skin-smoothers, check out our delicious 'cook-at-home' recipes on page 198

REN GUERANDE SALT EXFOLIATING BODY BALM
❋❋

SCORE: 9.33/10

This is a longstanding favourite with testers but when we duly dispatched another 10 of the big salty tubs to a fresh team they fell for it all over again. (NB: Because it's salt-based, avoid use after gardening – something of an 'ouch' factor post rose-pruning we have found...)

COMMENTS: 'Absolutely the best scrub I've tried – a gorgeous balm that leaves your skin soft and healthy, and no need to moisturise afterwards – five stars!' • 'bumpy areas much more smooth and didn't need a body cream as skin felt nourished and moisturised – my new favourite' • 'before this my legs looked between an elephant and an alligator's skin, but this is the best scrub I've used; got rid of dry areas and made me feel fresh and clean' • 'quite gentle, even on dry patches – works especially well as a foot scrub, leaving feet baby soft; I don't usually use a body scrub but have been converted to use this one' • 'the fragrance is natural and gorgeous – slightly minty and very refreshing – but not so overwhelming that you can't put on scent afterwards'.

AT A GLANCE

REN GUERANDE
SALT EXFOLIATING
BODY BALM

LIZ EARLE ENERGISING
BODY SCRUB

GREEN & SPRING
INDULGING
EXFOLIATING
BODY BALM

EMMA HARDIE
AMAZING FACE
NATURAL LIFT
AND SCULPT
BODY TREATMENT

ORA NATURALS
ARGAN BODY
SCRUB REVIVE

DR.ORGANIC
ROSE OTTO
BODY SCRUB

LIZ EARLE ENERGISING BODY SCRUB
❋

SCORE: 8.94/10

A definite body pick-me-up for the mornings from the perennially popular Liz Earle range, delivering an energising blend of essential oils (including geranium, peppermint, eucalyptus, sweet orange, patchouli and rosemary). It is designed to exfoliate and cleanse as well as improve circulation, they say at Liz Earle. The flip-top bottle of gel features finely powdered olive stones as the skin-buffing ingredient – so this is more appropriate for a shower than a bath, we suggest, otherwise you may find yourself soaking in a pile of fine grit.

COMMENTS: 'Minty and healthy-smelling scrub which rinsed away very well leaving skin softer' • 'skin felt lovely afterwards – I wanted to keep touching it and will buy this again' • 'body looked brighter especially when I applied this without water directly onto dry patches – I could see a visible difference' • 'it has a heavenly, fresh Mediterranean smell, and is the loveliest product to use first thing in the morning' • 'gives you a spa-like experience' • 'my skin is much smoother, cellulite less visible' • 'loved this and am glad to have found it'.

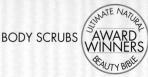
GREEN & SPRING INDULGING EXFOLIATING BODY BALM

✹✹

SCORE: 8.71/10

This sugar-based scrub in a tub offers a balm-type base of skin-nourishing oils 'including antioxidant rosehip' plus shea butter. (In our opinion the best scrubs leave a fine veil of lubrication on the skin.) Inspired by English country gardens, the fragrance is garlanded with rose, jasmine – plus touches of grounding vetiver and soothing chamomile – and was a universal rave, with testers.

COMMENTS: 'Lovely, uplifting but subtle scent of rose and jasmine' • 'skin definitely softer and I didn't need moisturiser – which is unusual, as I've just got back from holiday' • 'one of the nicest exfoliators I've ever used: the scrubby element wasn't harsh but at the same time very effective, leaving skin polished and fresh – I felt like I had been to a spa for a great massage' • 'skin glowy and hydrated after use' • 'really, really loved it – the smell is amazing!' • 'I suffer from unsightly red circular marks on my upper arms – I've had them for about seven years – but after three days of this, they looked less red and after seven days have disappeared. I've been able to wear a vest top for the first time in years during a recent bout of warm weather'.

EMMA HARDIE AMAZING FACE NATURAL LIFT AND SCULPT BODY TREATMENT

✹

SCORE: 8.44/10

Slightly random name (putting Amazing Face to a body scrub), but this pink paste is targeted for bodies. The colour is down to fine rose and china clays, which are mixed with exfoliating granules of organic red corn and Himalayan salt. To soften skin, Emma adds her signature moringa oil together with sweet almond oil.

COMMENTS: 'Skin was dry and suffering; now very dry areas massively improved, especially elbows and knees' • 'best body scrub I've ever used, leaving skin nourished and fresh' • 'the delicious fragrance evokes thoughts of holidays, spa treatments and happy days' • 'after using this my legs had a radiance that wasn't there before, and softness lasted a long time' • 'loved this – will be buying again; made me feel pampered and relaxed before bed' • 'I had awful rhino skin before using this whipped cream scrub; now it's 100 per cent better, and less spotty on chest' • 'luxurious, sweet scent: I'm a convert to body scrubs, after this'.

ORA NATURALS ARGAN BODY SCRUB REVIVE

✹✹

SCORE: 8.29/10

Packaging-wise, this is a bit of a lethal weapon (a really hefty glass jar), but inside, you find a gorgeously scented, loose scrub that gets its buffing action from sugar. The wake-up-call scent is down to red mandarin, grapefruit and lemongrass essential oils. Ora is a small brand created by a Brit-based New Zealander, following her travels to Morocco, homeland of the argan plant (*Argania spinosa*), on which the whole collection is based.

COMMENTS: 'Smells fantastic, and is brilliant at its job: left skin incredibly soft and moisturised as if I'd used body cream' • 'I love this stuff: couldn't wait to use it again – a wonderful aphrodisiac, lemony and zingy fragrance – sensory heaven' • 'my skin felt absolutely wonderful: I wanted to run around naked showing off to my husband!' • 'the skin on my legs was much softer compared to my arms, where I hadn't used the product – loved it'.

DR.ORGANIC ROSE OTTO BODY SCRUB

✹✹

SCORE: 8.29/10

Roses, roses all the way with this: a flip-top tube of quite intensely fragranced exfoliating cream, which gets its buffing power from pumice and crushed peach kernel stones. Another one for the shower rather than the bath – to avoid soaking in a pile of grit – although one tester loved the milky water. NB: This may not be the top choice for sensitive-skinned readers.

COMMENTS: 'A beautiful scent and nice to use' • 'the first product from a "normal" range (as opposed to Oilatum) that left skin feeling properly moisturised' • 'used in the bath it turned the water milky and rosy – Cleopatra eat your heart out!' • 'effective, gentle exfoliator that smoothed central-heating-dried skin' • 'skin refined and much smoother'.

WE LOVE

Jo loves the wonderful, grounding blend of essential oils in The Organic Pharmacy Cleopatra's Body Scrub (rose, rose geranium and ylang-ylang), and is a long-term devotee of Espa Detoxifying Salt Scrub. (And she really, really does buff every bath time, religiously!) Sarah is a devoted scrubber too, with a tottering pile of products by the shower: Odylique Coconut Candy Scrub is a longtime favourite. In extremis – when no scrub is to hand – she makes a sludge of sea salt and olive oil (need not be the best cold-pressed extra virgin), which works a treat!

SOFT SERVINGS

These moisturising body cherishers make ideal
gifts for friends – or keep them for yourself…

BODY BUTTER BLISS

We know from years of feedback that body
butters rank high on the list of readers'
favourite beauty treats. But, it's incredibly
simple to make your own butterlicious version
– and makes a lovely gift for a friend, too.
This formula is wonderful for post-holiday
skin. The beeswax transforms the oils into
a solid butter so it is less messy to use than
liquid body oils.

- 1 tablespoon calendula-infused olive oil
- 10g (½oz) beeswax
- 1 tablespoon coconut oil
- 2 tablespoons sesame oil
- 50g (2oz) grated cocoa butter

For the calendula oil, use the maceration
technique on page 51, or use Calendula
Macerated Oil from Neal's Yard Remedies.

Place all the ingredients in a double boiler
(see page 212) and heat gently until the
beeswax has melted.

Stir well, allow to cool slightly, and pour
the mixture into a sterilised jar with a screw
top. You can fragrance the body butter with
a blend of your favourite essential oils – stir
in up to 15 drops after you've removed the
mixture from the heat.

CUCUMBER BODY LOTION

This is super-refreshing in hot weather but it is a light lotion, so you might want to use a body butter on areas of drier skin. It also works well as a sinks-in-fast hand lotion, so keep it near the taps, and massage into hands after washing them.

- 5cm (2in) piece of cucumber, peeled and chopped
- 1 tablespoon witch hazel extract
- 1 teaspoon glycerine
- 1 teaspoon rose water
- 2 drops grapefruit seed extract
- 5 drops rose or lavender essential oil (optional)

Mash the cucumber in a pestle and mortar and add the witch hazel, glycerine and rose water. Or, whizz the whole lot in an electric blender or food processor for about 1 minute. At the last moment, drop in the grapefruit seed extract and essential oil – if you're using it – and stir or whizz again, for a beautiful pale-green lotion that smooths in easily. Kept in the fridge, this cucumber lotion will last for a couple of weeks.

TIP: Cucumber juice gives a boost to all skin types, so never discard cucumber peel without rubbing the inner side over your skin – it's great for necks, arms and the backs of hands.

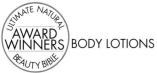
BODY LOTIONS
our award winners

We love slathering on body lotion, especially when it's full of delicious skin-nurturing ingredients. Of almost 50 trialled, our testers gave these four stellar scores

L'OCCITANE ULTRA RICH SHEA BUTTER BODY LOTION
✳

SCORE: 9.14/10

Shea butter is a cornerstone of the L'Occitane range: they've been working with a community project in West African Burkina Faso for decades. It's the star ingredient (at a 15 per cent concentration) in this super-scoring winner, with extracts of soothing calendula and nourishing sweet almond, plus a drizzle of honey.
COMMENTS: 'Skin felt softer with a natural glow; helped hard areas on feet, too' • 'ease of use a big plus: two or three pumps and legs and arms were moisturised and left feeling supple' • 'skin felt lovely and looked brighter' • 'leaves a sheen on my skin that makes it look glowy and fresh' • 'knees and elbows much softer after a week; no irritation or feeling of greasiness – will buy again' • 'beautiful smell – nutty, with a hint of lemon and coconut'.

REN MOROCCAN ROSE OTTO BODY LOTION
✳✳✳

SCORE: 9/10

Every time we send out one of REN's Moroccan Rose products, our testers fall in love, partly with the alluring fragrance and here with the soufflé-like texture of this cream in its generous pump-action bottle. With a nourishing blend of rose otto oil (from damask rose petals) and rosehip seed oil, rich in essential fatty acids, plus shea butter, it's one of Sarah's favourites.
COMMENTS: 'Perfect texture: velvety soft and scrumptious' • 'I have flaky/sore patches down the sides of my body but this definitely eased that problem – made riding my bike a lot more comfortable' • 'loved the gorgeous smell – often caught myself sniffing my arms at work' • 'one of the best body creams I've ever tried; have thought long and hard and there's not one negative thing I can say!'

AT A GLANCE

L'OCCITANE ULTRA RICH
SHEA BUTTER
BODY LOTION

REN MOROCCAN
ROSE OTTO
BODY LOTION

THIS WORKS
SKIN DEEP YOUTH ELIXIR

BAREFOOT SOS
DAILY RICH
BODY LOTION

THIS WORKS SKIN DEEP YOUTH ELIXIR
✳✳

SCORE: 8.71/10

This is Jo's favourite body treatment: a real de-ager that is actually more of a smoothing serum. As with all This Works products it features a glorious fusion of therapeutic essential oils including rose, patchouli, bergamot and clary sage, in a soothing base that incorporates aloe vera and chamomile.
COMMENTS: 'Lovely light body moisturiser that absorbs quickly; skin looks cared for and there are fewer little spots and bumps on my legs' • 'I loved this and noticed a great improvement in skin texture' • 'no cracking or stinging on my allergic, sensitive skin; definite improvement in silkiness right from the start' • 'lush smell reminds me of herbs and flowers' • 'would I buy this again? Hell, yes!' • 'parchment-paper effect on fine dry lines – gone'.

BAREFOOT SOS DAILY RICH BODY LOTION
✳

SCORE: 8.69/10

This sinks in fast, packing a turbo-charged punch of moisture. Originally created by a homeopath, the range is much-loved by anyone with challenged skin, including sufferers of eczema, psoriasis, dermatitis and general itching. Ingredients include shea butter, oils of jojoba, argan, macadamia and essential oils of orange blossom and lavender.
COMMENTS: 'Loved this cream: hard patches on elbows, knees and heels much improved' • 'I've tried so many body lotions – never satisfied – but this is amazing: excellent improvement in skin tone and texture after just three days' • 'loved the light, orange-blossom smell' • 'my skin is prone to dryness and itching but after using this I am the proud owner of silky-smooth, supple, irritation-free skin'.

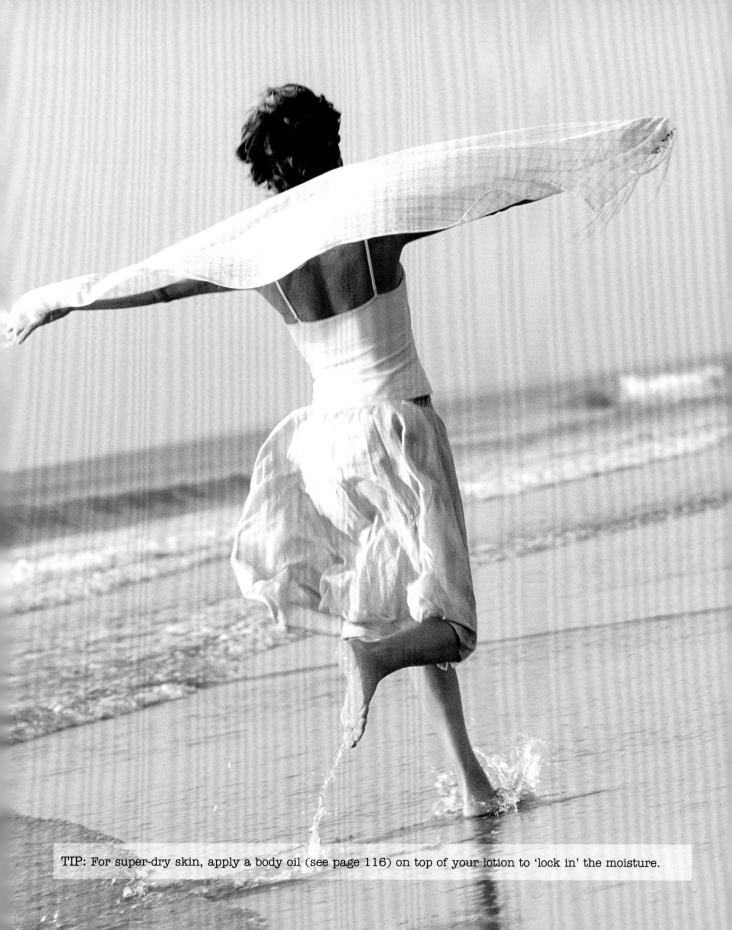

TIP: For super-dry skin, apply a body oil (see page 116) on top of your lotion to 'lock in' the moisture.

BANISH THE BLOAT

Whether it's the season for swimsuits or the season for LBDs, many women we know fret about how to get a flat(ter) tummy. So here, LA-based clinical nutritionist Kimberly Snyder shares her wisdom. Kimberly (whose clients include Hollywood A-listers such as Drew Barrymore and the Black Eyed Peas singer Fergie) gave us the best advice we've seen on slimming down and sleeking up, based on her book *The Beauty Detox Solution*, which we recommend unreservedly. Her writing is really down to earth and practical – inspirational, too – and by following her advice, you should see a difference pretty quickly. (NB: Anyone who suffers prolonged, continuous bloating should consult a doctor)

The bulk of your meals should be fibre-rich plant foods. To ensure you get lots of raw veggies, which are high in nutrients, vitamins and enzymes, make a big mixed salad for lunch and start dinner with a large green salad.

Try Kim's Glowing Green Smoothie for breakfast. Use organic ingredients and chop the veggies before blending. Blend 350ml (12fl oz) water, one head lettuce and a small bunch of spinach until smooth; gradually add 3–4 celery stalks, one apple/pear/banana, and the juice of half a lemon.

Eat animal protein, including dairy, only once a day. More is too 'acid-forming': your body should be slightly alkaline. Get protein from plant foods such as seeds, nuts, quinoa, millet and lentils.

Avoid or eat less cheese. Dairy is difficult to digest, so it can lead to bloating and weight gain.

Eat fruit only on an empty stomach, and never for pudding. If you eat it after heavier foods that take longer to digest, the fruit gets stuck and starts to ferment, leading to bloat.

Watch the salt. Too much sodium can cause bloating and puffiness. Add small amounts of high-quality sea salt (or Himalayan rock salt) directly to food; avoid processed foods. Drink unsweetened cranberry concentrate with fresh water – sweetened with stevia if wished – to help flush excessive fluids and salts. (That's a must before red-carpet events and awards, Kimberly says.)

Don't drink and eat at the same time. It dilutes gastric juices and digestive enzymes, and so impedes the digestive process. Just sip a little liquid and chew each mouthful thoroughly.

Avoid all fizzy drinks. The air bubbles in carbonated soft drinks release carbon dioxide in the digestive tract, creating bloating. NB: Excessive caffeine can also cause bloat.

Get to love raw apple cider vinegar. It acts as a prebiotic to feed the growth of probiotics (the 'good' bacteria in your gut), which help with optimal digestion, elimination and breaking down foods more efficiently – all important for a flat belly. Sip one tablespoonful diluted in a cup of warm water 20 minutes before meals. It's great in salad dressings too.

You can't be slim and trim – let alone healthy and happy – without exercise. Our bodies (and minds) thrive on being active. Do whatever you love: walking, running, riding, dancing, tennis, yoga, zumba – just do it. You don't have time not to! And use spare minutes to work out just that little bit more, says fitness expert Zana Morris, founder of The Library gym in London.

When you get up, take a minute to practise squats. With your feet flat on the floor, a shoulder width apart and pointed slightly out, drop gently down as if you are sitting, with your hips as low to the floor as possible. Stand up slowly, keeping your feet flat; don't bounce. Feel the weight on your upper thighs and the centre of your feet. Practise with a chair to start with (don't actually sit on it, you understand, but it will show you where your body should be). Repeat until the minute's up (set a timer on your phone). As well as keeping your whole body supple, this helps release natural growth hormone for fat burning and toning.

Do calf raisers as you wait for the kettle to boil. Stand on tiptoe as high as possible, arms above your head with fingertips reaching for the ceiling. Hold for a count of 10, then let arms slowly fall and return to standing flat on the floor. Then press your heels into the floor and raise your toes as high off the floor as possible. Hold for 10. Repeat these two steps 5–10 times.

Make use of time at the bus stop. (Or on the Tube.) When you're waiting in a queue, stand with your legs a hip width apart and slightly bent. Put all your body weight on one leg and hold for a count of 30. Repeat on the other leg. Increase the intensity by squeezing your gluteal (bottom) muscles. This is great for toning the thighs and bottom.

Sitting at work, try an exercise ball seat. Use it for short periods first as it really gives your core muscles an intense workout. It helps to strengthen your back – good for back problems – as well as reducing your waistline. (We like the Wellness Ball – Active Sitting by Technogym. It's not cheap but it is effective and is helping to solve a colleague's back problem.)

TIP: Sarah practises squatting when she is drying her hair upside down, and then does a yoga Warrior pose when she is styling it (with the fantastic John Frieda Volume Shine Airstyler – a heated round brush that you hold in position for half a minute or so, so it's perfect for working out upper arms as well).

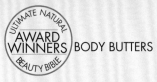
BODY BUTTERS
our award winners

The pleasure factor of body butter means we see some high scores in this category, and these impressed a new batch of beauty recruits, especially the top award winner. Testers lavished one side of their body with the butters for comparison and went completely soft on the following… PS: If you are wondering about the difference between butters and lotions (see page 110), the choice depends on your skin type: rich butters are fab for dry areas, particularly in the winter. But lighter, sink-in-fast lotions are fine for normal skin, with a butter to offer TLC on extra-parched bits

EMMA HARDIE NATURAL LIFT AND SCULPT BODY BUTTER
✳

SCORE: 9.17/10
Another super-high score for super-facialist Emma Hardie's range. This body nurturer is rich in skin-friendly omega 3/6/9 essential fatty acids for skin protection, alongside Inca inchi oil from Peru. The luscious cream scented with rose and jasmine dispenses through a clever cap: twist and it's open, twist again and it closes, which saves time removing the lid (and occasionally scrabbling for it under the bed, if you're anything like us). Emma advises applying this after a bath, when skin is still damp.
COMMENTS: 'My summer-desiccated skin felt rehydrated and moisturised and stayed this way for many hours afterwards' • 'oh, my goodness, the fragrance! Luxurious, expensive, divine – I loved it' • 'thick and velvet-like but in no way gloopy or sticky – generally, I don't get on with body butters but this was the perfect consistency' • 'this did appear to have much longer-lasting effects than my usual brand; my legs, especially, stayed less dry over the next few days' • 'within a few days all my stubborn dry areas had disappeared: elbows, knees and heel areas' • 'my husband said this was the best-scented body lotion he's smelt on me; he particularly commented that it had a natural fragrance' • 'my skin looks 300 per cent better – I suffer from dry skin due to an autoimmune

AT A GLANCE

EMMA HARDIE NATURAL LIFT AND SCULPT BODY BUTTER

DR.ORGANIC MANUKA HONEY BODY BUTTER

NEAL'S YARD BEAUTY SLEEP BODY BUTTER

DR.ORGANIC POMEGRANATE BODY BUTTER

GREEN PEOPLE BODY BUTTER

L'OCCITANE ULTRA RICH SHEA BUTTER BODY CREAM

disease, but this really delivers improvement and reduces itching' • 'gives a firmness and smoothness – and a little goes a long way'.

DR.ORGANIC MANUKA HONEY BODY BUTTER
✳ ✳

SCORE: 8.63/10
A small cheer echoes round *Beauty Bible* HQ when something like this happens: the Dr.Organic 'beauty steal' brand entered two butters in this category and they scored within a few micro-points of each other, even though they were sent to two different groups. We feel that underlines just how consistent our trials are. (We've always known it, but nice to have confirmation.) You can really smell the honey in this one, though otherwise the key skin-friendly ingredients are the same in both products: jojoba oil, glycerine, aloe vera, shea butter and sunflower seed oils feature in the line-up.
COMMENTS: 'Skin feels lovely and silky, a joy to apply – so luxurious' • 'I've used it on my dry heels which are much softer' • 'skin improved significantly; I no longer have dry patches on my legs and my body has a lovely glow; I'd buy this over and over' • 'really smells of honey: sweet and natural' • 'this is my new favourite cream; my skin is very dry and usually requires moisturising twice a day – but not now I have this product' • 'the honey smell is just glorious – almost good enough to eat'.

NEAL'S YARD BEAUTY SLEEP BODY BUTTER
✳ ✳ ✳
SCORE: 8.56/10

Soil Association certified with over 90 per cent organic ingredients, Neal's Yard's butterlicious option is recommended for pre-bedtime use. It blends shea and cocoa seed butters, sunflower seed oil, plus aloe vera to enhance the skin's own natural barrier and prevent moisture loss, while the aromatherapeutic addition of cypress, patchouli, ylang-ylang and clary sage aren't just lovely smells: they're active ingredients that help nudge you to the Land of Nod.

COMMENTS: 'A wonderful product, nice texture and scent: I usually avoid lavender fragrances as they remind me of old ladies, but this smells lovely as it relaxes and aids sleep' • 'gorgeous texture, rubbed in easily even on extra-dry areas; perfect for use at bedtime' • 'I'd buy it as a treat for a friend who was stressed' • 'so rich and smooth, afterwards the body feels cool and refreshed; skin is softer and feels healthier' • 'scaly patches have massively improved' • 'the nicest body butter I have used, with an amazing relaxing scent'.

DR.ORGANIC POMEGRANATE BODY BUTTER
✳ ✳
SCORE: 8.5/10

A gorgeous tangy fragrance from antioxidant-rich pomegranate is really what sets this apart from the Dr.Organic Manuka Body Butter entry opposite. We suggest when choosing between the two you're steered by your nose: if you like soft, sweet, honeyed scents, choose the former (unless you're vegan, of course, as it contains honey) – but if you prefer a fresher, more tart scent, this is your baby. (See also We Love, right.)

COMMENTS: 'After using for a week, noticed a gradual softening of harder skin areas – elbows, knees, heels' • 'very good value for money; I'll buy this again' • 'used it on arms and chest and the following morning skin felt beautifully soft and refreshed' • 'feels fabulous! Love the thick, creamy texture and the swift way it absorbs into skin – gorgeous, like spreading liquid chocolate onto the body' • 'tried this on my eight-year-old son who has dry skin particularly on his upper arms; we generally only use a cream prescribed by our GP, but with this his skin is noticeably softer and smoother. My skin is less dry, softer and plumper – including backs of hands. Fab!'

GREEN PEOPLE BODY BUTTER
✳ ✳ ✳
SCORE: 8.39/10

This is certified organic by the Organic Food Federation (with an impressive 99 per cent organic ingredients). We'd actually categorise it more as a body balm. It's a blend of oils – coconut, hemp seed, palm, sunflower, jojoba and pomegranate seed, together with fragrant essential oils of rosemary, lavender and lemongrass – which is solidified with beeswax. It softens in the hand, to be massaged into skin, and is great for dry, cracked bits, as the barrier allows them to recover. Green People recommend you smooth it in before bedtime, on legs, feet (then slip on clean socks), and other dry areas.

COMMENTS: 'Quite "green-smelling" rather than floral; could be used by men or women' • 'particularly good on dry legs leaving behind winter hosiery' • 'instant results – and I like an all-in-one product that moisturises and repairs skin all over the body from elbows to heels as well as hard cuticles' • 'my hands get really wrecked in the garden but this has been way more effective than normal hand creams' • 'as soon as I opened the pot I wanted to cocoon the whole of my body in this delicious treat'.

L'OCCITANE ULTRA RICH SHEA BUTTER BODY CREAM
✳
SCORE: 8.33/10

One of L'Occitane's classic bestsellers: enriched with 25 per cent cocoa butter, as well as moisturising linseed, marshmallow, sweet almond, apricot oil and honey (which gives a drippingly gorgeous fragrance). This luxurious body treat is quickly absorbed into skin but in L'Occitane's own trials was shown to hydrate enduringly for as long as 24 hours.

COMMENTS: 'Loved this body cream: smelt divine, was easy to use, quick to absorb and particularly effective on elbows, feet and knees' • 'will buy again – has replaced my regular body cream which I've been loyal to for years' • 'much better than other shea butter products I've used; absorbed very quickly for smoother, softer post-holiday skin' • 'with a texture like double cream this is a real luxury, leaving a delicate sheen' • 'this is fine for my sensitive skin' • 'dry areas felt soothed, smoothed and glistened with health – leaving the most soft, luxurious-feeling arms and legs I've ever had!'

WE LOVE
Jo has two body butters on the go at all times: the Emma Hardie body butter which tops the category here, and yet another from the Dr.Organic line: the Aloe Vera Body Butter, which she finds wonderfully cooling in hot weather. (She's a fan of the fresh scent, too.) Sarah's had a thing for Pure Lochside for a long time, revelling in the 95 per cent organic Calm And Soothe Luxury Balm; is devoted to Trilogy Ultra Hydrating Body Cream and yes, loves the Emma Hardie one, too (honestly, we don't confer on our favourites...).

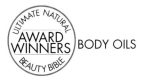
BODY OILS
our award winners

Luscious body oils rank high on our list of favourite indulgent treats. We road-tested dozens for this book – and our panel said these floated to the top

CAUDALÍE DIVINE OIL
✳

SCORE: 9.17/10

One of our biggest gripes about body oils is that it's way too easy to over-slurp them and get the oil everywhere. This super-high scorer avoids that problem as it mists 'dry oil' onto the body, spritzing on a lovely scent of rose, grapefruit, pink pepper, cedar and vanilla. To create the dry oil texture some synthetic ingredients are added (so, only one daisy here) to the blend of argan, hibiscus, sesame and Caudalíe's signature grapeseed oil.

COMMENTS: 'Gave skin a gorgeous, healthy, glow' • 'sinks in quickly so clothes didn't stick to skin' • 'the spray makes it easy to apply' • 'the best body oil I've ever used (and I've tried plenty)' • 'daily use helped to prolong my suntan' • 'fantastic, versatile product for face, body, hair and problem areas' • 'smells fabulous – rich, warm and lush' • 'used it overnight on thick, heavy, dry hair: it left no mark on my pillow and next day I ploughed a comb straight through hair – a marvel!'

REN MOROCCAN ROSE OTTO ULTRA-MOISTURE OIL
✳

SCORE: 9/10

Our testers fall time and again for the sublime rose otto scent of REN's bestselling bodycare range. The latest addition to the roll call of rosy favourites is this oil: another pump-action bottle (less mess), which infuses the realistic rose scent into a skin-nurturing blend of rice germ, jojoba, macadamia, argan and rose hip seed oils.

COMMENTS: 'Smell is gorgeous without being overpowering; I have used it twice a day and apart from my skin looking lovely and dewy, I'm still only halfway through the bottle' • 'gave an instant lift to skin which is in better condition, not so dry' • 'an absolutely fabulous product,

---

AT A GLANCE

CAUDALÍE
DIVINE OIL

REN MOROCCAN
ROSE OTTO
ULTRA-MOISTURE OIL

CINQ MONDES
SUBLIME BODY
AND HAIR OIL

ESPA SOOTHING
BODY OIL

TIP: These oils are real multi-duty body beautifiers. Use them to smooth skin from top to toe: soothe into sunburnt areas, add them to the bath, or pop a drop in your palms and stroke over flyaway hairs, frizz and split ends – and they're great for cuticles, too.

---

giving skin a youthful radiance and leaving it velvety smooth' • 'expensive but worth every penny' • 'great on legs before shaving'.

CINQ MONDES SUBLIME BODY AND HAIR OIL
✳ ✳ ✳

SCORE: 8.86/10

The certified-organic Paris spa brand Cinq Mondes takes its inspiration from Polynesian healing traditions. The blend of Tahitian noni and monoi oils is infused with uplifting orange and sweet vanilla essential oils. This is the only plastic-packaged contender – if you don't like glass in the bathroom. It's available by mail order – see Directory (on page 216) for details.

COMMENTS: 'Skin felt softer' • 'smells good: a fruity, slight coconut scent' • 'great multitasker: made my hair very soft and silky' • 'left skin sexy, glossy, glistening; vastly improved its texture and condition all over' • 'skin remained moisturised the day after use and didn't dry out the way it has with other body oils'.

ESPA SOOTHING BODY OIL
✳ ✳

SCORE: 8.78/10

One of ESPA's classics with a divine aroma of soothing sandalwood, rose geranium, myrrh and frankincense, which will be familiar to ESPA fans (and that includes us), designed to calm an overactive mind and prepare you for sleep. Testers commented on its age-defying powers.

COMMENTS: 'Everything about this is gorgeous – a perfect 10' • 'although it's rich, doesn't take long to absorb' • 'reduced fine lines and wrinkles and removed years' worth of hard skin' • 'a noticeable reduction in cellulite and stretch marks' • 'amazing smell – worth buying for that alone' • 'am now rationing the last bit as dreading when this runs out – I inhale before sleep and it's a great stress reliever'.

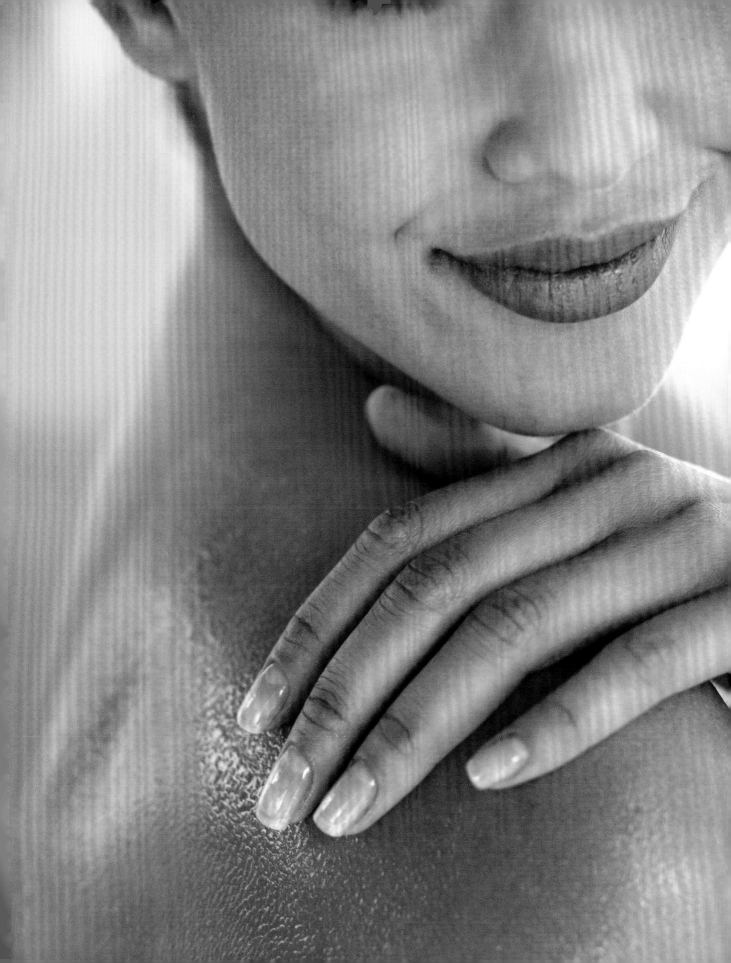

SMOOTH TALK

We all know what it looks like – orange peel-type dimpling if you are lucky, cottage-cheese type blobby cushions tethered like a button-back chair in more advanced cases. It invariably affects your thighs and bottom, sometimes upper arms and tum. But, according to our testers, there is hope for improvement

Cellulite is the constant companion of 80–90 per cent of post-adolescent women, according to surveys over decades. (About 10 per cent of men suffer, and that's down to different hormones.) And our *Beauty Bible* testers are certainly not immune. But two fascinating things emerged when we read the questionnaires from our latest trials of cellulite-busters.

One tester says: 'I'm a gym bunny with a muscular physique – and a cellulite problem. Nothing has shifted this orange-peel effect that is ruining all my hard work at the gym – UNTIL NOW! The difference to texture and firmness of my troublesome inner thighs is incredible.'

Another writes: 'I definitely saw improvement in texture and appearance of cellulite though, as a doctor, I'm wary about attributing it to this product: it may be the twice-daily massaging encouraging lymph drainage and blood supply. Having said that, skin's smoother, softer and improvement definite.' (To see the products that made such a difference, turn to page 120.)

So – our consumer surveys demonstrate three key facts, which bear out what we know from researching the subject for 25 years.

First, you can improve cellulite. Second, it affects all kinds of women, super-fit skinnies as well as plumptious couch potatoes. Third, massage is a key part of the process. Before we move on, just let us

say that the results of these latest trials – where our diligent testers trialled products on one leg only, then compared the results with the untreated leg after several weeks – amazed us. We are used to testers testifying to some effect but not the degree of improvement they reported this time round.

Interestingly, the last time we saw such good results was way back before cosmetics had to show ingredient labelling. A leading product was so successful that women bought it in suitcase-fuls. One of our testers then was a doctor's wife and he told us the product had a real effect. Then cosmetic labelling came in, the formula was tweaked (apparently the active ingredients would have made it liable to be licensed as a drug) and it no longer wowed our testers. Now, it seems that cosmetic companies have come up with ingredients that really do pack the same punch.

So what is cellulite? In a word, fat. And here's a fat fact: the female of the species is genetically programmed for fertility reasons to have lots of lovely fat cells on thighs, bottom, abdomen and upper arms. In our reproductive years, we usually have enough collagen – the main protein in connective tissue, which gives our skin its tone and bounciness – to keep the cellulite in check. When oestrogen starts to decrease, so does the supply of collagen and then the trouble starts.

Cellulite usually begins appearing from 25–35, although occasionally it affects teenage girls after puberty, often those taking the contraceptive pill. That may be because the pill blocks the production of oestrogen; younger women say that cellulite first appears with the pill. In the same way, a bit of dimpling often turns into full-blown blobs as oestrogen declines towards the menopause.

Another man/woman thing: the structure of collagen is different in us and them. In women, says Lionel Bissoon, author of The Cellulite Cure, it looks like a picket fence – with fibres going one way only – whereas in men it looks like a criss-cross fence – with cross-linked fibres: it's not rocket science to see which is stronger and better at keeping fat cells contained.

As we age or put on weight, fat cells get larger. (Women also break down fat less easily than men do.) Combine that with less supple collagen and the result is that the fat starts protruding through. The fibres anchoring the fatty tissue to the layers of skin above pull at the pockets of fat, creating the button-back chair look.

Another problem is the prevalence of junk food, with additives and pesticide residues even in our water supply. Some chemicals act as hormones, disrupting the functioning of the body, which may partly explain why the super-skinnies are affected too. Lack of essential nutrients, particularly the antioxidant vitamins A, C and E and trace minerals, is known to stimulate cellulite. Lionel Bissoon notes that in photos from the 1940s and 50s, pre-junk food, 'women had perfect legs'.

Other triggers are a sluggish digestion, food intolerances, gut problems such as irritable bowel syndrome, yo-yo dieting and stress.

WHAT YOU CAN DO

We don't have a magic cure but as well as massaging in targeted products (our Award Winners overleaf) we suggest:

Body brushing: our key weapon! Choose a firm brush but avoid bristles that scratch your skin. (Test by whisking it across the back of your hand. If you have sensitive skin, try one with rubber nodules.) Brush dry skin before bath or shower. Start at feet and work up legs, across hips, bottom and tummy with long, upward movements. Move from hands, up arms to shoulders and across your chest, working towards the heart. Avoid breasts or you may cause soreness, and skin problems or wounds. Do this daily and the difference is phenomenal.

Exercise lots: do at least five minutes of stretching every day, walk whenever you can, and aim for four sessions of toning exercise – yoga, pilates, dancing, swimming – every week.

Eat plenty of fresh foods, with lots of vegetables and fruit, organic if possible. (We actually have virtually no cellulite, which we put down to a principally organic diet and yoga.)

Cut out fatty sugary foods, which are stored as fat. Also dairy products, particularly cow's milk; consider a calcium/magnesium (ratio 1:2) supplement to compensate.

Eat some protein daily, especially if you're vegetarian. A protein breakfast (eg, eggs) can stabilise blood sugar all day.

Sip plenty of still, filtered water between meals. Our bodies are over two-thirds water and need it to work well.

Relax: de-stressing helps your whole body, so practise mindfulness and/or meditation. At the very least, just sit and breathe slowly, gently, rhythmically as often as possible.

Take a good multivitamin/mineral daily, and consider adding in extra vitamin C and natural vitamin E.

In desperation, slosh on the self-tan! We'll never forget meeting a Rubenesque swimsuit model at a fashion show who swore by camouflaging her cellulite with a fake bronze.

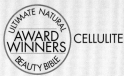

CELLULITE TREATMENTS
our award winners

Extraordinary, this: L'Occitane completely swept the board at the top of our cellulite-blitzing charts – one of the most stubborn and challenging categories in the book. The products were all trialled separately, rather than as part of a 'regime' – and it's a straight gold, silver and bronze medal for the French brand. (We're pleased to see an old favourite from Weleda appearing here, too.) Remember: testers applied these (as well as 30 others) on one thigh and buttock for comparison – so there was no chance that the effects might be an illusion…

L'OCCITANE ALMOND MILK CONCENTRATE (FIRMING & SMOOTHING)
✳

SCORE: 8.33/10

This is a whacking great heavy jar of luscious sweet-scented gel. It's excelled in previous trials and now this updated version, reformulated in 2012, scores highly again. Almond proteins work to improve skin firmness, while a 'mesh' from the almond extracts visibly tightens the skin and stimulates collagen production. The new formula also features a new patented complex of rose bud and almond extracts; a great firming action, our testers noted.

COMMENTS: 'Cellulite improved and skin looked better; smells lovely, texture gorgeous. A perfect 10/10' • 'after a few uses it was noticeable how much more elastic my skin looked; stretch marks were softer • 'really impressed with visible results; smells refreshing' • 'the fragrance is divine: almond-y but not in a sickly marzipan way; find myself sniffing my arm for a whiff' • 'good results: firmness improved – I didn't think any cream would smooth my dimples' • 'skin softer and the appearance of cellulite less noticeable; during the trial I had an ovary removed (ouch) and had several weeks of bed rest; however, there's

AT A GLANCE

L'OCCITANE ALMOND MILK CONCENTRATE (FIRMING & SMOOTHING)

L'OCCITANE ALMOND MILK VEIL (FIRMING & SMOOTHING)

L'OCCITANE ALMOND BEAUTIFUL SHAPE (EXPERT CELLULITE CONTROL)

THE ORGANIC PHARMACY RESCULPTING BODY GEL

INLIGHT ORGANIC FIRM & TONE OIL

WELEDA BIRCH CELLULITE OIL

a distinct improvement in skin of my left thigh compared to my right, which can only be this product. The smell's just gorgeous and really lifted my spirits, so my husband bought me the shower gel to cheer me up after the op'.

L'OCCITANE ALMOND MILK VEIL (FIRMING & SMOOTHING)
✳

SCORE: 7.88/10

In its pump-action plastic bottle this looks like a lotion but it really is a sinks-in-fast, lightweight 'veil'. Softening almond oil and almond milk nourish the skin, almond proteins and silicium (from horsetail) work to even and firm, but there's also a subtle illuminating effect when it's massaged into skin – so skin looks healthier in a soft-focus way. To be honest, testers loved this more for its skin-conditioning, firming, smoothing action than for de-dimpling – it certainly made them feel better about their bodies.

COMMENTS: 'Smells divine: very almond-y and feminine' • 'cellulite looks smoother, though it's still there; overall improvement in the look and feel of my skin' • 'dimples not so horrendous, but I'd recommend this for any part of the body: skin felt amazing, thighs smoother and little bumps on my arms have disappeared' • 'loved the golden shimmer on my skin'.

L'OCCITANE ALMOND BEAUTIFUL SHAPE (EXPERT CELLULITE CONTROL)

❋

SCORE: 7.71/10

And again! L'Occitane's third winner comes with a twist-open-twist-closed top, which dispenses a lightweight cooling gel that specifically targets legs. It contains almond tree bud extract (packed with flavonoids), natural caffeine, essential oils of immortelle, palmarosa and peppermint to instantly firm and smooth the appearance of 'orange peel', while working longer term on the underlying problem.

COMMENTS: 'Inside leg measurement and hips decreased, and tone of my skin was improved; firmness apparent' • 'cellulite much improved and has really boosted my weight-loss plan as it seems to help with water retention' • 'liked the texture: easy to apply, fast drying, cooling and skin feels much firmer' • 'definitely saw improvement in texture and appearance of cellulite, though, as a doctor, I'm wary about attributing it all to this product: it may be the twice-daily massaging that's encouraging lymph drainage and blood supply. Having said that, skin's smoother, softer and improvement definite' • 'dimpling/cellulite noticeably diminished'.

THE ORGANIC PHARMACY RESCULPTING BODY GEL

❋❋❋

SCORE: 7.31/10

This tangily scented gel with skin-smoothing pomegranate combines powerful natural actives from green coffee, horse chestnut, skin-firming kigelia – plus chilli, which delivers a perceptible 'warming' action when massaged into skin. The Organic Pharmacy remind users that upper arms can often benefit from the gentle firming action of a cellulite product, too.

COMMENTS: 'Reduction in measurement of thigh I used this on – an inch lost, fantastic for me' • 'exciting, vibrant, fun product to use with a lovely fruity, citrus smell' • 'skin looks smoother and cellulite not as pronounced' • 'really liked the smell – very fresh and pleasant – and sank into skin very easily' • 'I hadn't ever used any cellulite products previous to this as I was never convinced there'd be any effect on my skin texture, but it's improved – so I will continue using' • 'skin feels firmer and softer'.

WE LOVE

After L'Occitane's triumph, Jo thought she'd better put the three products reviewed here through their paces – and is thoroughly enjoying the almond-y experience (though too soon at the time of going to press to report on major improvements). Previously, her favourite product was Decléor Aromessence Sculpt-Firming Body Concentrate, a 100 per cent natural blend featuring five essential oils for massaging into problem areas. Sarah's anti-cellulite regime consists of body brushing (see page 119) and massaging in body oils – but these results may tempt her to add in a targeted product.

INLIGHT ORGANIC FIRM & TONE OIL

❋❋❋

SCORE: 7.3/10

From a small Cornwall-based brand started by an Italian doctor and homeopath, this oil incorporates meadowsweet and rosemary to encourage lymph drainage; purifying burdock, stimulating and toning ginger root and green tea; plus bitter orange leaf and jojoba oils for their effectiveness on skin elasticity. As with all cellulite treatments, it's recommended for use at least once a day, every day.

COMMENTS: 'Cellulite less dimply and skin smoother; stretch marks also improved which I'm very surprised by as I'm 54 and thought I was past any joy with them' • 'I thought an oil-based product would be messy but this proved me wrong. It has a spoiling, feel-good factor: you want to use it every day as it's not a chore' • 'overall my treated thigh looks better, less puckered and lumpy than my non-tester leg' • 'saw a real difference after the first time I used it: thighs tighter and in better condition'.

WELEDA BIRCH CELLULITE OIL

❋❋❋

SCORE: 7.25/10

Several times this affordable biodynamic oil has made its way into our books, by virtue of its impressive performance on testers' cellulite – and here goes again. It is 100 per cent natural, and blends plant actives including butcher's broom and rosemary in a blend of apricot, wheat germ and jojoba oils, to smooth skin's texture, plus a blend of essential oils known for their toning action.

COMMENTS: 'I'm a gym bunny with a muscular physique – and a cellulite problem; nothing has shifted the orange-peel effect that is ruining all my dedicated fitness work – until now! The difference this product has made to the texture and firmness of my troublesome inner thighs is incredible' • 'measurements remain the same, but there is an improvement to dimply cellulite on bum and legs, with softer skin, too' • 'I was a bit cynical about this oil; I used it twice a day on one leg and the same side of my bottom; after six weeks I noticed an improvement in texture; and firmness seemed a lot better – and I have now started to use it on both sides as I don't want to have odd legs!'

SUPER TONICS

From stubborn cellulite to unwelcome odour, there's almost always a natural solution to routine body dilemmas – and often the ingredients are right on your doorstep. It's that simple

IVY ANTI-CELLULITE OIL

Ivy is found in many of the effective cellulite treatment products on sale in stores. But since it grows almost like a weed in both the countryside and cities, this cellulite-control ingredient is easy for anyone to get their hands on. Just be sure to use the bigger leaves and to wash them first.

- 15 large fresh ivy leaves
- 120ml (4fl oz) grapeseed oil
- 1 teaspoon wheat germ oil
- 15 drops juniper essential oil
- 5 drops fennel essential oil
- 5 drops rosemary essential oil

First bruise the ivy leaves in a pestle and mortar, place in the bottom of a jar and pour the grapeseed oil over them. Add the wheat germ oil, then the essential oils drop by drop. Leave the mixture to macerate for a week, then strain the blend into sterilised jars. Massage into problem areas – usually hips, thigh, and derrière. Ideally, body-brush first to maximise circulation (see page 119).

TIP: If you have a butcher's broom (*Ruscus aculeatus*) plant growing near you, pick several sprigs and crush with the ivy leaves, before macerating in the oil. Butcher's broom, like ivy, is detoxifying, and can help shift cellulite.

LAVENDER DEODORANT

Remember: this isn't an anti-perspirant so it won't keep you 'dry' – it's a deodorant, to help destroy the bacteria that make sweat smell, well, sweaty; plus lavender is an effective natural antiseptic.

- 250ml (9fl oz) vodka
- 50g (2oz) lavender flowers
- 50g (2oz) fresh rose petals
- 10 drops lavender essential oil
- 10 drops rose essential oil

Pour the vodka over the flowers and petals and add the drops of essential oil. Allow to macerate for about three weeks, then strain into an atomiser. Use in place of your regular deodorant.

Because this contains alcohol, don't use on just-shaved skin, or you may find yourself hopping round the bathroom.

If you're worried about body odour, even while using this deodorant, the problem may be clogged pores. When your body can't eliminate wastes, a sweaty odour can result. Gently dry-brush skin before a bath or shower to exfoliate the dead skin that clogs pores. (For the how-to, see page 119.) This will improve circulation, which, in turn, will help your body detoxify more efficiently. It might not eliminate your need for deodorant – but you should be able to use less of it.

MORE PONG-BEATER OPTIONS

Lovage, freshly picked, can be used in place of lavender in the deodorant recipe featured here; this herb – which smells of celery – effectively cleanses and deodorises.

Citrus peel gives skin a fresh, clean fragrance – and the citric acid helps tackle bacteria on the skin's surface. (In fact, our friend Kathy Phillips, founder of This Works, simply strokes on a cut lemon.) Use citrus in place of lavender in the recipe on this page. To enhance the fragrance, add 5 drops of sweet orange and 5 drops of lemon essential oils.

Witch hazel is very effective for tightening underarm pores and deodorising. Used on its own, it can be drying on skin, so add 1 tablespoon of glycerine to 50ml witch hazel, and then add 10 drops of your favourite essential oils: rose, lavender, melissa (lemon balm) or citrus oils (above) all make a sweet-smelling, sweat-beating blend.

Rose water is astringent and soothing; it can be spritzed top to toe as a freshening mist (though it's a little less effective at tackling serious sweat odour than the other ingredients here).

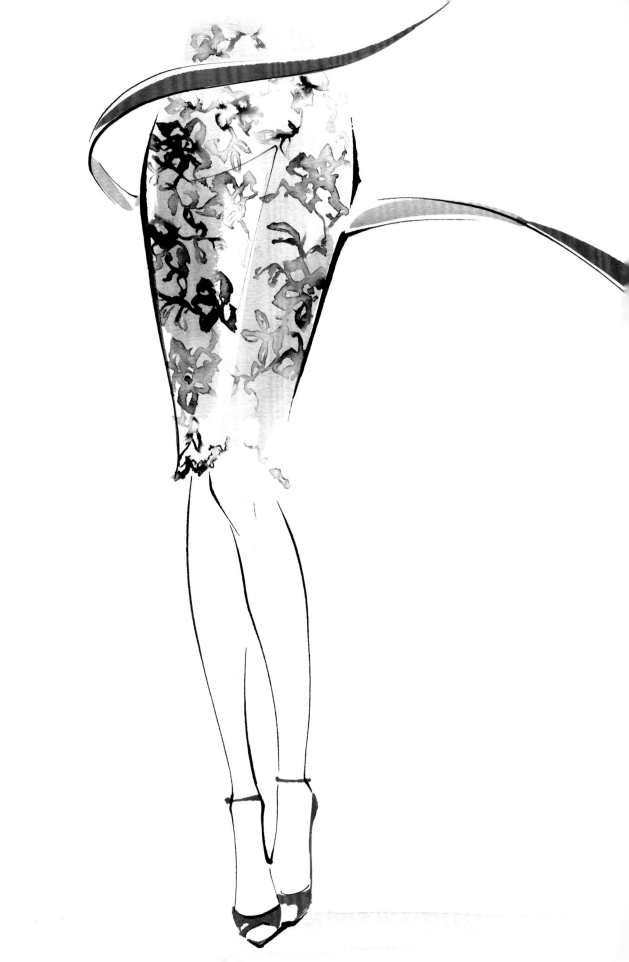

TLC for
HANDS
AND
FEET

Take care of your 'extremities' and they'll serve you well for a lifetime. Pretty them up and they'll cheer you instantly. So here are the tips, tricks – and treats – to do just that

How to have
HEALTHY, SHINY, STRONG NAILS

Here is a typical plea to our website, www.beautybible.com, from a woman with frail nails: 'I have suffered for many years with fragile nails but lately they seem a lot worse – very soft, brittle and peeling in layers. I feel so conscious of them and they make my hands look quite ugly. I have tried nail treatments, rub in cuticle oil, wear rubber gloves while washing up and have tried calcium supplements. I would greatly appreciate any advice you can give to help me achieve healthy, stronger nails.'

We thought the easiest way to help is to give you our best Dos – lots of them – and a few Don'ts. So here they are, but do be warned: it takes about three months for a new fingernail to grow in, so approach this as a long-term exercise, involving what you put in your body as much as what you put on your nails. You can, however, make a real difference to their appearance within two to three weeks – so plan ahead if you have a special occasion.

NB: The products we mention below are listed in the Directory (page 216). Do also look at our award-winning nail and cuticle treatments (page 128).

DO use a clear nail strengthener, such as Nail Magic, according to the directions. It will give your nails a slight shine, will help neaten them up so they look much better, and will help protect and nourish them.

DON'T buff weak nails, or let anyone else do it. The only buffing-type action that helps to increase blood flow is to rub them together, nail on nail, after you have oiled them.

DO file your nails gently with an emery board or crystal glass file in one direction, or towards the middle; don't saw from side to side.

DON'T try to file nails without polish on (or nail strengthener) to 'glue' them together.

DO wear gloves to wash up, garden, groom horses (in fact, a double layer of gloves are

needed here) and – perhaps surprisingly – if you work with paper as it dries out nails a lot.

DON'T use harsh, drying nail-polish removers: look for acetone-free versions with extra oils. See our Award Winner Fresh Therapies Eden Nail Polish Remover (page 135).

DO apply a hand and nail cream every time you wash your hands. Try Tisserand Signature Blend Intensive Hand & Nail Cream, which has impressed *Beauty Bible* testers (see page 138).

DO massage in nail oil every night. A good option is Dr.Hauschka Neem Nail Oil (see page 129). Neem is an Indian evergreen leaf that has ancient healing properties and has helped many a frail-nailed hand.

DON'T be tempted by gel nails: yes, they will look gorgeous for a couple of weeks but to get them to stay on – and take them off afterwards – the technicians have to abrade them quite roughly. Then you spend six months with nails falling off in layers and splitting down the middle, in Sarah's experience.

DO try a magnesium supplement, also omega 3 fatty acid and silica. Here's the thinking: calcium can't work without magnesium. Omega 3 fatty acids are essential for most body and brain functions including healthy hair, skin and nails. Silica is a vital mineral in general; in this case, it nourishes the nails and also ensures that nutrients get transported to the nail bed. (It's very good for lacklustre, thinning hair, too.) But remember: you have to go on taking these for several months, and preferably long-term. We take: Dyno-Mins Magnesium; Life-Flo Power Of Krill; and Solgar Vegetal Silica.

There seems to be a veritable epidemic of weak, splitting nails – judging by the number of times we are asked for help. We can't provide any quick fixes but we do have ways of boosting their health

DO get out in the sunlight to ensure you receive enough vitamin D. If you can't do that, or it's winter, consider supplementing with vitamin D3 – the most bioavailable form of the vitamin. We take: DLux 1000 Spray by Better You.

DO eat lots of oily fish (salmon, mackerel, sardines, tuna, trout etc); nuts and seeds (freshly ground flax seeds are particularly good), and olive oil. Remember to sip two litres of water or herbal tea in between meals.

DO eat enough protein: like hair and skin, nails are nourished by protein. Iron deficiency is a common cause, so if you are vegetarian, or eat little red meat, consider a gentle iron supplement such as Spatone 100% Natural Iron (to avoid stomach problems).

DO check out digestive problems. If you suffer bloating, constipation or diarrhea, or other symptoms of irritable bowel syndrome, you (and your nails) may benefit from a probiotic and/or digestive enzymes. Try Mega Probiotic ND by Science of Vermont and/or Super Digestive Enzymes by Life Extension.

DO try a 'green food': these are powders or pills based on chlorella, spirulina or other algae, which you add to yogurt, smoothies, or even soup. The results in terms of nail growth and strength for Sarah are startling. (They also make your gut alkaline, which helps with all sorts of things.)

And finally… **DON'T** abuse your nails by treating them as screwdrivers, staple removers, grout cleaners or for digging up flints in the field (Sarah again…).

NAIL AND CUTICLE TREATMENTS
our award winners

How can I have stronger, healthier nails? That always ranks in the top-five beauty questions we are asked at www.beautybible.com. The answer? A two-fold approach is best: there are great foods and supplements that will help boost nail health over time (see page 126) – but a daily massage with a targeted nail product will also pay dividends, delivering nails that are stronger, more flexible and less prone to snapping, splitting or flaking. Over a period of months our panellists trialled around 24 nail and cuticle treatments on one hand only – and these products nailed the highest scores

LIZ EARLE SUPERBALM
❋ ❋
SCORE: 8.38/10

This classic multitasker scored top of its class when our *Beauty Bible* testers trialled it as a nail and cuticle treatment. (It's done well in previous books, but we started from scratch for *The Ultimate Natural Beauty Bible* and it's very rewarding when similar scores are achieved time after time.) Superbalm blends plant oil nourishers including argan, olive, avocado, rosehip and hazelnut, with carnauba and beeswax, to create a soft but solid balm. Essential oils of neroli, lavender and chamomile deliver a wonderfully calming scent. Massaging your nails has never felt so relaxing.

COMMENTS: 'After one week, the cuticles on the hand I used it on were much less dry and felt softer' • 'my nails are looking greatly improved: smoother with fewer ridges and not so easily broken. My cuticles have not felt or looked so good in years' • 'smells gorgeous: very uplifting, slightly citrus, lavender, too – perfect' • 'nails are definitely stronger, cuticles healthier and easier to manage' • 'as time progressed I could actually wear nail polish which I don't usually get to do, due to the bitten

condition of my nails. This is a better alternative to nail-biting treatments' • 'my nails are now long and did not break as they usually do – they also grew quicker than normal' • 'even after a couple of days I could see such a difference between the two hands that I couldn't wait to use it on both – I'm glad I did one hand first or I wouldn't have believed how good it was' • 'I have also used it on my dry frizzy hair, parched lips and anywhere else in need of TLC'.

ARGAN 5+ PRECIOUS OIL ELIXIR
❋ ❋ ❋
SCORE: 8.28/10

Argan 5+ recommend massaging this into hands and nails in the morning to strengthen and hydrate. Argan oil has become ubiquitous in beauty – but the 'plus' in the name of this affordable brand refers to the fact they blend it with other African oils: baobab (trust us, it's the new argan), kukui, moringa and sacha inchi oils, for an intensely nourishing blend with a sweet, tropical scent. There's a small dispenser cap at the top which means you won't accidentally slurp it everywhere, although (like Superbalm) it has multiple uses: as a facial oil, hair oil and for dry skin just about anywhere.

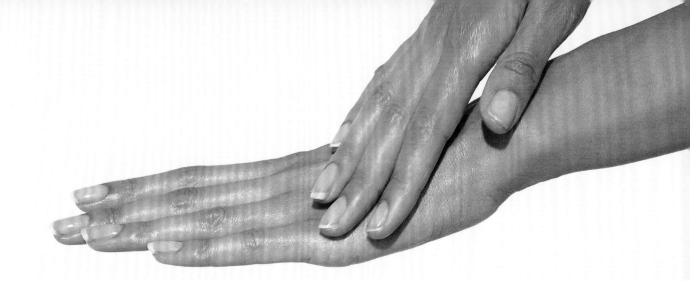

COMMENTS: 'My nails are much less brittle: it doesn't take long to notice results' • 'this really improved dryness of cuticles and also helped me stop picking at them as they were no longer dry and cracked: my manicurist has commented that my hands are looking much better' • 'also used this as a multi-purpose oil on dry heels, as a pre-wash hair conditioner and put a few drops in the bath' • 'it has helped strengthen my nails and I like the oiliness: it "feeds" my skin'.

VIRIDIAN ULTIMATE BEAUTY ORGANIC NAIL & CUTICLE OIL
✳✳✳
SCORE: 8/10
Targeted specifically at cracking, peeling or splitting nails, this blends jojoba oil with silica-rich horsetail (renowned for strengthening bones, teeth, hair and nails). Viridian – who are best known as a supplement company but also create some terrific beauty oils – then add repairing calendula and the anti-fungal, antibacterial oils of rosemary, lavender and lemon myrtle, delivering a citrus-aromatic scent. It comes with a dropper top for twice-daily application to nails (both fingers and toes).
COMMENTS: 'This has transformed nail strength and broken my habit of picking at cuticles' • 'I noticed the difference from the first week of using this and now have much longer and stronger nails' • 'my nails have grown quicker; great little product and am replacing my

Avon cuticle conditioner with this!' • 'like the bottle with the handy pipette dispenser – very portable, easy to use and helped my nails a lot'.

DR.HAUSCHKA NEEM NAIL OIL
✳✳✳
SCORE: 7.44/10
Neem leaf – a traditional Ayurvedic herb that has anti-fungal, healing properties – is the cornerstone of this product which also employs peanut oil, apricot kernel oil and an essence from a semi-evergreen tree, *Melia azadirachta*, which has antiseptic and anti-inflammatory properties. Chamomile adds a light, herbal scent. The biodynamic brand Dr.Hauschka also offer this oil in an alternative pen-style tool (with special nibs for pushing back cuticles), but our testers were perfectly happy with their liquid-in-a bottle option.
COMMENTS: 'Within a month nails were not so prone to snapping and appeared less dry – a real discovery for me' • 'you only need a tiny dab, but nails are 100 per cent stronger. No more splitting of layers, breaking or tearing' • 'I can now use my nails for getting labels off without breakages – I love this product, and it's very long-lasting' • 'adored the smell – like plants, but not overpowering' • 'am so glad to have discovered this and wouldn't be without it; to my surprise and delight, nails are a better colour now' • 'a lovely, simple product that does what it says on the bottle'.

♥ **WE LOVE**

Jo always carries Biodynamic Nail and Cuticle Oil, a wand-style pen from AEOS which dispenses a blend of spelt, poppy and sunflower oils with rose quartz gem essences. Whenever there's downtime (on a bus, waiting for a meeting), she brushes the oil onto nails and massages into cuticles. Sarah is a long-term devotee of Liz Earle Superbalm (opposite), which should, in her view, be known as Superb-balm. (But nothing saves her nails if she forgets to wear gloves with her horses or when gardening.)

TIP: When you apply the nail treatment, try actually rubbing your nails together – it makes a slightly clacky sound but really invigorates the nails by stimulating blood flow.

THE NAIL FILES

Rich in strengthening minerals, botanical horsetail gives a natural boost to dry and brittle nails. Use these night-nurturers to bring them back from the brink

NAIL AND CUTICLE NOURISHING CREAM

Frankly, the more often you can remember to use this, the greater the benefits to nails. Keep it on the bedside table and massage into nails before you drift off: you'll have smoother and softer cuticles by morning, and over time, nail growth and health will be truly transformed.

- 50g (2oz) freshly picked horsetail, or 25g (1oz) dried horsetail
- 150ml (¼ pint) olive oil
- 1 tablespoon beeswax
- 10 drops vitamin E oil
- 5 drops benzoin resin
- 15 drops lavender essential oil (optional, for fragrance)

Pick the horsetail and lay it on a cloth to wilt overnight. (This is best picked in spring, when the horsetail is flowering – but any time will do; if you can't get fresh horsetail, the dried version is the next best thing.)

Heat the horsetail in the oil in a double boiler (see page 212) and simmer for 30 minutes.

Grate or chop the beeswax (if you aren't using granules). Strain the horsetail and return the oil to the double boiler; add the beeswax and stir until melted.

Remove from the heat, and immediately add the benzoin and the vitamin E oil. (It's best to use a dropper for this.) Stir and pour into small sterilised jars and while it's still liquid, drop in the essential oil and stir with a chopstick. Allow to cool thoroughly before sealing.

Use nightly before bedtime for strong, flexible, snap-resistant nails.

> TIP: To whiten nails, particularly if they've yellowed from wearing polish, mix 1 teaspoon of lemon juice into 1 tablespoon of orange flower water. Keep in a clean, sealable container and once a day soak a cotton wool pad in the mixture to swipe over nails. Moisturise hands and cuticles afterwards.

NAIL BOOSTER OIL

Horsetail is very rich in silica, which is a miraculous nail-strengthener, and it also contains minerals such as iron, magnesium and potassium. After a few weeks' use your nails should be strong and flexible – the ideal combination. (You don't want nails so hard that they snap – which is the effect most commercial nail hardeners have.)

- 20g (1oz) fresh horsetail stems, finely chopped
- 2 tablespoons sweet almond oil – or, better still, neem oil (we use Neal's Yard Remedies)

Place the horsetail in a double boiler (see page 212) and add the oil; heat gently. Allow to cool and pour the whole mixture into a screw-top jar; stand for a week in the sun, and then strain the oil.

Use this oil nightly, ideally on unvarnished nails, and massage into cuticles, to stimulate blood flow.

For a deep nail-strengthening treatment, gently warm this oil in a double boiler, then soak nails for 20 minutes weekly. You can reuse it time and again.

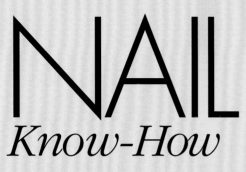

NAIL
Know-How

Whether you choose to have your nails short or long, *au naturel* or gorgeously polished (possibly with one of the 'free-from' polishes we review on page 134), it's vital to keep them looking in prime condition. So here's the lowdown from experts…

1 **Assemble your equipment.** A manicure should be a peaceful occupation and if you have to jump up every few minutes to get the next thing, you risk upsetting more than a bowl of water. So see our list, below.

2 **Remove any existing polish.** If you have weak nails, however, do this step after filing and shaping as the polish acts as a kind of glue to stop nails splitting while you file.

3 **File and shape.** Never use a metal nail file or a rough emery board, or you risk splitting and peeling. Don't saw to and fro; file in one direction from side to side or towards the centre. And please don't file the side walls of your nails or you weaken them. Shape nails into squovals – squares with gently rounded corners and a gentle curve.

4 **Soak and soften.** Soaking them in warm organic full-fat milk (if you have it, water if you don't) helps dissolve dead cells and softens cuticles, plus the natural fats are good for dry skin.

5 **Scrub grubby hands and nails.** We love using face or body scrubs on our paws to get them clean as a whistle, and soft (because you gently remove the top dead layer of skin as you scrub). Remove dug-in dirt by rubbing with a cut lemon. Apply cuticle remover.

6 **Push back cuticles.** Wrap a wisp of cotton wool round an angle-tipped orange stick and gently push the cuticles towards the nail base. We like this suggestion for a default cuticle pusher: wrap the rubber end of a pencil eraser in a tissue… NB: Never snip cuticles – just don't.

7 **Buff nails until they gleam.** Use a smooth, soft nail buffer (such as a chamois leather), never anything that abrades nails if they are weak. Do it gently and swiftly, and don't let heat build up: you want to smooth and strengthen the surface, not damage it.

8 **Moisturise and massage.** Our favourite bit, even if we do it ourselves – and we just drool if someone else gives us a really good hand massage because we all store so much tension in our hands. Rub in warm oil (almond, avocado, jojoba or light olive do nicely), all over your hands, particularly your nails to stimulate growth. Then layer over your favourite hand cream (see page 138 for our Award Winners). That's it for 'au naturel' but read on if you are going for the polished look.

9 **Wipe nails clean and apply a base coat.** Do make sure there's no oil or hand cream lingering and dry well before you apply a nourishing protective base coat, which will also stop polish discolouring the nail. Make sure you 'cap' your nail tips with the base coat and each succeeding layer of polish to help prevent chipping.

10 **Shake polish and apply.** Yvette Snowden, creator of Eve Snow (whose polishes are free of five chemical nasties), advises loading the brush carefully – you don't want blobs of polish everywhere. Aim for two thin coats. Now brush on with three strokes: a stroke down the centre of each nail first, then a stroke either side. Do one hand at a time, starting with the thumb. Keep hands flat, still and relaxed as you paint. Let the polish dry for a few minutes, then repeat for the second coat.

11 **Apply a top coat.** This gives a high-gloss finish and protects your colour. To make it last longer re-apply your top coat every few days, says Yvette. (The 'less toxic' ranges on page 134 also generally offer top coats, so choose one of these.)

12 **Drizzle a little drop of oil (any sort) on each nail.** This stops freshly polished nails sticking if you brush against or hit something. Now sit peacefully for as long as you can to let your polish dry perfectly hard.

> TIP:
> When we're sitting at our keyboards fretting and getting tense, we shake our hands vigorously – side to side, up and down – and abracadabra! The tension dissipates…

Nail tools

- Nail polish remover
- Crystal glass file or fine emery board
- Basin of warm organic full-fat milk
- Scrub (face or body, or mix your own with roughly equal amounts of organic brown sugar, olive oil and honey)
- Orange stick for nails with angled tip
- Cotton wool
- Cuticle oil/cream
- Soft nail buffer
- Hand oil
- Hand cream
- Base coat
- Polish
- Top coat

NAIL POLISHES
our award winners

The only truly 'natural' nail, of course, is one that's simply buffed and oiled. But many of us love polish for both the glam factor and also for nail protection. Happily, the manicure industry has made great strides on the subject of '3 Free', reformulating varnishes without the triple toxic 'nasties' of formaldehyde, toluene and phthalate (sometimes listed as DBP for di-n-butyl phthalate). There's even 4 Free now, which excludes formaldehyde resin, a possible allergen, and 5 Free, which doesn't contain camphor, said to be a potential skin irritant. For the first time, we trialled 3-Free polishes – plus some that go even further on the natural front – and discovered that you don't need to compromise on performance, durability or shades. (We trialled nail polish removers, too, but only one made the grade – find it in the box at the end.)

ORGANIC GLAM NAIL POLISH
❋
SCORE: 8.29/10

This range – from The Organic Pharmacy's as-glam-as-it-sounds make-up line – offers a boredom-defying spectrum of 36 shades with a high-gloss, professional-style finish and a fast-drying formula to boot. Our panellists tested the pretty ballerina-ish French Manicure Pink, one of those eternally classic nail shades. *COMMENTS:* 'I wash up a lot, garden and run round after three children so any nail polish that lasts more than a day is good in my eyes – I found this lasted four days before it started to chip (and I didn't apply a topcoat)' • 'I am an early years teacher so my hands get a lot of stick throughout the day but I found, impressively, that this still looked good after several days – shiny and glossy' • 'I had several comments from friends and colleagues about how nice my nails looked when wearing this polish' • 'it went on very smoothly; I initially only applied one coat which gave nails a slightly opaque, healthy looking sheen' • 'lasted exceptionally well, gave a fantastic "polished" look'.

AT A GLANCE
NAIL POLISHES

ORGANIC GLAM
NAIL POLISH

LIZ EARLE
STRENGTHENING
NAIL COLOUR

OPI
NAIL POLISH

KURE BAZAAR
NAIL POLISH

**NAIL POLISH
REMOVERS**

FRESH THERAPIES EDEN
NAIL POLISH REMOVER

LIZ EARLE STRENGTHENING NAIL COLOUR
❋
SCORE: 8.21/10

A new addition to the Liz Earle make-up line, this polish is designed – as the name implies – to strengthen nails with the addition of ingredients such as borage and avocado oils to the formulation. There are 12 wearable shades, each named after a rose; Pure Poetry – a rich burgundy – graced our testers' nails. *COMMENTS:* 'The brush gave good coverage and the bottle was easy to hold while I was painting my nails' • 'still wearing well with no chips two weeks later' • 'I have ridges in my nails and usually apply a ridge-filler first; I didn't with this polish and was really surprised at how well it disguised the ridges – much better than my usual polish' • 'I tested it with no base coat, only one layer of polish and no topcoat and the result was brilliant – a great product and definitely a time-saver' • 'very impressive – I've never kept a varnish on for six days without a base and topcoat – and even more amazing, it didn't stain nails'.

OPI NAIL POLISH

✳

SCORE: 8.14/10

OPI is almost a household name nail-wise, and we were delighted when they went 3 Free some years ago, committing to 'safe, effective and innovative products that promise beautiful results'. There's a staggering offering of 240 fashion-forward shades to choose from (many of them with names that invariably put a smile on our lips, such as Didgeridoo Your Nails). Slightly frustratingly, the shade our testers were sent turned out to be limited edition – but since our questions here focus on performance and durability, rather than colour, it didn't signify.

COMMENTS: 'By far the best nail varnish I've ever used; very good-shaped brush makes it easy to apply and one coat lasted nearly a week without chipping' • 'not an overwhelming smell; other brands linger for ages (and sometimes even give me a headache)' • 'a good-quality brush which has smooth bristles and no stragglers' • 'smooth application – seems to self-level' • 'you'd get a lot of manicures out of this generous-size bottle'.

KURE BAZAAR NAIL POLISH

✳✳

SCORE: 8.06/10

Kure Bazaar goes one stage further than other polishes we trialled, being 4 Free – and more than that, it's actually 85 per cent made of natural origin, based on wood pulp, potatoes, cotton and corn. (That's why we decided to bring in a one-and-a-half daisy rating, just for Kure Bazaar!) It's impossible to equate those ingredients with the smooth, glossy, quick-dry, chip-resistant polish you get in the bottle – but it's true. As they say, it couldn't be simpler 'to detox your nails'. Seasonal collections are released but our *Beauty Bible* testers painted on Rouge Flore, a classic pillar-box red.

COMMENTS: 'Loved this product which went on really easily; I've bought very expensive designer polishes (Chanel, Dior) previously, and they're not a patch on this' • 'transformed me from a boring fortysomething into a glamorous siren in no more than 10 minutes!' • 'this gave even coverage and a great shine' • 'I loved the fact this is non-toxic and will try other shades'.

TIP: Even with 3 Free or natural nail polishes, we recommend painting nails in a room with an open window or a through draught: this is because some products still smell of chemicals, even if the 'health hazardous' ingredients have been eliminated.

AND NOW FOR... NATURAL NAIL POLISH REMOVERS

To be honest, only one of the handful out there 'wowed' our panellists but this really did score a very high mark, considering the tough beauty challenge of removing nail polish... If you loathe that powerful, acetone scent, it's well worth switching to this remover, according to our testers.

FRESH THERAPIES EDEN NAIL POLISH REMOVER

✳✳

SCORE: 8.69/10

This high-scoring natural polish remover is a clear, lime-scented formula from a successful Hampshire nail salon owner. Nicola Dickinson set about creating a product using biodegradable food-and-plant-based ingredients. As a result, it's safe for pregnant women, children and anyone undergoing treatment for illnesses. It's also nail and cuticle nourishing: we're not surprised this has won a raft of other awards.

COMMENTS: 'I didn't believe a natural varnish remover would work – yet this was really effective and pleasant to use' • 'leaves nails feeling moisturised' • 'I used this on thick polish – yet it all came off easily' • 'removed black, sparkly polish with great ease' • 'a faint citrussy aroma – no chemical smell: a revelation!' • 'conditioning and nourishing; not like paint stripper' • 'I'll use this as a nail treatment as it smells and looks incredible'.

WE LOVE

Jo is a convert of Kure Bazaar's long-lasting, high-gloss polishes. And she's blown away by Crabtree & Evelyn Nail Polish Remover Wipes, which replace damaging solvents with a soy-based formula, yet are highly effective. Sarah is a recent fan of Eve Snow's gorgeous colours: her fave is taupe Film Noir.

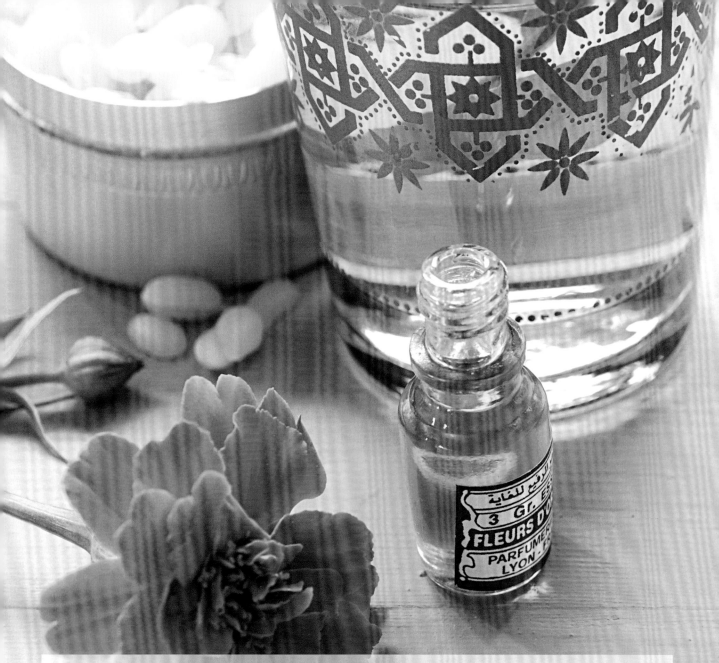

PEPPERMINT FOOT BALM

Use this balm at night for a skin-softening foot massage (see page 143); it's also incredible for smoothing rough skin on heels, ensuring feet are worthy of even the most elegant Manolo mules. In Chinese traditional medicine, it's believed that toxins and germs are excreted through the feet and that it's important to sluice them away before going to bed. So foot washing and nourishing is encouraged as a nightly ritual.

- The petals from 24 calendula flowers; or 10g dried marigold flowers
- 1 tablespoon avocado oil
- 90ml (3fl oz) sweet almond oil
- 20g (¾oz) beeswax
- 40 drops peppermint essential oil

Put the calendula flowers in the bottom of a bottle and pour the oils over the top. Place in direct sunlight to speed up the infusion of the calendula into the oils. After three weeks, strain through a sieve – mashing the calendula to squeeze out the last of the goodness. Then heat the oil and beeswax in a double boiler (see page 212); when the wax has melted, remove from the heat and allow to cool slightly before adding the peppermint essential oil and decanting into a sterilised jar.

EXTREME MEASURES

We often neglect the skin on our hands and feet but these hard-working extremities need as much TLC as the rest of the body. Keep them soft and healthy with soothing balms

MARSH MALLOW HAND SOOTHER

This makes a fabulous barrier cream for housework or gardening – it replenishes natural moisture and velvetiness, whenever hands are dry and rough.

- 200ml (7fl oz) still mineral water
- 10g (½oz) marsh mallow leaves (fresh or dried)
- 10 drops orange essential oil
- 10 drops lemon essential oil
- 50ml (1¾fl oz) sweet almond oil
- 10g (½oz) cocoa butter
- 10g (½oz) beeswax
- 4 drops grapefruit seed extract

In a stainless-steel pan, bring the water and marsh mallow leaves to a boil, then simmer for about 10 minutes. Allow to cool slightly. When the mixture is lukewarm, strain and return 40ml (1½fl oz) of the liquid back into the saucepan.

In a double boiler (see page 212), melt the oils, cocoa butter and beeswax. Reheat the marsh mallow liquid until it's almost boiling and add it to the beeswax mixture a little at a time. (The liquid has to be hot, otherwise the oils will set.)

Mix with a hand blender to create a creamy emulsion. Lastly, add the drops of grapefruit seed extract.

Divide into dry, sterilised jars; keep in the fridge to maintain freshness, but the jar that's in use won't need refrigerating.

HAND CREAMS
our award winners

How to make team *Beauty Bible* happy? Give us a gorgeous hand cream. And we've found that most women feel the same way – hand treats always make popular presents and tend to notch up impressive scores in our trials. So: a big hand please, for the winners from over 50 natural smoothers and soothers tested by our panels. The top-scoring products below include fragranced offerings (rose is always popular with *BB* testers) and one targeted at problem skins. Now there's no excuse for dry paws… and they'll help nails and cuticles, too

TISSERAND SIGNATURE BLEND INTENSIVE HAND & NAIL CREAM
✳

SCORE: 9/10

It always gives us a kick when the highest scorer in a category is also a beauty 'steal', but that's the case here: a blend of 14 essential oils (including orange blossom, rose, bergamot, geranium, sandalwood and lashings of lavender) infuse this rich-but-not-greasy flip-top tube of cream which is based on vitamin-rich kukui nut oil and skin-conditioning jojoba oil as well as shea butter, plus extract of chamomile to calm redness or chapping.

COMMENTS: 'This is better than my other hand creams: it leaves hands looking plumped and evens out skin tone with a nice, dewy sheen – radiant!' • 'not sticky at all and absorbed within seconds' • 'could smell a little lavender – a pleasant herby scent; great as a soothing night hand cream' • 'nails are nourished and less brittle' • 'loved the fragrance and found that at stressful times at work I could use it on my hands, cup them over my nose and take a few deep breaths to feel instantly calmer' • 'would highly recommend to everyone – another got-to-have product that I've discovered through *Beauty Bible*'.

JURLIQUE ROSE HAND CREAM
✳ ✳

SCORE: 8.94/10

We've a bit of history with this rose-fragranced hand treat from the Australian biodynamic skincare brand: it appeared in our first book and subsequently in others – each time trialled by a new set of testers. And it has happened again: our *Ultimate Natural Beauty Bible* panellists were similarly wowed by this rich, protective cream which infuses sweet almond, macadamia, safflower seed oils, skin-restoring carrot root extract, plus aloe vera and vitamin E.

COMMENTS: 'The "old lady" skin on my hands definitely feels more supple and looks less papery' • 'immediately transformed my reptilian hands into baby-soft ones; I've put this on my list for Santa this year' • 'have used this on my face under my eyes when skin has felt particularly dry – a really good face cream, too!' • 'feels hydrating but isn't at all greasy, smells divine and does what you need it to: skin looks so much clearer, brighter after use – am already planning on buying this as gifts for friends' • 'has lasting effects – moisturises hands like no other cream I've used' • 'like the fact that as you get near the end, the metal tube can be folded down, so every last bit can be used'.

BAREFOOT SOS BARRIER HAND CREAM

❋❋

SCORE: 8.86/10

The 'SOS' in the name refers to the fact that this range (originally formulated by a homeopath) is targeted at problematic skins – including those with psoriasis, dermatitis and eczema, as well as sensitive types. It is indeed more of a 'barrier' cream than others we trialled, shielding skin and preventing moisture loss with a blend of shea butter, macadamia, sunflower and jojoba oils, chickweed and mallow extracts, plus soothing lavender and frankincense.

COMMENTS: 'Worked miracles on my dry nurse's hands! Gorgeous fragrance, hands more moisturised, cuticles less ragged' • 'a pleasure to use: healed my dry, cracked hands (I have eczema) – if I could give a higher score than 10 I would' • 'smoothed in easily, no dragging' • 'skin looked softer, fresher, younger and felt comfortable for hours after use' • 'I would recommend to anyone looking for a natural hand cream that really works' • 'it's a real delight to smooth in'.

MV ORGANIC SKINCARE HAND RESCUE

❋❋

SCORE: 8.83/10

This hails from a little Aussie brand (one of Sarah's favourites), founded by Sydney-based beauty therapist Sharon McGlinchey, which has a couple of award winners in this book. This hand cream has a richer formula than most, and if slathered on thickly can work as an overnight hand treatment (ditto for feet, MV suggest). Active skin nourishers include rosehip (good for premature ageing, itchiness and sun damage), anti-inflammatory calendula oil, and benzoin resin, used for centuries to treat wounds, cracked skin and irritation. Tangerine and sandalwood oils give it a fresh fragrance.

COMMENTS: 'This is not just a hand cream: it's a "one-stop shop" for moisturising hands, nails, skin and it smells gorgeous and edible – love it!' • 'this has a fresh and citrussy scent, like walking through a field after it's rained' • 'I am not a hand-cream person but this has converted me and I will re-buy' • 'hands were cracked and peeling after a bout of flu; now they're

super soft' • 'I loved the orange, vanilla scent of this hand cream – it's the nicest I've ever used'.

EVOLVE PURE MOISTURE HAND LOTION

❋❋

SCORE: 8.8/10

Oh-so-fashionable antioxidant goji berry features as an ingredient in this British brand's pump-action hand cream. (NB: all other award winners come in tubes or jars.) Founder Laura Rudoe, formerly at NUDE skincare, set about creating affordable organic beauty options – including this, which delivers organic aloe vera and shea butter in a lightweight lotion scented with the Japanese yusu plant, a member of the citrus family.

COMMENTS: 'Very effective without leaving my hands feeling too greasy – would definitely buy' • 'I gave my dear mum, who's 92, some to try and she loved it and asked if I could get more for her' • 'loved the spa-like smell' • 'perfect light cream rubbed in beautifully smoothly and quickly' • 'used it after washing-up and gardening and instantly my dry, cracked hands were a lot smoother and nourished' • 'I can't believe the improvement in my skin condition, specifically an eczema patch – there's definitely a magic ingredient in this'.

CIRCAROMA REPLENISHING HAND CREAM

❋❋

SCORE: 8.61/10

We've history with this product, too – another previous winner, reassigned to a new team of testers, who fell yet again for its rose-drenched charms. Rose attar and rose water both feature, blended with essential oils of rose geranium and patchouli in a super-softening base of sunflower, almond, coconut and cocoa butter.

COMMENTS: 'I had always thought of hand creams as a boring necessity but this is a lovely product – skin looked smoother and results lasted all day even after much hand-washing' • 'this has been a bit of a miracle as my hands look smoother and actually younger' • 'lovely, subtle scent of roses that really lasted, but not in an overpowering way' • 'amazing product: a little goes a long way and without a doubt the best hand cream I've ever used'.

WE LOVE

Jo and Sarah are both addicted to slathering on Emma Hardie Amazing Face Hand and Nail Treatment Cream: rich, silky and packed with shea butter. Jo also loves Aesop Resurrection Aromatique Hand Balm, intensely scented with vetiver – one of Jo's all-time favourite essential oils. Sarah welcomes offerings from two other Australian brands, MV Organic Skincare Hand Rescue (left) and Lanolips Rose Balm Intense For Very Dry Hands and Nails. Lastly, we can't forget Liz Earle's Hand Repair, it's a classic.

FOOT TREATS
our award winners

Foot treats are very high on our list of priorities: buffers, scrubs, luscious creams and rich balms for nightly TLC. Our testers clearly love them, too: the words 'soft', 'smooth', 'refreshing' kept coming up in the Comments for these natural foot delights. And since the skin on our feet is highly absorbent (according to traditional Chinese medicine), we love slathering on natural nourishers. The winners here put a spring in our testers' steps, scoring really high marks from the 30 or so products we dispatched to our 10-woman panels

LIZ EARLE FOOT SCRUB
✳

SCORE: 8.89/10

It is pointless massaging even the richest, most luscious cream into feet if you haven't buffed away hard skin first. And that's what this winning scrub does, deploying natural pumice for its exfoliating action. However, the product is also infused with moisturising elements – avocado and wheat germ oils – so it nourishes as it scuffs. Real double-duty beauty! As with just about everything Liz Earle produces, it smells great with an invigorating fragrance of peppermint and rosemary essential oils. (If you're using this in the bath, as opposed to the shower, we suggest applying it last thing before emerging from the tub, otherwise you'll find yourself sitting in a pile of grit!)

COMMENTS: 'This had an instant cooling effect and the pumice filed away rough edges; my feet felt softer and smoother – great!' • 'I adored the clean peppermint smell' • 'my feet felt lovely and buffed' • 'this refreshed, smoothed and moisturised my feet – I was impressed with its effectiveness' • 'the thick, creamy paste left feet feeling soft and revived' • 'what an amazing smell; soreness and tenderness were completely gone after using this scrub, which made my feet feel as soft as a newborn baby's' • 'the skin on my feet felt really great after using this: fresh, and a little bit tingly, while the rough patches on the soles were left much smoother'.

AT A GLANCE

LIZ EARLE FOOT SCRUB

DR.ORGANIC
VIRGIN OLIVE OIL
FOOT & HEEL CREAM

MELVITA
EXTRA-SOFT
FOOT CREAM

SUTI FABULOUS
ORGANIC FOOT BALM

L'OCCITANE
SHEA BUTTER
FOOT CREAM

DR.ORGANIC VIRGIN OLIVE OIL FOOT & HEEL CREAM
✳ ✳

SCORE: 8.89/10

This actually tied with the Liz Earle scrub at the top of the leader board: it's a very affordable non-greasy option packed with emollients including aloe vera, organic olive oil and olive leaf, plus cassis and vitamins A, C and E. Dr.Organic promise it will soften and reduce calluses and dry, cracked areas of skin, while deodorising, too. The scent is pretty light (well, pretty and light actually), aromatic to our nostrils, with just a touch of lemon and thyme.

COMMENTS: 'I have diabetes, poor circulation and a skin condition – I was given a drug a few years ago which caused the skin on my feet to blister and then fall off; the regrowth had never been the same but this has made such a difference in the past few weeks – far and away above my expectations' • 'I have plantar fasciitis [pain and inflammation under the heels] and all I can say is I felt relief as soon as I applied this: the only way my feet could have felt better is if David Beckham was actually rubbing in the cream for me!' • 'a lovely refreshing smell – in fact, so nice I use this as a hand cream as well' • 'can't believe how inexpensive it is – please, please recommend it?' • 'the beautician who looks after my feet commented on how much better the condition of the skin is now' • 'left my feet refreshed, soothed and deodorised'.

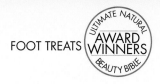

MELVITA EXTRA-SOFT FOOT CREAM
❋ ❋ ❋
SCORE: 8.25/10

Personally, we quite like a medicinal-smelling foot product (it feels like part of good hygiene, to us) – and this ticks that box as it is strongly scented with rosemary, lavender and mint extracts, chosen for their cooling, soothing action. Its nourishing qualities come from macadamia oil and nigella seed (black cumin) oil which also has antibacterial properties. This comes in a generous flip-top tube – a little too weighty for a handbag and on-the-go slathering, we'd say, but brilliant for the bedside.

COMMENTS: 'This is a must for anyone who suffers from tired, aching feet: blown away by the instant cooling action' • 'it reduced swelling and tenderness, although not all the soreness' • 'liked this for ease of application, rubbed in really well and wasn't too greasy; I also liked the refreshing smell' • 'my feet are looking the best they've ever done, especially my heels' • 'it was cooling and revived my weary feet' • 'a pleasant scent of mint and rosemary' • 'I work in retail and spend all day on my feet; this didn't remove soreness completely but eased it – as if my feet were given a gentle hug!'

SUTI FABULOUS ORGANIC FOOT BALM
❋ ❋ ❋
SCORE: 8.16/10

You'll find this glass jar of balm on Jo's bedside table: she ritually smooths it into feet before bed, after washing them. (Her Chinese herbalist gave her this advice years ago to help ward off colds and flu, and it really seems to work.) Suti is a small, British, mostly Soil Association certified organic brand, and its foot cream is a simple but effective formulation of shea butter, olive, avocado, pumpkin seed oils and beeswax, with

WE LOVE

Sarah, like Jo, uses the award-winning Suti Fabulous Organic Foot Balm featured here. But one thing we would ask is please use any product daily: it really helps prevent dry skin forming on your feet. Jo also recommends the extraordinarily effective Micro Pedi, a foot-sanding gizmo that has dramatically extended the time between her Margaret Dabbs Medical Pedicures, because of its effectiveness at (gently) blasting away dry skin. Sarah recommends it too, as well as a good old-fashioned foot buffer from any high-street chemist.

essential oils of eucalyptus, peppermint and lemon to stimulate circulation in weary feet. It's very rich and probably not suitable for daytime use (except very sparingly), but Jo recommends it for rich slathering on before sleep.

COMMENTS: 'I've quite dry skin on my feet but have never used a product which moisturises so deeply; the hard areas on the soles of my feet are in much better condition – amazing' • 'a real joy to use; it's a long time since my feet have looked this good' • 'a lovely pepperminty, rosemary fragrance – very refreshing' • 'a real treat for tired feet at the end of the day' • 'luxurious, and kept feet smelling fresh'.

L'OCCITANE SHEA BUTTER FOOT CREAM
❋
SCORE: 8.13/10

L'Occitane's shea-butter-rich products have performed well in categories across the whole book. Here you will find their foot cream, which comes in an aluminium (toothpaste-style) tube and features a 15 per cent concentration of their signature shea butter, with lavender and arnica extract chosen for their anti-inflammatory properties. They say it can be applied to tired feet and ankles over tights – but only the sheerest, we'd say, and with a very light touch.

COMMENTS: 'This is a joy to use: my feet felt lovely and warm after use' • 'the skin on my heels is much smoother after an overnight application' • 'this eased swollen feet after a day standing and walking' • 'feet felt just great straight after I put on this cream, and stay much softer after a few days' use' • 'it reduced soreness and refreshed feet after being on them all day' • 'I loved the fresh herbal smell – like walking through a Mediterranean garden'.

FOOTLOOSE AND FANCY FEET

We have learnt the importance of giving our feet lots (and lots) of TLC to keep them looking and feeling good. And we urge you to do the same. They work very hard for you, so keep them happy – and you will be too

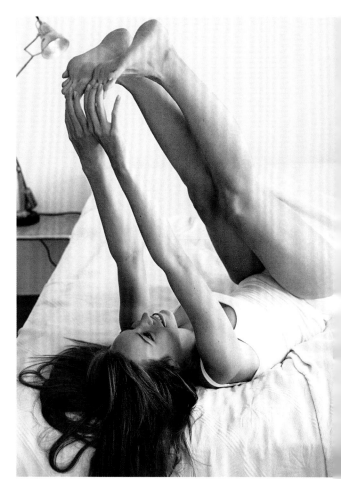

Most of us are (literally) on our feet a good part of the day and with every step we take, our feet have to absorb the stress of up to twice our body weight. About 75 per cent of people have some kind of foot problem during their lives. And if your feet are hurting, your back may well be too – and vice versa. (Not to mention the way it shows in your face…)

Investing in your feet is so worthwhile. Spend a little time, a little money, keeping them in good shape, and they will happily carry you around, looking and feeling great. Neglect them and not only will they look unattractive but you're storing up problems in the short and long term.

Maintaining your feet isn't rocket science and doesn't take much time – unless you're starting from seriously untended, when you will need to invest a bit more at the beginning.

The key is daily care – and some professional help.
● **For unloved feet,** please see a qualified podiatrist and get them checked over. Do this every two to three months ideally (and definitely if you have problems such as corns or calluses) but at least twice yearly. ● **Keep them hydrated:** the biggest problem is dry feet, according to podiatrists. Moisturise daily with an intensive product after bathing, massaging it in firmly (see panel right). ● **For thickened or callused feet,** you need more than a balm (which only improves the surface); use an intensive foot oil, such as Dr. Organic Virgin Olive Oil Foot & Heel Cream. ● **Exfoliate at least twice a week;** apply to dry feet before your bath or shower. (We tend to use our body scrubs but you can find targeted foot scrubs such as Liz Earle's on the previous page.) ● **Use a foot buffer on dry feet once or twice a week,** not more as that can result in a build-up of dry skin. (Sarah uses a standard foot file but Jo loves her MICRO-Pedi, see page 141.) ● Always keep toenails cut straight across. Use a buffing block to remove staining, then polish if you wish. ● **Apply cuticle oil to toenails** as well as fingers to keep them soft. ● **Treat your feet to a pair of FitFlops.** We love them and so do experts. They help your posture as well as supporting your feet and legs. And they now come in a range of styles and colours.

A HEAVENLY FOOT MASSAGE

● First make sure your feet are warm: soak them for 5–15 minutes in a footbath of warm (not too hot) water. Add a handful of Epsom salts – or bath salts – to soothe feet. (Or do this massage after soaking in your night-time bath.)

● Dry your feet thoroughly – especially between the toes – with an absorbent towel.

● Sit in a comfy chair with one leg crossed over the top of the other and the sole of that foot facing you.

● Apply your favourite product (see our Award Winners on page 140).

● Your thumbs are your massage tools. Move them over the bottom of the raised foot in a circular movement, kneading as hard as you can with comfort. Concentrate on one small area at a time, and gradually work back from the tips of your toes towards your heel.

● As you rub, pay extra attention to any area that feels 'crystallised' or knotty. Reflexologists say the instep reflects your state of stress, so if you are having an anxious time, massage that until it feels soft and supple. Warning: it may be sore to start with.

● Turn your foot right-side up so you can work on the top. Work with your thumbs in the same way as before, but more gently as this bit can be sensitive.

● Then pull on each toe and wiggle them from side to side between your thumb and forefinger.

● Now massage your ankles and calves, again using your thumbs but in bigger circles.

● Switch feet and repeat the whole massage. Spend as much time as you can – ideally 10–15 minutes, but even a couple makes a big difference we find, especially at the end of a long day or if you have been gallivanting around in high heels!

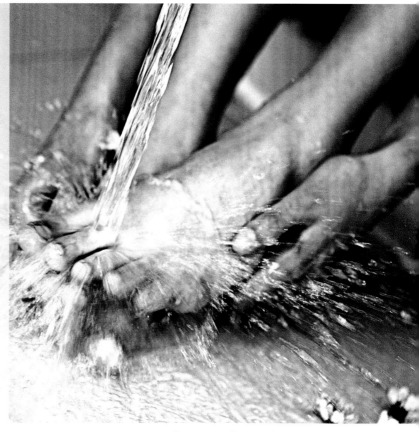

KICK UP YOUR (HIGH) HEELS

We all know high heels are really, really bad for our feet – and toes and calves and back – but parties bring out the Louboutin-lovers in all of us. We stand by these tips for minimising the pain and suffering, given to us by podiatrist Dr Charlotte Hawkins, who loves heels herself.

● First, stand up straight. High heels shorten the calf muscles, tipping the body forward (so your bottom tends to stick out…) and putting pressure on the back and neck. Standing tall, with chest and top of head floating upwards, shoulder blades down, compensates for this.

● Cushioned gel inserts may help, but the downside in pointy-toe shoes is even less room for toes, which may make things worse, so try out inserts around the house first. (We think wearing new high heels around the house first is a good idea anyway.)

● If you are wearing high-heeled boots, support your feet and legs with in-flight socks to reduce swelling and fatigue.

● Wear low heels to and from the event or get a lift both ways and try not to stand all night. At the end of the evening, massage feet and calves, and if you can, lie down with your feet up a wall for a few minutes.

● Put a thick book or catalogue under the mattress at the foot of the bed to help swollen feet and ankles.

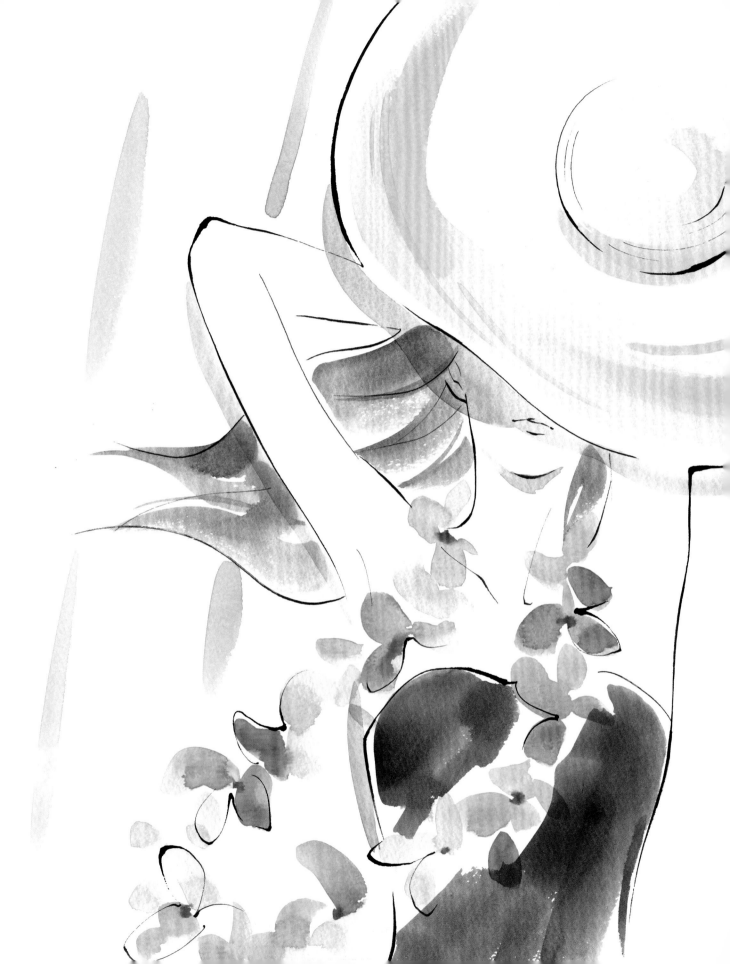

Just let the
SUN SHINE

Contrary to popular thinking, the sun isn't the enemy. Treated with respect, it's a health-giving life force. Here's how to bloom – not burn – beneath those rays

GOLDEN RULES

A sea change has taken place recently on the hot topic of exposing your skin to the sun. Official medical advice now is that you should abandon yourself regularly to UV light – but not for long. Here we decode the safety enigma

A little bit of history: for centuries, the vogue for lily-white skin held sway. Lauded as a thing of beauty in itself, pallor also implied refinement because nut-brown maidens obtained their ruddy glow from working in the fields. Until the start of the 20th century, genteel ladies covered up from head to toe. The effect was often accentuated with lead-based cosmetics – or arsenic after it was discovered that lead was toxic.

Then, in the early 20th century, doctors discovered the therapeutic effects of sunlight. By 1913 sunbathing was a desirable activity, confirmed a decade later by fashion designer Coco Chanel sporting a suntan (apparently she got sunburnt accidentally on the French Riviera).

Deep copper tans from holidays frazzling on Mediterranean beaches became de rigueur but then, in the late 1970s, the hole in the ozone layer was discovered, and with it came the increased risk of skin cancer. Since then, the sunscreen market has grown hugely, fake tans are a staple on many women's shelves – and, to cancer experts' fury, sunbeds have become a billion-dollar business.

Then, most recently, the issue of vitamin D deficiency hit the headlines and things became topsy-turvy. Used to being told we should slather ourselves in a high SPF and stay out of the midday sun, a consensus of medical experts warned that unless we got enough sunlight on our skin – the most important and efficient method of absorbing vitamin D – our bones would suffer. Rickets, which had disappeared in the UK, was diagnosed again in children, osteomalacia (bone pain) and osteoporosis (brittle bones) in adults.

Furthermore, experts claim there is accumulating evidence that vitamin D deficiency is linked to an increased risk of many chronic diseases. According to health campaigner Oliver Gillie (www.healthresearchforum.org.uk), these include 16 types of cancer, multiple sclerosis, diabetes and schizophrenia. It's a contributory cause of heart disease, raised blood pressure, inflammatory bowel diseases, polycystic ovary syndrome, period problems, infertility, infections, dental decay and depression.

For more northern lands (as opposed to sunny climes), the problem is worse in the dark winter months, with up to 69 per cent of the population in Scotland at risk of low levels of vitamin D. But although levels should naturally be higher in summer, a large proportion of the UK population is still deficient – mainly because we have heeded medical advice and slopped on the sun preps from head to toe.

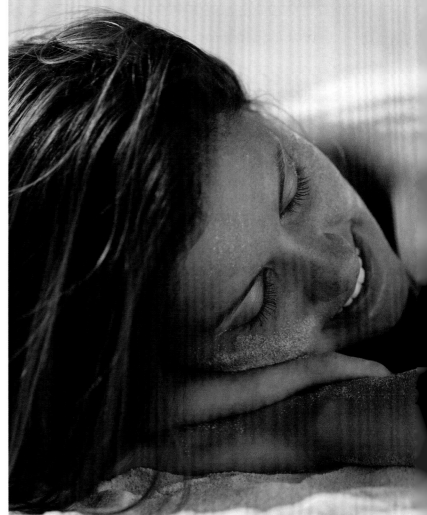

SO WHAT TO DO?

A little sun does you good. A consensus statement from Cancer Research UK and six other key bodies including the British Association of Dermatologists now advises 'regularly going outside for a matter of minutes around the middle of the day without sunscreen', as the time it takes to make enough vitamin D is less than it takes for skin to burn.

Exactly how long for is a moot point. It varies with 'a number of environmental, physical and personal factors', says the statement. However, it adds that 'when it comes to sun exposure, little and often is best, and the more skin that is exposed, the greater the chance of making sufficient vitamin D before burning. People should get to know their own skin to understand how long they can spend outside before risking sunburn under different conditions.'

Oliver Gillie is more prescriptive. From May to August, he recommends that 'a white-skinned person in the UK needs at least 20 minutes three times a week of sunbathing in bright midday sunlight with few clothes'; they can spend even longer in the midday sun before May and after August, and before midday and after 3pm during high summer.

Sunbeds are not a safe alternative. Apart from the horrific burns that have resulted from using them for too long, Cancer Research UK warns that people using a sunbed once a month or more can increase their skin cancer risk by more than half.

Certain groups have a higher risk of vitamin D deficiency. People with darker skin need longer UV exposure to produce the same amount of vitamin D. Older people make it less easily, and obese people have lower levels. Other vulnerable people are those who wear whole body coverings, pregnant women, skin cancer patients and children.

The British government recommends vitamin D3 supplementation for those at risk. As well as eating vitamin D-rich food (oily fish, eggs, butter and cheese and some fortified foods), the Department of Health advises a 10 microgram (400 international units) supplement for adults at risk, with seven mcg (280iu) for all children aged from six months to five years.

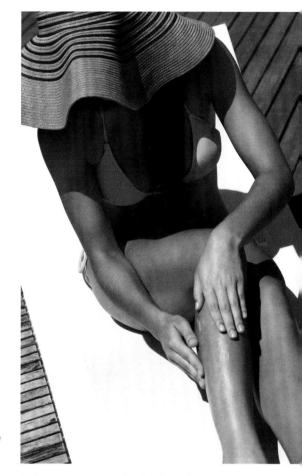

Other experts advise higher doses. Oliver Gillie and others believe we should all take a supplement, particularly in the winter. Amounts are discussed in detail by the Vitamin D Council (www.vitamindcouncil.org). If you suspect your levels are low, ask your doctor to measure them – it's a simple, cheap test and most doctors now will agree. If you are below optimal levels, discuss supplementation.

But remember, the human skin is not designed to fry. Apart from skin cancer, the other concern is skin ageing: the sun is the most supremely efficient ageing agent causing lines, wrinkles, sagging, brown spots and croc-type skin. (Jo never puts her fair complexion in the sun if she can avoid it.) So: do use sun preps (SPF20–30), top up every two hours if you are in the sun, and stay in the shade from 11am to 3pm (10am to 4pm in very hot countries) – except for your few minutes of sun exposure. Wear big-brimmed hats and wraparound Jackie O sunglasses. And keep hydrated to avoid heat stroke.

THE SELF-TAN COMMANDMENTS

A gorgeous honey glow can transform your face and body (camouflaging cellulite a treat) and give your whole psyche a lift. But even the best self-tanner can't work miracles on dry, rough or (let's be honest) hairy skin, so do follow these really simple instructions for a perfect golden patina

1 **Plan ahead.** If you need a pedicure or manicure, to de-fuzz anywhere, or touch up your hair colour, do it before you plan to apply the self-tanner. They can all remove the product.

2 **Scrub up.** Self-tanner builds up on dry skin leaving darker patches, so do exfoliate thoroughly from top to toe, particularly creased places such as elbows, knees, ankles and heels. On your face use a gentle exfoliator and, if possible, a skin brush such as Clarisonic to whisk away surface debris. Avoid oil-based products which can leave a streak-causing slick. Afterwards, rinse off the scrub and dry thoroughly so that not a drop of water is left on your skin. See our award-winning face scrubs (page 66) and body scrubs (page 106).

3 **Moisturise your skin.** In an ideal world, you would scrub and moisturise your body for three days ahead of applying self-tanner. One day ahead may have to suffice in our time-pressed lives. So, after exfoliating and drying as above, apply a light lotion and let it sink in thoroughly. Pay particular attention to nostrils and other crease-y places as above.

4 **Get your gloves on.** We swear by those sponge mittens. Self-tanner goes on more evenly and our hands don't end up orange.

5 **Start at the feet and work up.** Apply about a teaspoonful of self-tanner at a time, rubbing into the skin with circular movements.

(If you are using a liquid product, remember to squeeze it on to your hands over the bath or sink to avoid staining the floor or towels, etc.)

6 **Leave your face till last.** Apply the self-tanner carefully with fingertips or a teeny cosmetic sponge, concentrating on the bony areas that would naturally tan – forehead, nose, cheekbones and chin – then stroke the product out into your hairline. Remember to do your neck and under your jawline.

7 **Allow double time to dry...** then dust any self-tanned areas with talc-free powder. This avoids any of the product transferring onto your clothes. Avoid showering or taking a bath for six to eight hours – and make sure you don't get in a sweaty situation!

8 **Take emergency action.** If you see any streaks or splotches, rub half a lemon on the area until it starts to fade out, then buff skin gently with a damp towel.

9 **Prolong your tan.** Use a gentle (natural) cleanser on face and body, and keep your skin moisturised. Don't use peeling agents, such as retinol, or over-the-counter acne treatments which strip your skin.

10 **Start over.** When your tan has faded, refresh your skin, starting with exfoliation, and repeat the steps all over again (unless, of course, you are using a gradual daily tanner).

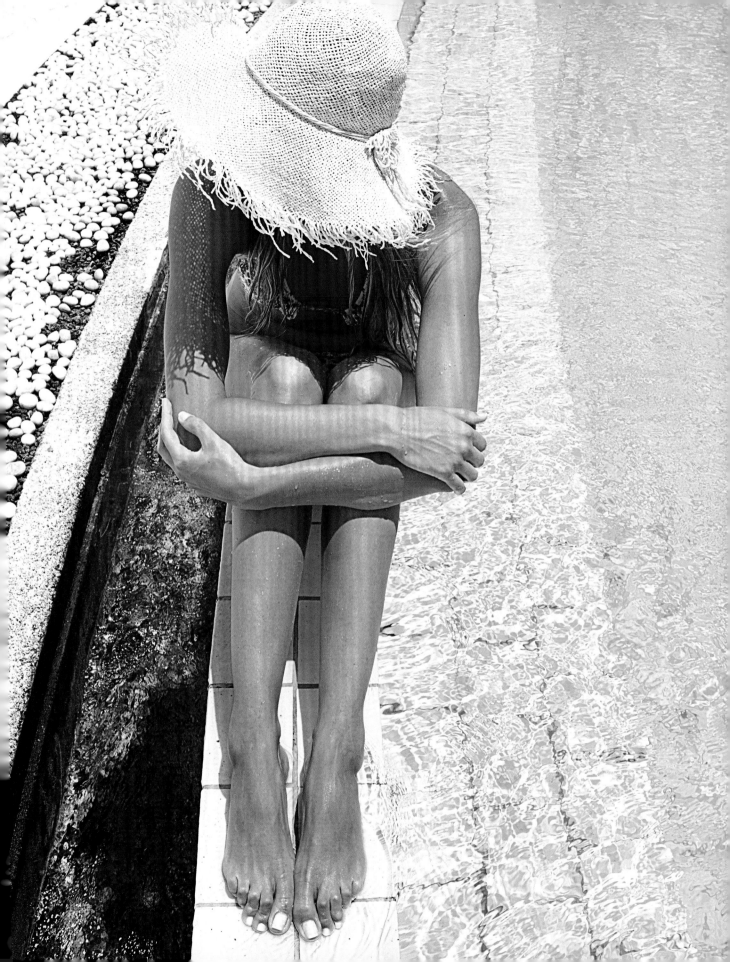

SELF-TANNERS
our award winners

These are an optional extra to your beauty regime but have become popular as a safe way to tan. There are now plenty of self-tanning formulations around that are 'more natural' and include fewer synthetic chemicals. However, although the self-tanning ingredient DHA (dihydroxyacetone) can be naturally derived and approved organic, it still provokes debate (see page 152). But how natural are the results? Some of these award winners multitask on faces and bodies, while others target just the face or the body. Find out here which ones our testers gave glowing results

FOR FACE AND BODY
JANE IREDALE TANTASIA SELF TANNER & BRONZER
✻

SCORE: 8.17/10

From a pioneering mineral brand better known for its make-up comes this tinted product said to be moisturising enough to apply to face or body straight from the tube. As well as the self-tanning DHA, it contains tyrosine and monk's pepper to stimulate synthesis of melanin in the skin, plus copper gluconate to ensure an even colour. (Personally, we'd like to have a little whinge about what seems an entirely unnecessary plastic outer carton around the nozzled tube. Jane Iredale, please note.)

COMMENTS: 'The best-smelling self-tanner I've ever used: a gentle citrus aroma which faded after the colour developed' • 'this has everything you'd want from a fake-tanner: easy to apply (you can see where you've put it), not streaky at all, lovely colour, very realistic, no streaks' • 'it gave a really natural tone on my naturally very fair and freckly skin' • 'I am hopeless with fake tan but this product really suits me – and no stained hands the next day' • 'healthy result without the fake-tan look' • 'a pure delight: it's so easy to apply with no streaking, a beautiful aroma and the colour built up to an extremely

AT A GLANCE

FOR FACE AND BODY
JANE IREDALE TANTASIA SELF TANNER & BRONZER

THE ORGANIC PHARMACY SELF TAN

FOR FACE
ST. TROPEZ SELF TAN SENSITIVE BRONZING LOTION FOR FACE

FOR BODY
GREEN PEOPLE SELF TAN LOTION

TANORGANIC SELF TAN

ST. TROPEZ SELF TAN SENSITIVE BRONZING LOTION

natural all-over tan – love it as it doesn't smell or feel like any other tanning product I've used'.

THE ORGANIC PHARMACY SELF TAN
✻ ✻

SCORE: 7.25/10

The Organic Pharmacy tell us that the DHA in this tube of self-tanner is natural (from sugar beet), and the organic certification body Ecocert are certainly happy enough to have approved that as such. It's a moisturising formula that is enriched with aloe vera, coconut, jojoba and sesame oils, but untinted (so you'll need to feel rather than see where you've applied it).

COMMENTS: 'Loved this, very easy to use and a great result' • 'the colour was a really good natural brown; lots of people commented on how well I looked' • 'very natural, light bronze shade' • 'goes on so smoothly and feels velvety; I like the natural honey gold' • 'this is a really good product all round'.

FOR FACE
ST. TROPEZ SELF TAN SENSITIVE BRONZING LOTION FOR FACE
✻

SCORE: 8/10

This range was previously known as St. Tropez Naturals, so if you loved that range you can find it again here. (Both the face and the body options did well with our testers, as they did in their previous incarnations.) The breakthrough with the new products is that they are specially formulated for sensitive skins, so even those with eczema and easily irritated complexions can experience the natural-looking golden results from this luxurious lotion, which – though not tinted – has a subtle iridescence that lets you see where you've applied it.

COMMENTS: 'I'm very, very happy with this product: it's extremely pleasant to use and gave a fantastic, natural-looking result' • 'smelt like a moisturiser and gave an attractive light glow within an hour' • 'my husband said the colour was very subtle and looked healthy – I am impressed with this' • 'easy-peasy to apply and the end result looked amazing and totally natural – I wish all self-tanners were like this' • 'perfect consistency: a cinch to rub in – behaved like my usual moisturiser'.

FOR BODY
GREEN PEOPLE SELF TAN LOTION
❋❋❋
SCORE: 8.14/10

With natural DHA, plus organic rose, geranium and sandalwood, this certified-organic pump-action lotion was highly rated for its pleasant aroma (and lack of 'biscuit tin' after smell). It is lusciously skin-softening, too, with olive and sunflower oils. (PS: Green People submitted this twice, and it got an almost identical mark from each of the teams of 10 testers!)

COMMENTS: 'The best self-tanner I have ever used, no fake smell' • 'it sank in while I dried my hair – not at all sticky or tacky' • 'took time to develop but gave a lovely golden tone; very natural and pretty on my fair, freckly skin with no streaking' • 'faded very evenly' • 'several people have said I look very well, or very nice, so it made me feel good' • 'left my skin feeling really soft – should be called a moisturising self-tan lotion' • 'this shows me self-tanners have come a long way from the era when they'd give you orange "knee pads"' • 'so good to apply: like having an aromatherapy massage, then gorgeously scented limbs, and relax'.

TANORGANIC SELF TAN
❋❋❋
SCORE: 7.75/10

A tall, slim, glass (beware) bottle of deliciously orange-scented Ecocert-certified liquid, this lightly tints the skin while hydrating it with aloe vera juice and hyaluronic acid. The liquid adds a touch of pretty shimmer, too, and is said to be just fine for sensitive souls. (Or rather, bodies.)

COMMENTS: 'I'm in love with this product which is hands down the best fake tan I have ever had; for the first time ever I was streak-free after applying self-tanner' • 'I rarely use false tanners on my body as they invariably end up making my skin look patchy and streaky, but this product has changed my mind' • 'a beautiful golden brown that makes me look like I've spent five days on holiday'.

ST. TROPEZ SELF TAN SENSITIVE BRONZING LOTION
❋❋❋
SCORE: 7.65/10

This is the body version of the winning face product and comes in a much bigger flip-top tube. With a texture that seems to melt into skin (Jo loves), it delivers grape and mango seed oils and avocado butter along with the naturally derived tanning ingredients. Like the face alternative, there is no 'guide' tint.

COMMENTS: 'Was impressed by the lack of chemical false-tan smell you often get from these products' • 'I'm pale and an eczema sufferer; this looks natural and faded evenly – and I experienced no irritation even after a second application' • 'would recommend to anyone who wants a discreet zap of colour – great for out-of-season tanning or to perk up pale skins' • 'loved this fragrance – it smelt natural and next day there was no scent at all (and there's nothing worse than when it gets a little warm and you smell the aroma of your fake tan wafting around!)' • 'gave a sun-kissed effect on legs, very healthy looking – not streaky – and realistic' • 'loved this: I always manage to achieve the stripy-deckchair look with dark knees and ankles, but now I've discovered a product that actually works!'

TIP: Don't pay a blind bit of notice to the self-tanners that claim to offer an SPF. It will be minimal and may last only a couple of hours. You still need to apply sun protection. There, rant over.

Rumbles in the
BEAUTY JUNGLE

Some cosmetics ingredients continue to be the subject of debate among scientists and consumers. Here we explain the latest thinking about the hot topics

NANOPARTICLES They may look like glitzy Christmas baubles in blown-up, colour-enhanced images, like the one pictured right, but in fact nanoparticles are infinitesimally small particles – at least 500 could fit across the diameter of a human hair. Cosmetics manufacturers like them because they allow a much finer finish than bigger particles. In mineral sunscreens, nano-sized titanium dioxide and zinc oxide become transparent on the skin, preventing a chalky veil, but still absorb and reflect UV light.

The debate centres on how deeply the particles can penetrate and be absorbed by the skin, or access the body in other ways. One of the reasons for using them in moisturisers, for instance, is that they can deliver nutrients such as cell-regenerating peptides deeper into the outer protective layers of the skin. But most experts say they are not absorbed into the bloodstream. In some products, they have a special coating that keeps them on the surface.

Turning to powder make-up, recent research showed that, when inhaled, the nanoparticles in these products tend to clump together in the upper airways, rather than making their way to the lungs as single particles would. Researchers hypothesise this might also pose health problems (such as affecting breathing).

While the market is expanding rapidly, the scientific evidence for their use in cosmetics – unlike pharmaceutical drugs – is not. The long-term effects of nanoparticles accumulating in the skin, for instance, is a question mark.

While there are no regulations to stop the use of nanoparticles in beauty products, new regulations in the EU (and also in Australia) mandate that any nano-sized ingredients must now be labelled with (nano) after it in the ingredients listing – a victory for campaigners.

In general, natural products are less likely to contain nano-ingredients but please get used to reading the label if you are concerned. Nanoparticles are forbidden in organically certified products.

DHA, THE SKIN-COLOURING COMPOUND Dihydroxyacetone (DHA) is the most widely used active ingredient in self-tanners. Following mutterings for some years, a big investigation by America's ABC News unleashed headlines worldwide. After reviewing all the evidence, a panel of leading medical experts voiced the concern that if DHA enters the bloodstream, it could theoretically alter and damage DNA, which could in turn lead to the development of cancers and malignancies. 'We simply don't know the relative risk but it is a concern,' consultant dermatologist Dr Nick Lowe told us.

The danger is principally linked to spray tanning booths, according to the FDA (US Food and Drug Administration), which has not licensed them. If users are not properly protected, spray tan may get into the body via exposed mucous membrane – eyes, nose, lips and mouth – or inhalation. If you use a booth, ensure you are properly protected.

Regular fake tanning by any method (spray, cream or lotion) may allow a small amount of DHA to get through the skin barrier into your bloodstream. 'Regular "tanaholics" are more at risk than the occasional user where the risk is zero to minimal,' says Dr Lowe.

However, over-exfoliating beforehand for a smoother finish will make the skin barrier more vulnerable, as it is in people with eczema and similar skin conditions. If you're self-tanning, always follow the directions carefully and don't get it in your eyes, nose or mouth. Choose creams and lotions rather than mists or sprays.

Organic products are not potentially less harmful. Although the DHA in them is usually derived from organic beetroot or sugar cane, it is identical in chemical formula (a three-carbon sugar) to synthetic or non-organic versions.

METHYLISOTHIAZOLINONE (MI): A NEW WORRY

MI is a synthetic chemical preservative, now widely used in cosmetics, including skin- and haircare, sun preps, deodorants, wipes and moist toilet tissue, as well as make-up and shaving products. It has caused an unprecedented rise in cases of eczema (acute allergic contact dermatitis). Reactions may include itching, redness, blistering and swelling where the product was applied and may spread to adjacent sites. They may not appear until a day or so later.

Some decades ago, MI was used with a preservative MCI (methylchloroisothiazolinone) that triggered wide-scale allergic contact dermatitis. MCI was thought to be the culprit, so regulators allowed MI to be used on its own in cosmetic products at a higher concentration from 2005. It wasn't until 2009 that dermatologists realised the potential problem and started patch testing for MI. Since then, patch centres have found 10 per cent or more of patients are allergic to MI and MCI. The products most often implicated are moisturisers (affecting face and hands) and moist tissue wipes (anogenital areas). Shampoos may cause eczema at the hairline and on eyelids. If you are affected, do see your doctor and also write to the manufacturer.

(Organic products, of course, do omit other synthetic chemicals.)

NB: You should always wear sunscreen over a self-tanner. In one study, DHA-covered skin had more free radical damage during sun exposure than bare skin.

PARABENS These very widely used preservatives, which protect products against the growth of microbes, became public enemy number one in 2004 when a small study detected parabens in breast tumours. Although parabens do have weak oestrogen-like properties – and oestrogen is linked to the development of some breast cancers – the study did not show that parabens actually caused cancer or were harmful in any way. It also did not look at paraben levels in normal tissue.

Most experts have concluded that the small amounts of parabens in cosmetic products and the weakness of their oestrogen-like activity made it 'implausible that parabens could increase the risk associated with exposure to oestrogenic chemicals', as the FDA puts it. Parabens are accepted as being mostly non-irritating and non-sensitising but a small number of people (estimates vary from 0.5–3.5 per cent) are allergic to parabens and may develop eczema-type symptoms or rosacea if they use them. People with unexplained skin irritation should see their doctors to identify the allergen. Another synthetic preservative called MI (see above) may be a culprit.

However, many mainstream brands have now dropped parabens in response to public perception of the (hypothetical) risk. Most natural ones do not use them and organic certification does not permit them.

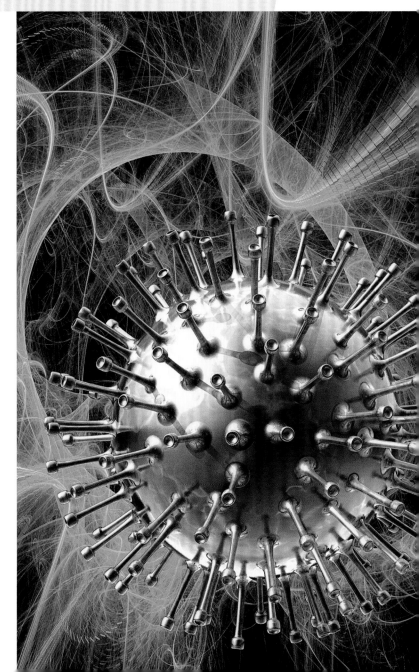

FACIAL SUNCARE
our award winners

Our face-saving formula? Big hats, Jackie-O sunglasses and lots of SPF. Like us, many of our testers prefer 'more natural' sun products – not least because some chemical sunscreens can trigger sensitivity – and these three shone out from the rest

L'OCCITANE ANGELICA RADIANT UV SHIELD SPF40
✳

SCORE: 8.23/10

Featuring hydrating and toning angelica from the Drôme region of France, this high-protection illuminating milk has a very light and silky texture with a pretty scent from the organic angelica plants. The sun protection is down to titanium dioxide. However, it comes in a pump-action glass bottle, which would be heavy to lug to the beach and, of course, you need to beware of glass around swimming pools. NB: Unlike one tester below, please don't rub the milk in too hard, or you risk lowering the SPF. *COMMENTS:* 'I loved the "smell of summer" fragrance – like fresh-cut grass! And good moisturisation, without making my skin look like it was covered in chalk, as many sunscreens do' • 'easy to apply and rubbed in well, ideal for people who hate a heavy-duty SPF moisturiser, or great over an ordinary day cream' • 'sunk in well over my usual moisturiser, leaving a healthy glow' • 'a good make-up base' • 'feels very comfortable on the skin' • 'I love this! The lotion was silky and easily absorbed, felt lovely on my skin and didn't leave any white ghostliness – gorgeous' • 'a light, fresh, sunny fragrance' • 'liked the benefit of having a flattering dewy sheen, while knowing my skin was protected'.

ÉMINENCE TROPICAL VANILLA DAY CREAM SPF32
✳ ✳ ✳

SCORE: 8.07/10

Don't be put off by the idea that this is over-whelmingly vanilla-y: it has more of a subtle, sweet, tropical scent. We tested it as a summer suncare product but, in fact, this Hungarian brand recommend the cream (which comes in a tub) can be used all year round. The SPF32 is

AT A GLANCE

L'OCCITANE ANGELICA RADIANT UV SHIELD SPF40

ÉMINENCE TROPICAL VANILLA DAY CREAM SPF32

L'OCCITANE IMMORTELLE BRIGHTENING SHIELD SPF40

> TIP: Mineral sunscreens (titanium dioxide or zinc oxide) can be nano-sized particles; if you prefer to avoid these, check the ingredients' list, as new EU regulations mean that nanoparticles have to be labelled.

suitable for on- and off-beach use, offering a good base for make-up (but remember to top up if you go in the sun). It features shea butter, corn germ oil, aloe vera and antioxidant green tea, and has a combo of zinc oxide and a cinnamon-derived sunscreen. It's certified organic by the Hungarian organic body. *COMMENTS:* 'Cream completely disappeared after application; skin felt soft, smooth and complexion more even – gorgeous fragrance' • 'this instantly improved the appearance of my skin, which felt less greasy by the end of the day' • 'sugary, vanilla smell – lovely' • 'feels like a luxury – I'm enjoying wearing this sun product' • 'I'm really in love with it and now interested in finding out more about the other products in the Éminence range'.

L'OCCITANE IMMORTELLE BRIGHTENING SHIELD SPF40
✳

SCORE: 7.94/10

Well done to L'Occitane, with this second winner in the same category. The Brightening range features their signature age-defying immortelle essential oil, along with Bellis perennis (daisy) extract, which both work together to help even out skin tone. This SPF40, which comes in a handy plastic pump-action dispenser, is also ideal for anyone trying to stop age spots, or prevent them from getting worse. Again, the active sunscreen is the mineral titanium dioxide, but this formulation sinks right in, leaving a lovely dewy sheen. *COMMENTS:* 'Amazing: the cream went from being completely white and opaque in my hand to invisible on the face' • 'skin appeared smooth, clear, well-moisturised, with no oily patches – felt wonderful, very light' • 'really like the gentle glow this gives' • 'has a subtle smell of summer; felt very comfortable to wear'.

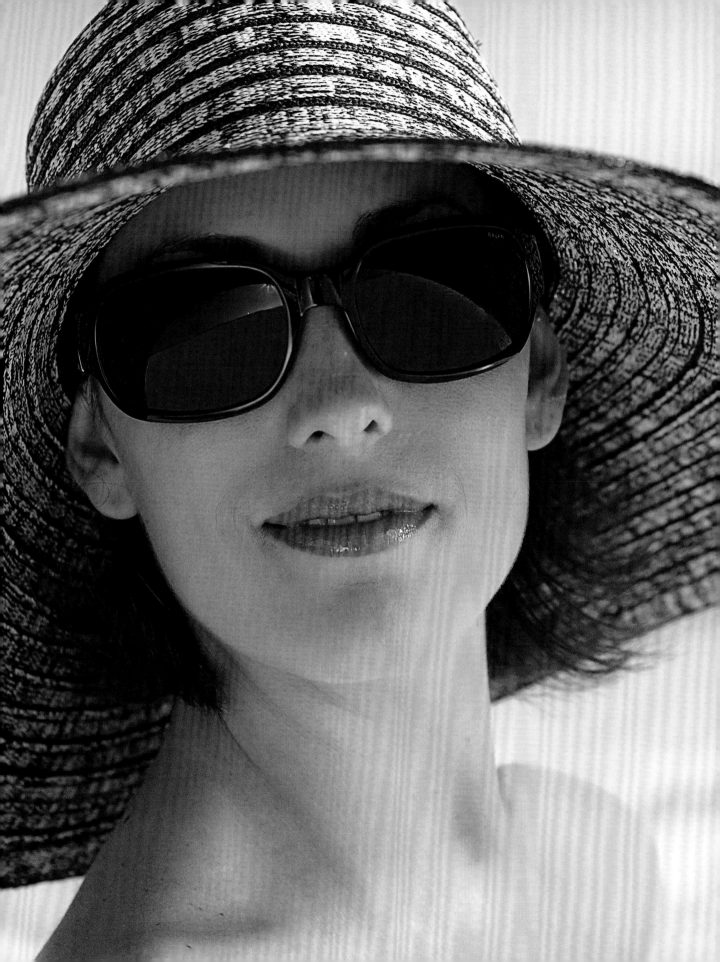

BODY SUNCARE
our award winners

We trialled pretty well every all-natural sunscreen on the market for this section, as well as some 'more natural' versions. Most of the all-natural ones (not really to our surprise, based on past experience) didn't do well. 'Too chalky' or 'too ghostly', our testers commented. As we know, it's exceptionally hard to come up with something people want to use if you are only including mineral sunblock ingredients. So the award winners below have done a stellar (make that solar…) job

GREEN PEOPLE SCENT-FREE SUN LOTION SPF25

✳

SCORE: 8.55/10

A triumph for Green People in this category. We've often dispatched their suncare to testers in the past – not just 'green' fans and natural testers, but the real L'Oréal/Piz Buin-slathering brigade – and it has consistently done well. But to have two winners topping the list when we sent out over 25 natural sunscreens is stupendous. The sunscreen ingredients in this (to shield skin against both UVA and UVB rays) are titanium dioxide, edelweiss extract and a chemical from natural cinnamic acid. Of all the options in the Green People sunscreen range, this highest scorer was also great for sensitive skins and is scent-free – quite a rarity in a category where you can be 20 paces away from your neighbour on the beach and still get strong whiffs of faux coconut…

COMMENTS: 'Love this and am going to switch to it straight away; I felt as if I'd just used a moisturising body lotion: lighter than other suntan creams and simple to rub in' • 'glided on easily and sunk into skin within seconds; comfortable, but not oily' • 'no apparent smell which is a good thing for people who prefer their own fragrance – and men, especially' • 'compared favourably with my usual Ambre Solaire milk' • 'I enjoyed using this: it is easy to apply and feels moisturising on the skin' • 'excellent hydrating effect, not sticky'.

GREEN PEOPLE SUN LOTION SPF15 WITH TAN ACCELERATOR

✳

SCORE: 8.36/10

This second Green People sun prep offers a lower level of SPF than the top-scoring product's SPF25, so is more suited to less sunny days, or for later on in your holiday when your skin has acquired some natural melanin protection. (It may also suit those with naturally darker skin.) It is water resistant, moisture retaining – and the tan-accelerating action is down to a natural carob-derived ingredient, which 'gives you 25 per cent more tan', according to Green People. This features the same sun-protection complex as the Scent-Free lotion, alongside organic aloe vera, green tea and avocado extracts (more than 80 per cent of the ingredients in the formula are of organic origins). In common with the rest of the range, trial sizes are available – good for popping in a bag, or for checking out whether it suits you as well as it suited our testers.

COMMENTS: 'This is very effective with a lovely fragrance – probably down to the combination of avocado and edelweiss' • 'I'm usually reluctant to wear sunscreen if I have formal or nice clothes on, as I don't want them to get greasy stains or the smell of sun cream on them – but this absorbed quickly so I have no hesitation about using it' • 'lovely and silky with a cooling effect which I liked' • 'rubbed in evenly and with minimal effort'.

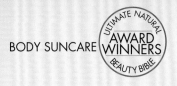

NATIO SUNSCREEN LOTION SPF30+

✻

SCORE: 8.15/10

Sun-scorched Australia, not surprisingly, produces some highly effective suncare, including this flip-top lotion, from a brand that's a household name there. It is said to be water-resistant for up to four hours, and uses synthetic sunscreens in a base of botanicals including vitamin E to help counteract some of the sun's harsh drying effects on the skin.

COMMENTS: 'More like a nice body cream than a sun lotion; very easy to use with a slight perfume' • 'smells light, fresh and felt comforting' • 'did a good job at protecting exposed bits of my weather-beaten chest on a sunny day by the coast' • 'I was a bit wary of using this Natio product as I have eczema, but I had no reaction – skin actually felt more moisturised' • 'the cream completely disappeared without leaving chalky or coloured residue; left skin with a sheen but wasn't greasy'.

JASON FAMILY NATURAL SUNBLOCK SPF45

✻

SCORE: 8.05/10

Every year we trial products for *YOU* Magazine's summer-sun special, and perennially this flip-top (again) product does well. It makes a good choice for all the family as it contains the higher SPF level that many mums prefer to shield children's vulnerable skins. The formula includes chemical sun filters, something to bear in mind if using on sensitive skins. Natural ingredients include cucumber and aloe extracts.

COMMENTS: 'A good moisturiser: skin felt soft after application' • 'so simple to use and I only had to reapply once: I normally burn very easily but this product prevented my skin from catching the sun while leaving it feeling soft and smooth' • 'smells of coconut, which is nice, and left me in a holiday mood' • 'absorbed easily with a couple of strokes and didn't feel heavy, even though it has a high factor'.

LIZ EARLE MINERAL SUN CREAM SPF20 MEDIUM PROTECTION

✻

SCORE: 7.72/10

We worship the water that Liz Earle walks on (and so do many of our testers), but when the Liz Earle suncare range first came out, it just wasn't that great. Fact. Since then it has been reformulated and made into a more user-friendly, skin-friendly product – and as a result, our *Beauty Bible* testers enjoyed using it. Of the five award winners featured here, this is the only one which just uses minerals as protection – zinc and titanium dioxide – rather than adding nature-based or synthetic chemical screens. Antioxidant green tea, pomegranate extract and pro-vitamin B5 also feature.

COMMENTS: 'Felt more like I was using a luxurious body cream than applying sunscreen' • 'very impressed: no horrible white sheen, no nasty chemical smell; left skin feeling and smelling lovely – plus I tried this on my face (delicate, easily upset skin) and I can attest it was fine for that' • 'I used this Liz Earle product a couple of years ago but gave up as it was so hard to rub in; really pleased to report it is now very easy to apply'.

WE LOVE

If Jo's ever taken out by a sniper, it'll be someone from the sun-prep industry in revenge for the revelation that no, she doesn't use suncare; she relies on common sense, covering up, sitting in the shade in the middle of the day, and sloshing on extra virgin olive oil – and she never burns. Sarah doesn't sunbathe, and in the UK seldom wears sunscreen, except on her face. But in West Australia (where she goes every year) or other hot spots, she slops on SPF30.

AFTER-SUN
our award winners

After-sun is often an afterthought for many holidaymakers. But, in fact, it's just as important an element of your beach regime as sunscreen. After-suns that feature antioxidants can help neutralise some (only some, we say) of the damage caused by UV exposure. And nourishing ingredients will replenish skin frazzled by a day of sun, sea or swimming pools. Finally, they're brilliant, of course, for soothing sunburn. Our testers put dozens through their paces – and warmed to these the most

LIZ EARLE BOTANICAL AFTERSUN GEL

❋

SCORE: 8.89/10

This very lightweight and cooling gel based on aloe vera also features refreshing cucumber and antioxidant vitamin E, plus moisture-attracting glycerine. The sinks-in-fast gel formulation contains lavender, too – apply before bedtime and it will help to induce a night of restful sleep. (To our nostrils, there's also a pleasant mintiness to the fragrance.)

COMMENTS: 'This felt like a cream rather than a gel – and definitely made skin feel colder' • 'I'd give this an 11 if I was allowed! It smells gorgeously of lavender and cucumber, and lingers delightfully – the best after-sun I've ever used, instantly takes the heat out of burning and sore skin' • 'this smells really classy – it reminds me of a high-quality spa; I will be buying it for my forthcoming holiday to the Caribbean – it really is lush!' • 'you only need to use a small amount, so it's quite economical' • 'I am by nature a scaly creature – my skin constantly seeking moisture – but this seemed to make it instantly hydrated, it was a real beauty revelation to me and a delight to use; the bonus was the gel also worked brilliantly even after an hour and a half of hot yoga!' • 'would I buy this? Yes, yes, yes'.

AT A GLANCE

LIZ EARLE BOTANICAL
AFTERSUN GEL

DR.ORGANIC
ALOE VERA GEL

GREEN PEOPLE
HYDRATING AFTER SUN

JASON SOOTHING 98%
ALOE VERA GEL

DR.HAUSCHKA
AFTER SUN LOTION

DR.ORGANIC ALOE VERA GEL

❋❋

SCORE: 8.86/10

This affordable product by a high-street brand, which has impressed many of our testers (and us), demonstrated the soothing action of 'double-strength' aloe vera gel. It's also useful for insect bites, general skin irritation, itching and any kind of dry, damaged skin, they tell us (and aloe is a well-known and scientifically proven traditional remedy for all-round skin soothing). That's the kind of multitasker we like. NB: Although some ingredients are certified organic, the finished product is not.

COMMENTS: 'This left my skin feeling soft, cool and not sticky, unlike some after-suns I have tried' • 'it has a lovely, fresh scent that lingers and uplifts the senses, making you feel more positive' • 'this is fabulous for post-waxing, too – really soothing, cooling and moisturising; every woman should own a tube of this' • 'the gel is thick enough to hold in the palm without going everywhere – which is a problem I've had with other aloe vera gels' • 'this gave a strong cooling sensation that is ideal for refreshing skin after a day under the sun' • 'my favourite of all the products I tested; I went on holiday to Hawaii and after a week or so suffered mild sunburn, so I used this gel to soothe and cool; my skin felt very soft and hydrated, and there was no peeling'.

GREEN PEOPLE HYDRATING AFTER SUN
✺✺✺

SCORE: 8.25/10

The packaging trumpets '94% organic' (and we like that refreshing precision) plus, the ingredients are Fairtrade, so Green People tell us (something we feel passionately about). You'll find this in our bathroom cabinets (see We Love, right), and we know for a fact that the minty, creamy lotion really does take the heat out of over-exposed skin. It's deliciously skin-quenching, too.

COMMENTS: 'I prefer this to my normal L'Oréal after-sun; loved the mint-fresh scent – almost made me wish I had sunburn' • 'this glides on without dragging whatsoever; my skin felt so smooth, lovely and soft – and I awoke next morning with silky skin' • 'my husband suffers from itchy skin on his arms, and after applying this it was much better, with no irritation. It works for me, too: never mind an after-sun – it's actually replaced my usual body lotion' • 'I often get allergies to various products, but this helped to moisturise, cool and repair my skin – and those are Big Benefits' • 'I burned my arm on the oven door recently and immediately applied this – it cooled and took out the redness' • 'I like the fact that the ingredients in this after-sun are organic because the last thing you want is an allergic reaction to chemicals on top of sunburn'.

JASON SOOTHING 98% ALOE VERA GEL
✺

SCORE: 7.84/10

Aloe vera-based after-suns have done very well in this particular trial, as you can see. This option from Jason is another instant cooler, with a very high percentage of organically certified aloe vera, and a useful pump-action bottle which makes it simple and un-messy to apply. Alongside the aloe vera, Jason include soothing, nourishing allantoin and vitamin B5, to enhance the condition of skin – making it ideal as a post-shaving treatment, too. Like the Dr.Organic product, this is a real 'beauty steal'.

COMMENTS: 'I wanted to hate this product! I've tried aloe vera gels in the past and found them to be sticky, thick and smelly – so I was very pleasantly surprised, amazed and delighted when I discovered that my skin felt comfortable, cool and hydrated, with a lovely clean, fresh, citrus smell' • 'an absolute bargain – this is a new "must-buy"' • 'I definitely see this as a multi-purpose product – not just for the sun' • 'I found this to be especially good for the back of the neck where the sun made most impact'.

DR.HAUSCHKA AFTER SUN LOTION
✺✺

SCORE: 7.6/10

We were gutted when Dr.Hauschka withdrew their sun protection line a few years ago – but pleased they kept this after-sun in the skincare range. Sweet almond oil, shea butter, carrot root extract, apricot kernel oil and calendula all feature in the ingredients list – and so does a very special 'ice plant' extract, from a succulent that's very efficient at storing water in its leaves. Translate that to an after-sun, and you've got a highly effective moisturiser.

COMMENTS: 'Really enjoyed using this: skin felt soft, cool, and no tightness' • 'took any redness out of my skin; and my arms, neck, chest and face looked lightly tanned; impressed and will use again' • 'kept skin moisturised, which prevented peeling' • 'a delight to use as the lotion glided easily onto skin and came out of the tube in just the right amount per squeeze' • 'this is 100 times better than any other after-sun I've bought in the past'.

WE LOVE

Jo is super-careful not to get burned but has given the Green People Hydrating After Sun (which did well here) to guests – and has watched as the redness fades from their sunburnt skin. Although Sarah is outside with horses and gardening, she never sunbathes, sloshes on sun preps and avoids the midday sun when in hot countries and hasn't burnt for decades (fingers crossed).

TIP: Aloe vera is nature's own after-sun. We keep a pot on windowsills (and in stables, in Sarah's case) not just for sunburn, but minor grazes, cuts, stings and so on. If you find a fresh leaf, simply slice, squeeze, slather and soothe.

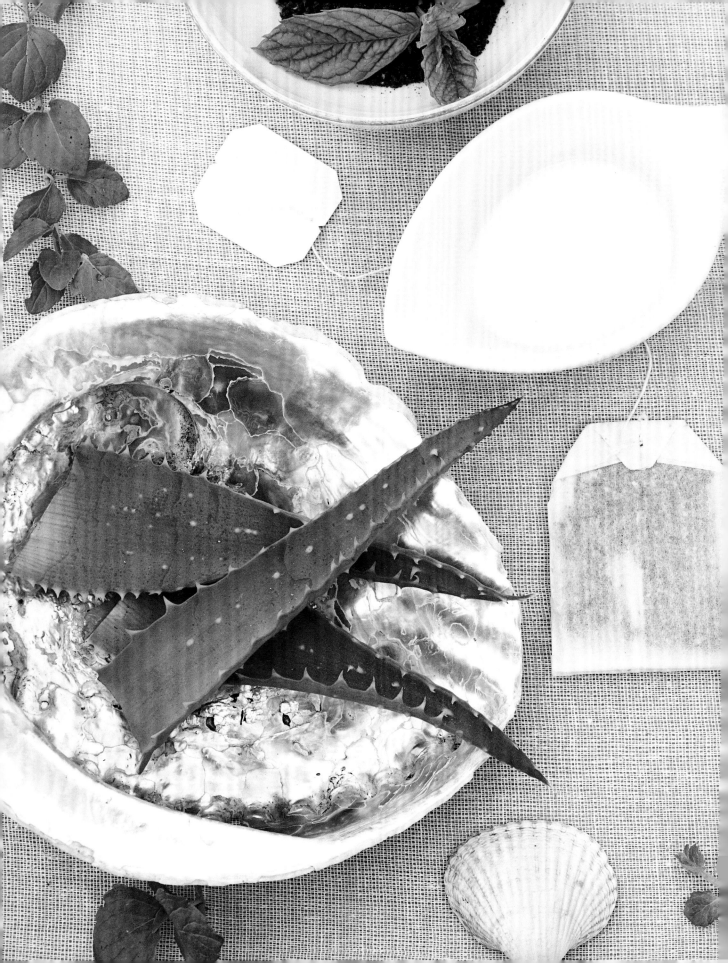

AFTER-SUN SKIN COOLERS

As much as we might try to avoid sunburn, sometimes we all make mistakes…
These calming DIY treatments take the heat and redness out of frazzled skin

MINT AND BLACK TEA SUNBURN SOLUTION

Used straight from the fridge, this easy-to-prepare mint and tea lotion will take the heat out of sunburn in a flash.

- 110g (4oz) fresh mint leaves
- 3–4 black tea bags
- 1 litre (40fl oz) boiling water

Pour the boiling water over the mint leaves and tea bags. Cover and allow the solution to stand for 10 minutes.

Strain and cool, then transfer to a glass jar or bottle and store in your fridge, where it will keep for several weeks. Apply to the sore skin areas with cotton pads.

ALOE VERA AFTER-SUN SOOTHER

The light, gooey gel in aloe vera is instantly cooling and healing. All you need is one aloe vera leaf. Just slice it in half horizontally and slide it slowly over the affected area.

MORE AFTER-SUN SKIN-SAVERS

• Smearing yogurt (preferably straight from the fridge) onto your skin as soon as it turns pink can help unburn your sunburn, cool the area and re-establish the vital pH balance, so it heals faster. Use plain, full-fat organic yogurt, if possible. Let it sit on your skin until it warms up, rinse with tepid water, then reapply.

• Sunburn can also be cooled with mashed strawberries: apply and leave for five minutes to take the heat out of skin. Or, even more effectively, on a face that's caught the sun, mash 1 tablespoon of yogurt with two strawberries, and smooth onto the face for instant relief.

• Witch hazel, cucumber juice and apple cider vinegar all work to calm overheated skin. Simply add 1 tablespoon of any of these to 1 cup of water. Put in a spritzer bottle to carry with you, then you can spray onto skin as required. (Although, of course, with sunburn prevention is always better than cure.)

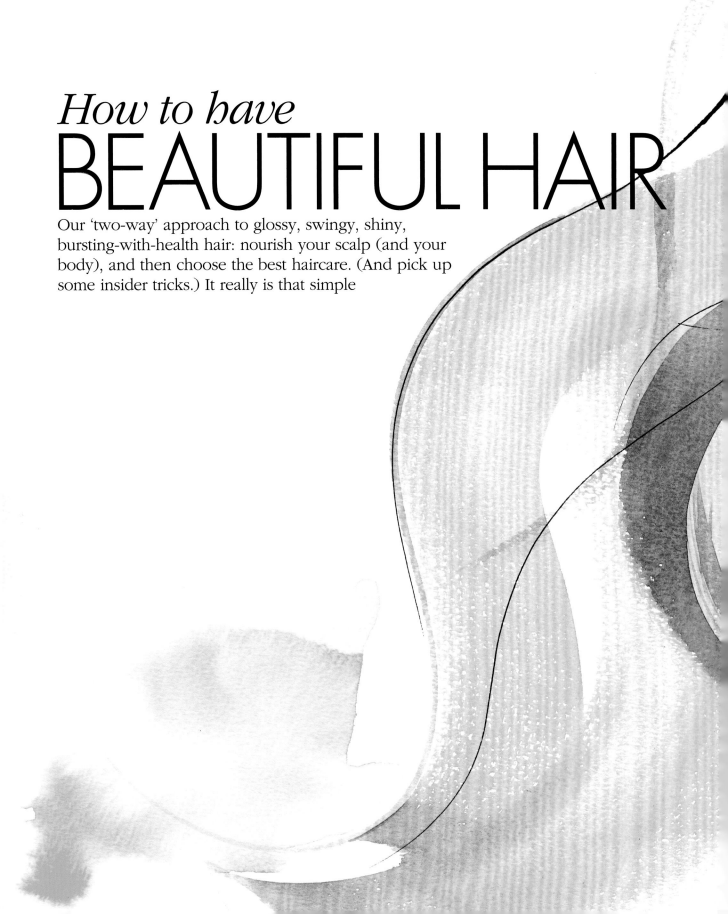

How to have
BEAUTIFUL HAIR

Our 'two-way' approach to glossy, swingy, shiny, bursting-with-health hair: nourish your scalp (and your body), and then choose the best haircare. (And pick up some insider tricks.) It really is that simple

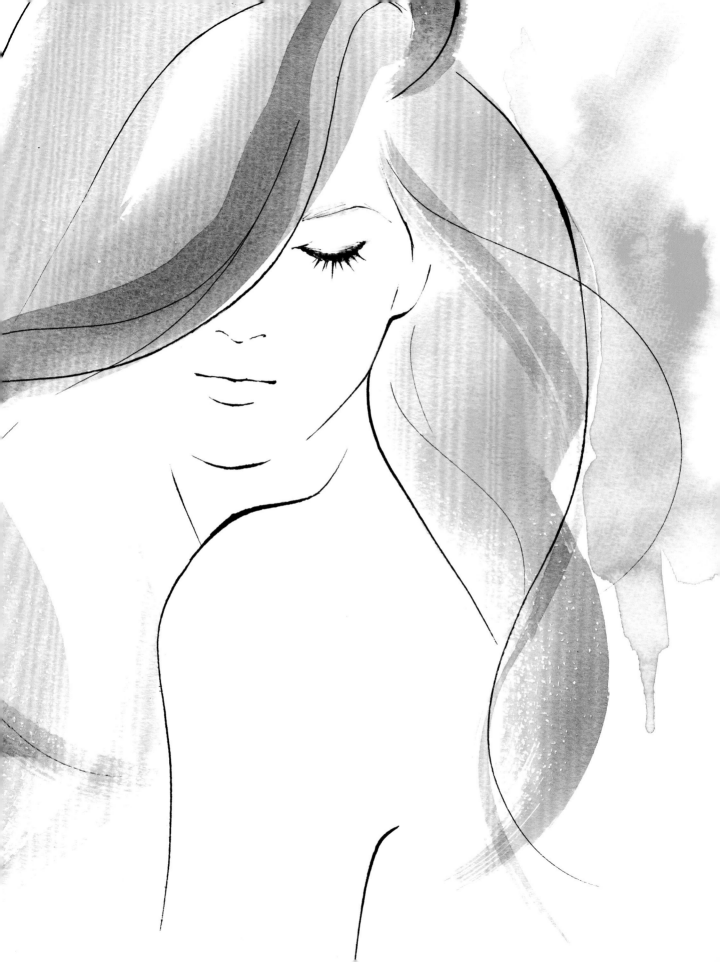

How to have
GORGEOUS HAIR

We've all known bad hair days – and even weeks – but there are some simple ways to make your locks look more luscious. Read these top tips from experts (and us!) and go cherish, nourish and flaunt your crowning glory

1 **Go with the hair nature gave you.** 'Don't fight nature,' advises John Masters, the world's first organic hairdresser and one of our hair heroes. 'If you have curly hair, find a way of styling that enables you to live with the wave. If you have straight hair, just think about all the women who spend ages trying to achieve what you are naturally blessed with.'

2 **Get a good cut.** Our years of experience have told us: the best investment you can possibly make is in a fantastic haircut. The very best you can afford: it's worth it every time.

3 **Go ionic!** We love hair-smoothing ionic driers and – most of all – Sarah loves her ionic Volume Shine Airstyler (by our favourite hair genius John Frieda), like a big, round brush crossed with a Carmen roller. Switch on this styling tool and hot air gushes through, smoothing, lifting, waving – it's THE key to salon styling at home. (We don't really understand the science of ionic styling, but basically it seems they produce a stream of negative – that's good! – ions, which reduce static and frizz, neutralise the dulling ions that build up on hair and attract dust and grime, and seal the hair strands locking in moisture. Ionic styling tools also use less heat. What we notice is how smooth and shiny they make your hair.)

4 **If your hair isn't dirty, don't bother shampooing,** just spritz it with water from a mister (we use a plant spray) and re-style.

5 **Feed your follicles:** hair is made of a protein called keratin (the same as skin and nails). So you need a protein-rich diet, which is great for general health too. Feast on fresh oily fish, lots of different coloured veggies especially dark green leaves, pulses (peas, beans and lentils), natural live yogurt, cold-pressed oils (olive, hemp and walnut), seeds (linseed, sunflower, pumpkin and sesame), and if you eat red meat, small portions twice weekly will provide hair-helping iron too. And go nutty! Almonds, walnuts and Brazil nuts are fabulous nutrition for hair.

6 **Avoid too many cow's milk products, especially if you have dandruff or other scalp problems:** also reduce caffeine, sugar, salt and hydrogenated fats. (For dandruff, try a neem-based shampoo.)

7 **Drink lots of still, pure water:** we know we keep saying it, but it works! (And don't smoke, you know that, too…)

8 **De-stress your tresses:** tight scalp, neck and shoulders can affect blood supply. So give yourself a head and neck massage, working your fingertips firmly into the tissue. We love it: it revives flagging styles, peps you up generally and is a great headache buster. If you don't have a willing pair of hands to give you a shoulder massage, try one of those wooden rollers – they are very effective.

9 **Look for sulphate-free hair care:** these harsh detergents (listed as sodium lauryl or laureth sulphate) dry out scalp and hair, irritate skin conditions, and possibly attack the follicles potentially causing hair loss. There are now many more sulphate-free hair products, which foam beautifully – and naturally. (See our Award Winners on page 164.)

10 **When you treat your face to a mask, treat your hair too (and your hands).** Turbo-charge a hair mask with a hot towel round your head. Then make like a princess and slumber on a silk pillow: result – silky, shiny, smooth hair (and no sleep wrinkles on your face).

> **TIP:** Dry your hair upside down to enhance volume, ruffling with your fingers, then smoothing with a vent brush. Set the style with a shot of cool air.

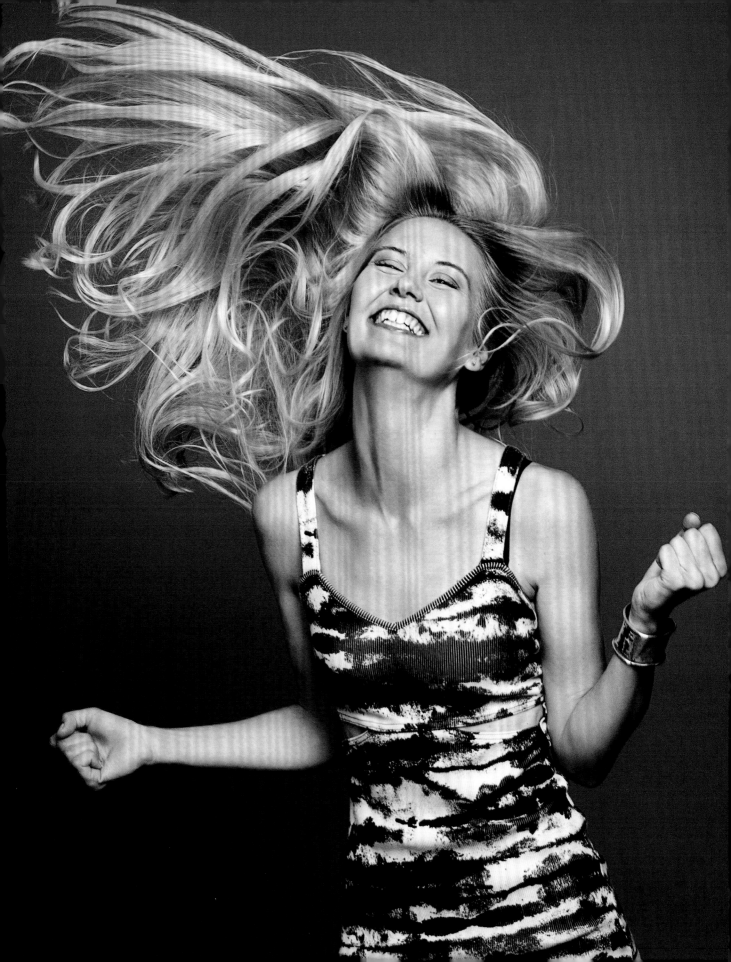

SHAMPOOS
our award winners

Brands recommend you use 'matching' shampoos and conditioners, and in some cases we sent out duos to testers. In other instances (a reflection of real life), products were trialled with the panellists' usual conditioners. But whether you match or mix, the results prove that natural shampoos have come a long way since our previous books. The top five here all delivered on cleansing, volume, manageability and shine…

LIZ EARLE BOTANICAL SHINE SHAMPOO
✹

SCORE: 8.71/10

Echoing the way that Liz Earle has one cleanser for all skin types, the brand offers only one shampoo, formulated with gentle cleansing agents together with natural vitamin E, shea butter (to cleanse without stripping hair), apple and orange extracts and a gorgeously fragrant blend of essential oils. With over 89 per cent natural ingredients, this was trialled separately to the winning conditioner from the same range.

COMMENTS: 'I've had numerous problems with irritation after using other shampoos, even those which claim they're good for a sensitive scalp, but this is very gentle, and left my hair looking great; I'll be switching to this in future' • 'didn't expect to find that this shampoo would reduce the itchiness of my scalp, but it seems to have done the trick' • 'this didn't produce a big lather but was very effective and left hair feeling thoroughly cleansed' • 'gave my normally flat hair more volume' • 'lovely herbal scent' • 'I've been disappointed by natural shampoos in the past but this surpassed all others by some margin – a great shampoo for all the family'.

OGARIO HYDRATE AND SHINE SHAMPOO
✹

SCORE: 8.71/10

Ogario's hair mask came top in its category (see page 172), but it was a different group of testers who put this popular shampoo through

AT A GLANCE

LIZ EARLE
BOTANICAL SHINE
SHAMPOO

OGARIO
HYDRATE AND SHINE
SHAMPOO

L'OCCITANE
AROMACHOLOGY
REPAIRING SHAMPOO

GIELLY GREEN
VOLUME SHAMPOO

GREEN PEOPLE
INTENSIVE REPAIR
SHAMPOO

its paces. Ogario is a small independent North London hairdresser, so for two of its products to do so incredibly well (against dozens of competitors) is really notable. A blend of eight essential oils in this delivers the uplifting scent testers raved about, while the brand's Protein Protect formula makes it particularly appropriate for dry or coloured hair. (Sarah keeps a bottle at the hairdresser…)

COMMENTS: 'Hair felt wonderfully fresh, shiny and more manageable, too' • 'I've had some good comments on how glossy my hair is looking' • 'lovely fragrance: smells of fruit and honey' • 'I've occasionally had a problem with an itchy scalp but didn't suffer with this shampoo, despite using it every day' • 'suited the hard water in my area; loved the aroma and couldn't wait to wash my hair with it' • 'delivered a natural, healthy shine; a beautiful, quality product' • 'will definitely buy again' • 'this really made my highlighted hair really shine' • 'fab uplifting smell – received comments from the family after I emerged from the shower'.

L'OCCITANE AROMACHOLOGY REPAIRING SHAMPOO
✹

SCORE: 8.17/10

This was sent out to testers with the matching conditioner as a duo, so maybe it's a little tricky to establish which of the two excelled, or whether it was the synergistic use of them. But who really cares…? Both products feature the same blend of five essential oils (lavender,

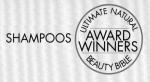

ylang-ylang, sweet orange, geranium and angelica), that deliver the scent which testers enjoyed. They also include the same 'repairing complex'; in fact, L'Occitane promise '83 per cent less broken hairs when brushing'. Both products are packaged in chunky plastic bottles with a convenient small flip-top opening, which makes for controlled pouring.

COMMENTS: 'My hair is fine and difficult, and I like my usual shampoo – but now I'm a total convert to this one: hair looked and felt better, thicker, and in visibly better condition; the best shampoo I've ever used' • 'love the addictive fragrance' • 'mane very soft and silky after use' • 'hair felt fabulous, squeaky clean and bouncy, with a lovely gloss' • 'economical to use as only a small amount is needed' • 'love this shampoo: I don't have to wash my hair so often, and it feels so full and shiny' • 'didn't irritate my scalp – I have psoriasis – which was a huge plus'.

GIELLY GREEN VOLUME SHAMPOO
✳

SCORE: 8/10
Gielly Green have done well in *The Anti-Ageing Beauty Bible*, but for this book the eco-minded London salon (which also has a cute Blow Dry Lounge outpost in department store Fenwick of Bond Street) put forward their products all over again. Result: fresh success. Flat hair is a widespread woe among our readers, and this is a good bet for the limp-tressed with its formula of naturally thickening ingredients, plus shea butter, rosemary and olive oils, and a blend of citrus essential oils for a zesty scent.

COMMENTS: 'Lovely, glossy, bouncy hair and I loved the citrussy smell' • 'would I buy again? Yes, yes, yes!' • 'my coloured hair feels fabulous; I also have the limpest locks and this made a huge difference – my hair didn't feel weighed down and even in damp weather it looks great after using this' • 'I still have some

of this shampoo left, even though I've been using it for three months, so it lasts for ages' • 'delivered volume and manageability; a great product' • 'hair continued to have good volume even after I'd slept on it' • 'this shampoo is amazing: my hair looks good all the time, is not as heavy and greasy; and my hairdresser commented on how healthy it had become, too'.

GREEN PEOPLE INTENSIVE REPAIR SHAMPOO
✳ ✳ ✳

SCORE: 7.92/10
One promise Green People make is that this concentrated formula lasts about three times as long as other shampoos – since many products are mostly made up of water, and we can add that easily at home, we'd like more brands to follow their lead. (Huge amounts of money and petroleum are wasted transporting beauty products around the globe which could be manufactured to more concentrated recipes.) On an ingredients note, this formula contains pineapple fruit extract, wheat extract, aloe vera juice, green tea extract, plus plenty of essential oils, including lavender, sandalwood and rose geranium.

COMMENTS: 'A total hit for my problem hair: loved the really clean and natural smell, loved that my hair looked shiny and bouncy (well, as bouncy as thin, fine hair can), loved that a little really does go a long way as it lathers up so well' • 'foamed up in a really nice way which I was surprised about as it doesn't contain SLS, but despite the foaminess it was easy to rinse out and didn't sting the eyes' • 'nice, natural smell that reminds me of a beauty spa' • 'hair is in very good condition, is more manageable and definitely looks better – I'd recommend this as I've used a lot of shampoos over time but this one is the best, and I've already purchased another bottle. It's a real winner for me'.

WE LOVE

As with Liz Earle Botanical Shine conditioner, we have been known to sneak her one-bottle-suits-all shampoo into our West-End uber hairdresser (and since Liz does the same, we've even suggested they sell it there!). Jo's also a longstanding fan of Odylique Gentle Herb Shampoo, which she's prescribed to many itchy-scalped friends (and their children), with great results. Sarah sends up frequent thanks for Clean shampoo by Phylia de M, the staple product she uses to keep her dry-ish mane gleaming, as well as the brand's conditioner (see page 169).

CONDITIONERS
our award winners

These are the products we turn to for everyday hair manageability and gloss. (For deep treatments, see Hair Masks on page 172.) There are plenty of natural and more-natural options out there, but not that many shining stars we've found in the past. So we're delighted, after putting over 25 conditioners through their paces, to bring you these hair-boosting high-scorers

PHYTO PHYTOBAUME VOLUME EXPRESS CONDITIONER

✳

SCORE: 8.61/10

Calling fine- and limp-haired women: this 'volumising' option is for you. As the brand name suggests, Phyto is a botanically powered haircare range: this conditioner includes elderberry extract (to restore softness and suppleness), red algae extract (to plump) and an unpronounceable plant ingredient called gleditschia (we looked it up: it's a small, thorny tree), that 'thickens' hair. This is one of four conditioners in the Phytobaume range (delivered in lightweight, flip-top, portable tubes), and is designed not to weigh hair down – by contrast, it actually encourages long-lasting volume.

COMMENTS: 'Definitely added more volume than my normal moisturising conditioner' • 'loved how sleek and glossy my hair looked after using this – a lot more hydrated, and less frizz. The volume seems to have stayed, too' • 'this has a natural and delicate scent, very fresh' • 'I've had comments from people asking if I'd coloured my hair as it has that "newly dyed" shine to it – but it must be this conditioner' • 'wow! My hair has never been shinier or healthier looking; so many people have been commenting and I'm very chuffed' • 'love the volume and shine, plus being able to use a tiny amount' • 'it's been easier and quicker to look after my hair as I haven't needed to heat and style it in order to look nice'.

AT A GLANCE

PHYTO PHYTOBAUME
VOLUME EXPRESS
CONDITIONER

L'OCCITANE
AROMACHOLOGY
REPAIRING
CONDITIONER

JOHN MASTERS
ORGANICS CITRUS &
NEROLI DETANGLER

LIZ EARLE
BOTANICAL SHINE
CONDITIONER

OJON
RARE BLEND
DEEP CONDITIONER

L'OCCITANE AROMACHOLOGY REPAIRING CONDITIONER

✳

SCORE: 8.5/10

L'Occitane only moved into haircare relatively recently – but look how well they're doing! This high-scorer features a patented 'anti-breakage' ingredient from the angelica plant, combined with essential oils (lavender, geranium, sweet orange and ylang-ylang), which deliver the scent our testers loved. In L'Occitane's trials, 92 per cent of testers felt this conditioner left their hair 'supple and perfectly detangled' – and our testers could only agree. (It's a great choice for long hair, then.) And this is light but effective, they also commented.

COMMENTS: 'Loved the fragrance – totally addictive (it's the ylang-ylang)' • 'hair healthy, shiny, very easy to style' • 'very pleased with the smooth, glossy finish – and no tangles' • 'I'd definitely recommend as a general conditioner; the smell is addictively gorgeous' • 'I find most conditioners for dry hair have a thick consistency, but this was different: light and runny – so I was pleasantly surprised to find it really conditioned right to the dry ends of my hair'.

JOHN MASTERS ORGANICS CITRUS & NEROLI DETANGLER

✳✳

SCORE: 8.25/10

We've a soft spot for this gentle New York hairdresser who's been banging the drum for more natural haircare since way before it was fashionable. His pampering botanical products are available internationally but if you're in Manhattan it's worth a trip to his fab flagship store. You can perhaps guess from the name on the flip-top bottle that this has an utterly divine smell – from lemongrass, lemon and grapefruit – and it also features wheat and soya proteins, together with coconut oil, to help with comb-ability and shine. (The neroli actively works to nourish a dry scalp, too.)

COMMENTS: 'Really detangled my hair' • 'this smells divine – gorgeous and definitely citrussy – and does a great job of conditioning and detangling my hair (as promised)' • 'didn't irritate my sensitive scalp at all and I also noticed my hands felt softer after using it!' • 'made an immediate difference to the feel and manageability of my hair: love, love, love'.

LIZ EARLE BOTANICAL SHINE CONDITIONER

✽

SCORE: 8.11/10

This has done well in previous *Beauty Bible*s, and now it has done well again when we trialled it for this book: here are comments from another new batch of converts to Liz's popular haircare. The conditioner actually comes in three options – for Fine or Oily, Normal and Dry or Damaged Hair (it was this last one we trialled). All feature a signature ingredient from Kenya called yangu seed oil, which is hand-collected by a forest tribe in Kenya as part of a community trade project that is close to Liz's heart. In addition, the formula contains shea butter, aloe vera, and a delightful collection of sense-awakening oils including patchouli, cedarwood, lemon and geranium.

COMMENTS: 'A good defrizz factor; the fruity, not-too-sweet scent is very pleasant'

• 'manageability was much better: my hair was bouncy, had body but was not frizzy – and I could blow-dry it smooth without using my usual straighteners' • 'my hair detangles much more easily and feels silkier; I'll buy this again' • 'I don't need to wash my hair so often with this product' • 'definitely noticed less frizz – left to its own devices my hair would usually be a horrible messy mass' • 'I noticed the difference from the very first use: my hair was noticeably shiny, soft and nourished'.

OJON RARE BLEND DEEP CONDITIONER

✽

SCORE: 8.06/10

The Ojon brand gets its name from an oil used as a hair treatment for over 500 years by communities in Central America. Here, the signature ojon oil is blended with oils from murumuru, monoi and kukui nut, plus something called 'rouge oleifera extract' (from the fruit that surrounds the ojon nut). This sweet-scented rich conditioner can be used as a weekly or bi-weekly treatment, they tell us – or even more frequently on super-dry and damaged hair. Intriguingly, when the tube is squeezed, two different coloured streams of ingredients deliver a striped product. (Fun!)

COMMENTS: 'Lovely musky-sweet fragrance' • 'I was asked if I'd been to the hairdressers – yet the only thing I'd done is use this product; hair definitely looks better than normal' • 'I really love this: might seem gimmicky to have a two-tone product, but it really works' • 'left a beautiful high-gloss finish which surprised me as I have coarse hair; it is now softer and easier to style' • 'my daughter even commented my hair was looking better and asked what I was doing; it's rare I get compliments from anyone in this house so this conditioner must work wonders'.

WE LOVE

We're both fans of the Ojon range, but also admit to sneaking tubes of **Liz Earle Botanical Shine Conditioner** into the hairdresser with us, for our regular weekly blow-dries (as does Liz herself). Sarah is devoted to **Phylia de M** organic haircare, developed in California, and its conditioner simply called **Condition**. Other favourite natural options are **Kai** (the heavenly fragranced brainchild of La-La-Land lady Gaye Straza), **Ogario** (which did well in Hair Masks, page 172), and **Intelligent Nutrients**, developed by the founder of Aveda, Horst M Rechelbacher.

TIP: If you're going to massage your scalp, always do it during the conditioning phase of the hair-washing process: you want to get detergents (even gentle 'natural' ones) off the scalp quickly, as they may dry it out. If you're worried about conditioner weighing down your hair, massage with fingertips on a wet, product-free scalp instead, then condition the ends only.

MANE ATTRACTIONS

For healthy, shiny hair, ditch the chemical cleanser for a gentle shampoo soap turbo-charged with herbs your hair will love

HERB-BOOSTED CASTILE SHAMPOO

Castile is the gentlest 'shampoo' you can buy; it's basically a pure liquid soap, which cleanses gently and efficiently and isn't packed with chemicals that you may not care to expose your scalp to on a regular basis.

- 10g (½oz) dried chamomile (for blondes), rosemary (for brunettes) or marigold (for redheads), depending on your hair colour
- 125ml (4fl oz) water
- 125ml (4fl oz) Castile liquid soap
- 1 tablespoon glycerine
- 2 drops essential oil to match the herb of your choice

Turbo-charging the power of Castile soap with different herbs can help maintain hair health and very, very subtly enhance your natural hair colour.

Use chamomile for fair hair, rosemary for dark hair and marigold for red hair.

Make a strong infusion (see page 213 for technique) of the herbs and the water. Then add to the liquid soap and glycerine in a plastic jug or bottle (a clean, empty shampoo bottle is ideal); drop in the essential oils and leave to thicken overnight.

Shake well and use like regular shampoo, and then, of course, rinse well after use. If you want to stick to your usual commercial shampoo, you can still boost its power with the herbal infusion.

HAIR-BOLSTERING BOTANICALS

If your hair is normal... try chamomile (for blondes), sage (dark hair), elderflower, fennel, horsetail, nettle and rosemary.

If your hair is dry or damaged... these herbs should help: marshmallow, comfrey, linden flower, parsley, sage (dark hair).

If your hair is oily... use lemon balm, lavender, peppermint, rosemary, yarrow or thyme.

TIP: Did you know raw egg works in place of shampoo? Wet hair, massage beaten egg into your scalp and hair, then rinse out with cool or warm water (but not hot, or you'll end up with a scrambled scalp...). Eggs are great natural shine-boosters.

HAIR MASKS
our award winners

Once a week. All year round. Without fail. That's our prescription for a shiny, swingy mop, whatever your hair type (unless you're lucky enough to have perfect hair). Whether you need to nourish dry ends, smooth frizz, tame flyaways or boost shine, masks can work wonders. Our testers slathered their way through dozens of natural formulas and awarded impressively high scores to the following tress de-stressers

OGARIO RESTORE AND SHINE HAIR MASQUE
✻
SCORE: 8.5/10
Beauty Bible fell in love with this mask when we discovered it at a Cosmetic Executive Women product demo evening. The brand comes from a North London hair salon, and the mask is a huge boon for hair – packed with avocado, olive oil, aloe vera, nettle and horsetail, together with sage (which is rich in vitamins A, C and E). Just a sniff of this rich, unctuous creamy mask perks you up – thanks to an essential-oil blend of lemon and lime, with a touch of lavender. Don't stint: as with many hair masks, more is more, so slather on generously and comb through for gleaming shiny, healthy hair.
COMMENTS: 'Gorgeous smell – lemony, citrussy, which is so very refreshing' • 'less frizz after using this product' • 'hair feels smoother and more manageable, and lasted longer between washes – I'm a bit lazy so if I can leave it for three days I will, and I could with this' • 'glossy, super-soft, lovely smelling hair after the treatment' • 'noticeably less frizz' • 'I loved the smell and could have kept my nose in the jar all day; just makes you feel as though you're being pampered' • 'I'd recently bleached and coloured my hair which left it slightly frazzled – this got it feeling like normal hair again, so thank you for sending me this wonder product' • 'a good, thick mask that delivered smooth, manageable hair – it dealt with the damage from constant straightening very well'.

AT A GLANCE
OGARIO RESTORE AND SHINE HAIR MASQUE

AVEDA SUN CARE AFTER-SUN HAIR MASQUE

LOUISE GALVIN NATURAL LOCKS DEEP CONDITIONING TREATMENT

KORRES ALMOND & LINSEED NOURISHING HAIR MASK

PHYTO PHYTOJOBA INTENSE HYDRATING BRILLIANCE MASK

AVEDA SUN CARE AFTER-SUN HAIR MASQUE
✻
SCORE: 8.19/10
This treatment is specifically designed to put back into hair what the sun, sea, salt (and chlorine) take out – in under five minutes. But our testers trialled this deliciously rich, intensive mask 'out of season', and found that it worked its reglossing magic in winter, too. (Fact: central heating dries out hair almost as much as the sun does – so we prescribe masks all year round.) Aveda's haircare has been a long-time leader that has consistently scored well with our testers since we started this series of books. This blends morikue protein (from Brazil nuts), tamanu oil, shea butter, coconut, sunflower and palm oils, plus natural antioxidants from green tea. (Plus, if you are going on holiday, the hand tube format is very travel friendly.)
COMMENTS: 'I was so impressed: this was easy to work through my very thick curly hair; gave fabulous gloss, curls softer, hair was less flyaway and more manageable: I could blow-dry it to smooth sleekness' • 'helped enormously to moisturise my brittle, dry, coloured hair – a definite winner' • 'made my fine, soft, can't-do-anything-with-it hair much easier to style, with more staying power' • 'as soon as I run out of this I'm buying more!' • 'my hair is very soft and fine – a nightmare – usually I can't even use conditioner on it, yet with this I found I could manage my hair very well indeed; my style seems to hold for longer

between washes, so I'm happy, thanks' • 'hair now in great condition – so shiny and healthy'.

LOUISE GALVIN NATURAL LOCKS DEEP CONDITIONING TREATMENT

✸✸

SCORE: 8.14/10

Louise Galvin's haircare performed incredibly well in our book *The Green Beauty Bible* – and here she goes again, wowing a fresh bunch of testers. Louise is a (second-generation) A-list colourist with a passion for the natural environment, reflected in her signature haircare line: this pump-action bottle dispenses a luscious blend of hair nurturers including vegetable proteins (from soya and wheat), sweet almond oil, fennel seed extract, plus honey (for extra silky softness), among other ingredients, all of which help to shield against environmental damage and leave hair naturally gorgeous. COMMENTS: 'Nice, clean fragrance and made my dry, coarse hair more glossy than usual' • 'this had a good de-frizz factor in a very humid summer' • 'made my hair very soft and silky' • 'after the second application this transformed my hair from straw-like to softer and much healthier' • 'I've used some natural products which made my scalp itchy and flaky, but this didn't – it's great, and has encouraged me to use other products in the range' • 'very impressed: it left my hair soft and natural – and I have frizzy, kind of Afro hair…'

KORRES ALMOND & LINSEED NOURISHING HAIR MASK

✸

SCORE: 8/10

This squeezy, recyclable tube of goodness is specifically targeted at dry, damaged hair, with (as the name implies) almond and linseed oils. More than that we can't really say, as the packaging is all Greek to us. (Not surprising, really, since this brand originated in an Athens homeopathic pharmacy – though it's now a global player in natural skin/hair/bodycare

and fragrance.) We'll leave it to our testers, then, to tell you what you really need to know. COMMENTS: 'I love to eat almonds and linseed: why shouldn't I want them to take care of my hair? I love how soft it feels after using this mask' • 'definite de-frizz factor – hair much less flyaway than usual' • 'it has a luxurious and expensive fragrance that leaves hair smelling like you've been to a salon' • 'gave hair a soft gleam that was really pleasing; after a gentle blow-dry, my hair was sleek, and stayed looking that way for days' • 'would recommend to anyone with frizz' • 'absolutely adored it: no other intensive conditioners that I've tried have got rid of my split ends like this did – can't imagine anything else that could be better'.

PHYTO PHYTOJOBA INTENSE HYDRATING BRILLIANCE MASK

✸

SCORE: 7.88/10

As the name suggests, this features lashings of jojoba oil to nourish and moisturise hair – and comes in a large tub, rather than a metal tube. The dominant ingredient, however, is angelica root extract, which helps to strengthen hair. Sweet orange oil restores shine and adds a fruity fragrance. The French Phyto range has become something of a cult with healthy-hair seekers since hairdresser Patrick Alès created it in 1969. Jacqueline Kennedy Onassis – whose hair was always gleaming and voluminous – was an early adopter of the Phyto range, apparently, helping the brand to fame in the US. COMMENTS: 'Comment from my mum: she loves it and her hair has "definitely lost the frizz factor"' • 'left hair feeling glossy and clean – and you don't need much' • 'hair looks glossier, less dull – it got rid of frizz completely' • 'smells gorgeous – very luxurious, like a high-end perfume' • 'damaged, brittle hair looks more youthful' • 'this kept my hair in a healthy condition without any build-up – I look forward to trying more products from this range'.

WE LOVE

Jo's become utterly devoted to the Ogario mask (featured left) for keeping her bleached-blonde hair super shiny. Sarah sloshes conditioner (Phylia de M, Ogario, Kai or Intelligent Nutrients) onto dry hair, wraps it up in a hot towel and leaves for some time. (She does the same with masks.) When the haystack rears its un-pretty head, she resorts to Ojon's Damage Reverse Restorative Hair Treatment, a solid oil that you melt in warm water and apply liberally – it never fails.

TIP: Even oily scalps need hair masks: simply avoid the roots and comb the product through the drier, 'older' hair and massage into split ends – which always benefit from an additional moisture boost.

STYLING PRODUCTS
our award winners

Even wannabe natural beauties don't necessarily want to go *au naturel* and abandon hairstyling products, in our experience. Although there aren't, as yet, that many almost-natural formulas, we put those that do exist through their paces fairly comprehensively, coming up with top suggestions for the various product options. (We really don't suggest you go in for your own trial and error: there were some absolutely dismal scores in this category, which don't make it to these pages)

BEST HAIR GELS
AVEDA BRILLIANT RETEXTURING GEL
✳
SCORE: 8.33/10

A seriously decent score for this flip-top tube of gel which, of course, has that wonderful, grounding Aveda scent to it. Natural ingredients include organic aloe, chamomile and calendula. It is recommended for medium to coarse hair and, as with all hair gels, you smooth it through wet or damp locks, then heat style or tousle dry.
COMMENTS: 'I seldom use a styling gel, thinking it will be too heavy, but this has made it much easier to manage my sometimes frizzy, over-processed hair, defining my style and giving shine' • 'really thrilled: this gave my hair the exact tousled look I like without making it sticky or rigid' • 'made it easier to achieve what my younger daughter calls a "windswept" look – I call it "body and texture"' • 'loved the fresh scent' • 'so impressed with the results: I blow-dried and straightened my hair as usual and I have to say it looked much improved' • 'feels natural, not hard and crisp like some gels'.

INTELLIGENT NUTRIENTS STYLING GEL
✳ ✳ ✳
SCORE: 7.19/10

The Intelligent Nutrients brand is created by Horst M Rechelbacher, the founder of Aveda, so its credentials are immaculate. Organically certified by USDA (see page 214), this features aloe, glycerine, agave extract, and some natural gums which are a wholesome replacement for petrochemicals. It also includes hair-protective antioxidants and some fab-smelling essential oils, including rosemary, cardamom, cinnamon, chamomile, lime and bergamot.

AT A GLANCE

BEST HAIR GELS

AVEDA
BRILLIANT
RETEXTURING GEL

INTELLIGENT NUTRIENTS
STYLING GEL

**BEST
VOLUMISING
TREATMENT**

AVEDA
PURE ABUNDANCE
STYLE PREP

BEST HAIRSPRAY

LAVERA
VOLUME & SHINE
HAIRSPRAY

**BEST
HEAT-PROTECTOR**

OJON
RARE BLEND
PROTECTING
TREATMENT

**BEST
FRIZZ-SMOOTHER**

AVEDA
SMOOTH INFUSION
GLOSSING
STRAIGHTENER

COMMENTS: 'Love this – truly a wonder for my flat, fine, lanky hair; adds bounce and fullness while leaving hair sleek, and "defines" my long bob, so I look like I've just stepped out of the hairdresser's • 'even by the second day my hair still has body and lift – fantastic stuff!' • 'pleasant, minty-cinnamon fragrance with a dash of citrus – wanted to eat it on an oatcake!' • 'really easy to work through hair, made it easier to style and delivered a good, gentle hold – a salon-type finish'.

BEST VOLUMISING TREATMENT
AVEDA PURE ABUNDANCE STYLE PREP
✳
SCORE: 7.17/10

This 95 per cent naturally derived product offers a boost to the fine-haired, featuring a strand-thickening formula of acacia gum, rice bran, acai oil, organic aloe and passion fruit. The fragrance gives off lovely whiffs of ylang-ylang and palmarosa. Aveda also include wheat amino acids and morikue protein for thermal protection. Massage into wet hair, or spritz to revive day-old dry hair, before styling.
COMMENTS: 'My limp hair was easier to style; it added lift and body – I would definitely recommend to friends' • 'what a difference: I raved about the volume to my hairdresser who tried not to tell me he'd told me so!' • 'had a defrizzing effect and hair was bouncy and voluminous – nothing short of miraculous, really' • 'made my hair less flyaway and static; gave more "guts" to blow-dry and added hold' • 'love the fragrance – wafts of fresh rosemary and geranium' • 'hair was shiny after use'.

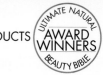

BEST HAIRSPRAY
LAVERA VOLUME & SHINE HAIRSPRAY
✹✹✹
SCORE: 7.43/10

From a long-respected, pioneering German brand, this hairspray – with organic bamboo, aloe vera and camellia extracts – is free from petrochemicals such as propylene glycol, a widely used ingredient for fixing hair. The pump action might take a couple of tries to get the correct dispensing technique which will give what Lavera call an 'extra-strong hold'. This natural hairspray takes a bit longer than usual to dry, Lavera say, so allow extra styling time.
COMMENTS: 'So simple to use: the container fitted in my hand and the spray worked each time with no clogging; misted onto hair for great hold all day with no sticky residue. Brushed out easily, too' • 'left hair with a lovely sheen' • 'pumps out a light mist, a cinch to use – not like a gloopy old-fashioned hairspray; natural hold – but enough for my fine, straight hair' • 'sprays evenly, gives a really healthy-looking shine and my style stayed put all day and evening' • 'my hair's heavy but this held the waves, and gave a light, natural gloss' • 'hold lasted all day in the heat'.

BEST HEAT-PROTECTOR
OJON RARE BLEND PROTECTING TREATMENT
✹
SCORE: 8/10

Hairdryers and straightening irons sure give hair a pounding. This lightweight mist helps to shield against some of heat's worst ravages, with a long list of natural ingredients including ginseng, honey (not sticky, we swear), lemongrass, Tahitian monoi, marula oil, kukui oil and Ojon's signature ojon oil. It does contain quite a few synthetics (including silicones), but since it's the only high-scoring heat protector, we felt it deserved a place.
COMMENTS: 'Very easy to apply; gave a lovely natural shine' • 'it was noticeably easier to run my fingers through my hair after first use; more than lived up to the manufacturers' promises and hair now in better condition' • 'took this on

---

TIP: To avoid exposing your hair to too much heat, get it as dry as possible before you start styling. Check out the Aquis Lisse microfibre towel: wrap it around your hair or use it to tousle-dry before styling; it absorbs an impressive amount of water, cutting out time with the dryer.

holiday to Spain and used it every day before going in the sun; really moisturised my curls – even though that's not what it's for!' • 'the scent reminded me of Guerlain Shalimar' • 'hair easier to style, for sure'.

BEST FRIZZ-SMOOTHER
AVEDA SMOOTH INFUSION GLOSSING STRAIGHTENER
✹
SCORE: 7/10

Frizz appears to be one of our readers' biggest bugbears (along with eye bags and nails that break easily). And now, a large section of the haircare industry is dedicated to keeping flyaways at bay. Of the more natural options, this offering from Aveda (and the third of the brand's winners here) is the one that performed best in our trials. It also works well to tame curls into soft waves, and has heat-protective powers (thanks to a hydrolysed wheat protein complex). Guar bean and plant-derived cellulose also feature, along with a smoothing 'plant infusion' – and as a base note in the aromatherapeutic blend, there's certified-organic sandalwood. Do also see the shampoos, conditioners and hair masks section (from page 166), as the panels reported good defrizzing results there, too.
COMMENTS: 'Made a big difference to the frizz factor' • 'I found it easier to blow-dry my hair, and it seemed to take less time than normal' • 'left hair less frizzy until the next wash, even in wet conditions' • 'very easy to use: just run through wet hair, which seemed to take less time to dry; great at defrizzing and I didn't have to use straighteners' • 'made hair soft and more manageable, not as frizzy, and more shiny' • 'brilliant: kept my hair dead straight even on humid, rainy days – usually when it gets damp, it will rebel'.

WE LOVE

Sarah won't travel without her ionic drier (see page 164) and John Frieda Volume Shine Airstyler, also ionic – to smooth and shine – allowing her to achieve a nearly salon-finish blow-dry at home with minimum effort and time. (She has recommended it to more friends than she can count.)

GLEAM TEAM

Home-made hair masks work a different way to conditioners: they're best applied before shampooing, left on the hair for a little while, and then washed out. Almost all of these are good enough to eat…

HAIR MASK FOR DRY HAIR AND SCALP

This will leave hair soft and manageable but isn't to be used like a normal post-shampoo conditioner: smooth it in before washing, leave on for 15 minutes (at least), and rinse well. It's great for coloured hair, too.

- 1 teaspoon avocado oil
- 1 teaspoon almond oil
- 1 teaspoon olive oil
- 1 egg yolk
- 1 tablespoon honey
- 1 teaspoon fresh lemon juice

Beat the ingredients together well, then massage into hair and scalp. Ideally, wrap your hair in clingfilm (it not only prevents drips, but the 'trapped' warmth of the scalp boosts the activity of the mask) and leave for 15 minutes. Shampoo and rinse well (you may need to shampoo twice) then condition as normal.

CLAY MASK FOR OILY HAIR AND SCALP

Clay has a gentle exfoliating and hydrating action that is good for dandruff or oily scalps.

- 3 tablespoons green clay or white clay (aka kaolin: for resource, see Directory on page 216)
- 1 egg yolk
- 1 teaspoon honey
- Water, to mix

Add the egg yolk and the honey to the clay in a bowl, and blend. Pour in the water drop by drop until you get to a mask-like consistency that can be massaged into the hair and scalp. Leave on for 30 minutes, and rinse before shampooing and conditioning as normal.

APPLE JUICE DANDRUFF BLITZER

Dandruff shampoos are harsh, medicinal and can be stimulating to the scalp, whereas we believe it should be soothed and calmed. Apple has an antiseptic action and you can use this as a rinse to help rebalance the scalp and tackle your dandruff problem.

- 1kg (2.2lb) fresh apples or 600ml (1 pint) bottled apple juice (no sugar)
- 600ml (1 pint) purified, mineral or tap water
- 125ml (4fl oz) apple cider vinegar
- 5 drops tea tree essential oil
- 2 drops lavender essential oil

Juice the apples (or take the bottled juice) and mix with the water. Add the vinegar and essential oils, drop by drop, and swish. Once you've rinsed and/or conditioned the hair, use this as your final rinse. Contrary to expectation, it doesn't leave your hair sticky!

BANANA MASK FOR ALL HAIR TYPES

Rich in vitamins and minerals, banana will soften and add shine to dry ends. NB: If you have long hair, you may need more yogurt.

- 2 tablespoons honey
- 75ml (3fl oz) natural yogurt
- 1 mashed banana

Mix the honey into the natural yogurt, then combine with the mashed banana to make a mask-like consistency. Damp your hair very slightly (not a complete drenching) and coat the hair with the mixture. Leave the mask on for up to an hour; then rinse, shampoo and condition as normal.

INVIGORATING MINT TEA RINSE

Why not drink a refreshing cupful, while you're at it? It is very uplifting.

- 2 large handfuls fresh mint leaves
- 600ml (1 pint) boiling tap, mineral or rain water

Pour the boiling water over the mint and leave to stew. When the liquid has cooled, strain the mint. Wash hair as normal and use the mint tea as a final conditioning rinse; comb while still wet and dry hair as usual.

TIP: Nasturtium is widely used by French herbalists for all kinds of scalp problems, from weakened hair to a scalp that's out of whack. Just make a simple decoction of the flowers, leaves and stems of the plant: take several really good handfuls, cover (just) with water and boil for 10 minutes. Strain and use the liquid as a final rinse.

Colour me
GENTLY

Globally, over half of women colour their hair; in the UK, it's an astounding 72 per cent, with men increasingly coming in on the act. It's a huge market worth billions but this really is beauty at a (potential) cost to health. However, natural strategies may help

We colour our hair. We have done for years and almost nothing would persuade us to change because we love the results. Jo has lots of blonde in her naturally dark hair – her mop is nearly as fair now as when she was a toddler – and Sarah has caramel and blonde tones in her dark hair, plus a 'permanent' tint to cover her partial grey.

And that tint is more likely to be the problem, according to research. Two of the most commonly used ingredients in tints – PPD (para-phenylenediamine) and PTD (para-toluenediamine) – are known contact allergens, which have 'excellent skin penetration qualities', according to consultant dermatologist Dr David Orton, a leading researcher. They may cause allergic eczema-type reactions – redness, itching and possible blistering of the face and scalp – also swelling and, rarely, hair loss. (One well-known actress of a certain age who habitually restored her auburn hair to its original colour told us the dye was responsible for thinning.) In rare cases, reactions including asthma, contact urticaria and anaphylactic shock have been reported.

However, the problem is not limited to PPD, which was first patented in 1883 and now features in up to 90 per cent of hair colours, with higher concentrations in darker colours. There are, in total, 27 chemicals listed as skin sensitisers in one report by the European Commission: 10 extreme, 13 strong and four moderate.

The number of people affected is tricky to establish. According to statistics from the European Academy of Dermatology and Venereology Conference 2013, one per cent suffers an allergic reaction. But, according to other data, the number suffering some adverse hair dye reactions is much higher.

In one UK questionnaire-based survey, nearly half the 1,800 subjects had used hair dye once or more, mostly women who had first coloured their hair around 25. Of those, 14 per cent reported eczema-type reactions, and three per cent said they had experienced swelling under the skin. Interestingly, most of the respondents coloured their hair blonde, or had highlights; fewer used dark brown or black dyes, which contain more PPD. (This reflected the ethnic mix of the respondents.) Over half had their hair coloured professionally.

Temporary henna tattoos, where PPD is added (sometimes 20 times the amount advised by manufacturers) to give a deeper black dye, appear to make users more likely to have allergic reactions to hair dye containing PPD. 'These tattoos are best avoided,' says Dr Orton.

Reduce the risks with natural measures

More people are dyeing their hair, they are starting much younger (16 was the average age in one Danish study), and the proportion of men is increasing. According to Dr Orton, serious hair dye reactions in children have now been reported. Although consumer self (patch) testing has been held out as the key safety measure for consumers, few people do it and theoretically it may increase the risk of sensitisation. The validity of the results is now considered so unreliable that the Scientific Committee on Consumer Safety (SCCS) may now recommend the current test is discontinued. Meanwhile, we have a few suggestions to reduce the risks:

Explore natural dye products: these won't give the same coverage for grey as PPD-containing products but are certainly worth trying if you have suffered a reaction. The website www.skinsmatter.com gives a list of brands offering natural dye products, warning however that some others going under a natural banner are not free of problem ingredients. (NB: Plants may cause reactions too, of course.)

Try the natural haircare and recipes in this book: they won't have the same effect as hair dyes but they will enhance the condition and appearance, which you might find is quite good enough.

Colour your hair with conventional products as seldom as possible: we know the temptation of keeping the colour fresh but try to limit colouring sessions to every six to eight weeks rather than every one to four. Fill in roots and soup up lights with a product such as Color Wow, a mineral powder-based brush-on powder that is very clever indeed.

Don't use hair dye to colour your eyelashes. Your eyes are precious and we have first-hand experience of allergic reactions.

If your hair is mostly grey, go with it. Consider growing out the grey and adding blonde lights, if necessary. (One friend has done this, having been 'red' for decades: the softer shade framing her face has taken off years and greatly enhanced her skin.)

Try this nutritional 'cocktail'. Dr Paula Baillie-Hamilton, a researcher into environmental chemicals, recommends the following measures to help protect against the risks of hair dye. About half an hour before your appointment, take extra antioxidant vitamins C (1g) and E (400iu) plus soluble fibre as psyllium husks (3g), in addition to your usual supplements. Take another 500mg vitamin C as soon as possible afterwards.

If you do have a reaction of any kind, seek medical help. Ask for patch testing to confirm the cause and to exclude an allergy to cross-reacting chemicals.

Watch out for new developments: at least one company (Wella Professionals) has been working on a formula which is 'significantly' less likely to cause an allergic reaction. And new patch tests may be available.

RINSE BRIGADE

Worried about chemicals in conventional dyes? These botanical washes encourage highlights in blonde hair and add depth to brunette shades

CHAMOMILE AND RHUBARB HAIR BRIGHTENER

Used once a week, this will keep the summer lightness in blonde hair or lift mousey shades.

- 25g (1oz) dried chamomile flowers
- 25g (1oz) rhubarb root powder (see method)
- 200ml (7fl oz) boiling mineral, purified tap or rain water
- 1 tablespoon olive oil

In a pestle and mortar or herb chopper, grind the chamomile flowers to a fine powder. Combine them with the rhubarb powder in a bowl. (To make your own, cut fresh rhubarb root crosswise into small pieces and spread on a baking sheet. Dry in a low oven (110°C/225°F for 2–3 hours. When cool, grind to a dust.)

Add the boiling water to create a paste, and then mix in the olive oil with a spoon.

Using clips or grips, section off your dry hair and smooth the paste from root to tip of each section. Wrap your hair in clingfilm and allow the treatment 45 minutes to work. Rinse thoroughly with warm water, then shampoo and condition.

TIP: Although lemon juice isn't great for hair condition, it's fantastic for creating highlights. Don't pour it all over: select some 'chunks' or big strands, and work a cotton pad dunked in lemon juice through to the tips. (Be careful not to get lemon juice on your scalp as it can burn in the sun.) If you use a mirror, you can work on the same streaks repeatedly for a sun-kissed effect.

SAGE DARKENING TREATMENT

It's hard to find a botanical, back-garden hair colourant that will cover grey hair – but this comes closest. Used regularly, it will gradually darken grey hair, although it won't ever cover it completely.

● 100g (4oz) chopped fresh sage leaves, or 50g (2oz) dried sage leaves
● 250ml (9fl oz) apple cider vinegar
● kaolin powder, to mix
● 1 egg yolk

To make the rinse, simmer the sage in the vinegar for 10 minutes and then strain while still warm. Allow to cool. Then using a tea strainer, or a sieve, sift in the kaolin until the mixture has a mask-like consistency.

Gradually beat in the egg yolk. If your hair tends to be dry and frizzy, you can also blend in 1 tablespoon of olive oil to the mixture, at this stage.

Using clips or grips, section off your dry hair and smooth the paste from roots to tip of each section. Wrap your hair in clingfilm and leave the treatment on for anywhere between 30 minutes and 1 hour. (A warm towel over the clingfilm can help speed up the treatment slightly.)

Rinse with cool-to-warm (but not hot) water, and shampoo and condition; use once a week.

ELDERBERRY RINSE FOR DARK HAIR

If elderberries are not currently in season, try the sage darkening treatment, left. Or freeze when plentiful.

● 3 handfuls elderberries
● 600ml (1 pint) apple cider vinegar

In a saucepan, add the elderberries and vinegar. Bring to the boil and simmer for 30 minutes. Remove from the heat; allow to cool before straining.

Use as the last rinse, after washing your hair. NB: You can also use leftover red or white wine for this recipe – if you don't always finish a bottle, keep a 'slop' carton and pour the leftovers into this for use in your hair rinse.

THAT DE-FUZZY FEELING

Shaving is the most common form of depilating legs and armpits, even bikini line, but there are other effective – and more natural – ways of removing hair (though we might pass on the ant egg oil for the moment…)

If you wonder whether you read that right – you did. In Asia and the Middle East, it appears that ant egg oil is a time-honoured natural way of preventing unwanted hair growth and reducing existing hair, dating back to the Ottoman Empire. It's still used today and is available online: we have not trialled it yet but who knows…? In some Indian communities, a paste of the golden spice turmeric, made with water or cream and sometimes also gram (besan) flour, is applied to facial hair. When the thick paste is removed, it apparently brings hairs with it. Other DIY remedies include a mask made with white of one egg, sugar (one tablespoon) and cornflour (half a tablespoon), which makes a thin mask that, when pulled off firmly, also pulls unwanted hair. (We haven't tried these either.)

There are, however, other better-known natural options, such as waxing, sugaring and threading. Many people claim that using waxing or sugaring long term, instead of shaving or depilatory creams, weakens hair growth so much it may eventually almost disappear.

WAXING This well-known and widely available method of depilation can be used on any part of the body or face. The wax mixture (which may contain synthetic chemicals) is spread thinly over the skin, then a cloth or paper strip is pressed firmly down and ripped off, bringing with it hairs embedded in the wax. It's very effective and because it removes hair at the root most people do not see regrowth for at least two weeks. It may, however, be tricky to get very short hairs to stick to the wax. But a new formula of wax, developed in Australia, offers a solution. Outback Organics, which offers organic after-waxing products, has launched Outback Gold, a peelable wax – actually a mix of beeswax, Brazilian pine resin and minerals – that incorporates a synthetic polymer (so not completely natural), which 'shrink-wraps' hairs as it dries. Therapists can remove even teeny stubborn hairs (this works, we have tried it). The technology means the wax can be used at lower temperatures, so it's much comfier, especially on the bikini line.

Some people wax at home but the majority is in-salon. By the way, if you ever see a therapist using a metal palette knife to apply the wax to your skin, shout 'No!' – because metal conducts the heat so efficiently, you may well get burnt.

SUGARING A warm (not hot) sticky paste of sugar, water and lemon juice is spread on the hairy area – again you can use it anywhere – and then pulled off. Apparently it's been in use since the 2nd century BC, probably using honey then. But the consumer debate about the merits of waxing versus sugaring is waged thick and furious online. The main difference is that sugaring fans say it sticks to the hair not to the skin, so is less painful and unlikely to irritate sensitive skin (although histamine reactions have occurred in some people, which can be prevented by taking an antihistamine). Many people make their own sugaring solution at home or buy at-home kits, using a strip to remove it, but professionals tend to use a rolling technique to remove the sugar.

THREADING Thought to have originated in India 6,000 years ago, this technique is becoming more popular in the West for facial hair removal. Having it done is fascinating: the therapist uses a thin cotton (or polyester) thread, which is doubled and twisted. Holding both ends, she (invariably it's a woman) rolls and loops the cotton, incredibly quickly, over the areas of unwanted hair, plucking out lines of hairs at the follicle level. The advantage for eyebrows is that, as opposed to waxing or sugaring, threading is said to give more control, so brows can be shaped precisely.

WARNING There are occasional reports of skin problems resulting from these methods. These are mostly sensitivity reactions, such as redness, irritation and/or soreness, but bikini waxes (and shaving) have led to serious infections.

Brazilian waxes may increase the risk of spreading infections such as sexually transmitted infections (STIs) and bacterial infections, caused by the waxing creating tiny skin tears in vulnerable areas that allow in bacteria. Always seek out a salon that uses fresh wax for each treatment.

Also, beware of waxing your face if you are using a topical product containing a retinoid because skin is extra susceptible to being burned.

If you wax or sugar your skin at home, be very careful to establish the correct temperature to heat the product and use a thermometer to confirm it. And, of course, always follow product directions to the letter.

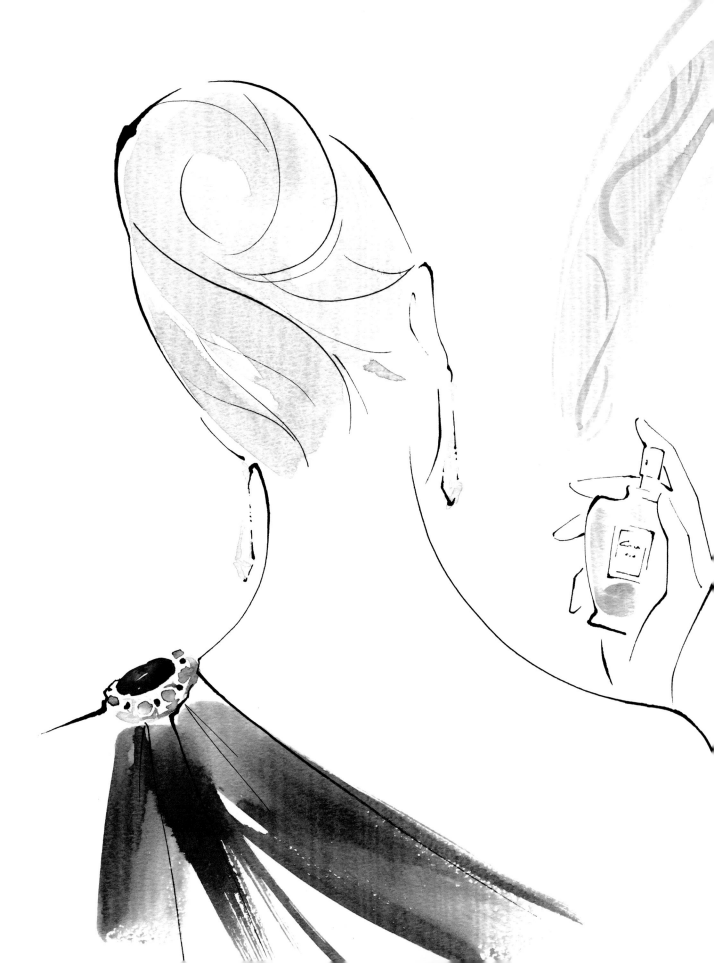

Naturally perfect
PERFUME

A spritz, a zoosh, a caress: discover the best 'natural'
scents from around the world – and maybe even
become a dab hand at creating your own

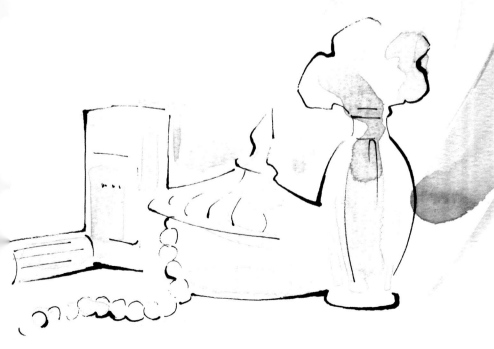

THE PERFECT
NATURAL SCENT FOR YOU

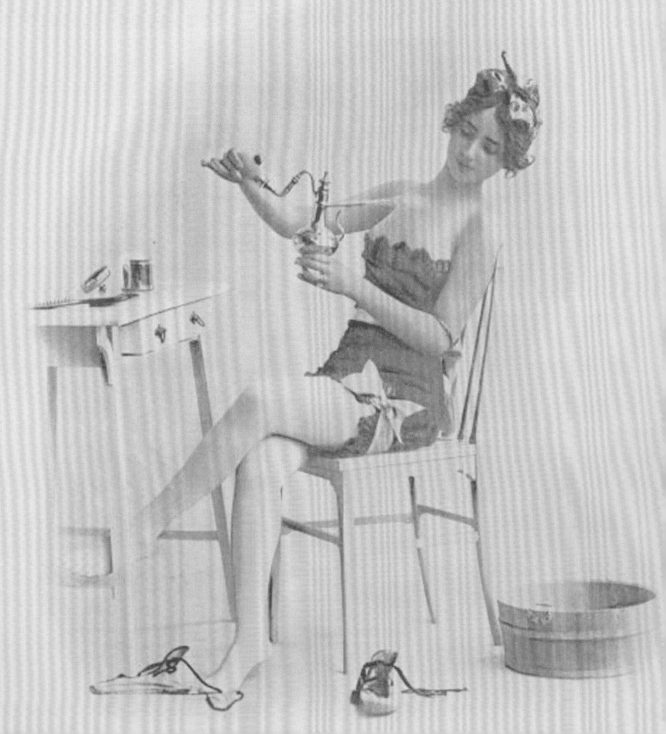

When you're looking for a new perfume, the same rules apply when you're choosing more natural scents as to the 'mainstream' fragrances which abound in every department store, every pharmacy, every Duty Free in the world. (Hard to find the more natural fragrances there, we'll tell you.) To avoid making mistakes – which equates to a waste of money, as that bottle languishes unworn on your dressing table – follow these simple guidelines

Most of the time now, most of us hurtle through life. Which is certainly not conducive to finding a new fragrance. In fact, choosing a new fragrance when en route from your desk to the school run, or in five lunch-hour minutes, is a recipe for disaster. So schedule in time to park, to stroll, then spritz, sniff, let it dry down, and sniff again…with each one you try.

● **Plan to shop in the morning, when your nose is fresh and the department stores are blissfully empty.** Do it at your leisure, just as if you were buying a book or music. Consider making a special expedition just to seek out a new perfume. (And if you're looking just for naturals, that may mean a pilgrimage to a large natural foods or organic store in a big city.)

● **Don't eat spicy foods or garlic the night before.** They can alter the nature of a scent on your skin.

● **Apply a totally unscented body lotion or oil to your arms/wrist, where you'll be trying the perfumes.** This gives fragrances something to 'cling' to; one of the downsides of natural perfumes is that they tend to last more fleetingly on the skin. Fragrance evaporates more quickly from dry skin; if you like to wear naturals, keep the skin you apply it to well moisturised.

● **Don't wear any scent** or even perfumed deodorant; they can clash with what you're sampling.

● **Wear a freshly washed T-shirt or other cotton top to shop in.** Fragrance clings to clothes and influences what you're smelling, and traces of the scent/scents you already wear will be detectable on cashmere jumpers, wool jackets or anything made of silk, in particular.

● **If possible, dress the way you'd dress to wear the type of scent you're searching for.** A long evening dress might be a challenge on a busy street (well, anywhere really) but you could take a gorgeous scarf and earrings with you.

● **Don't instantly start spritzing your skin.** Ask at the counter for special absorbent 'scent blotters', if they're not on display. Spray scents on to the blotters to establish which of them appeal to you at first whiff.

● **Smell a maximum of four fragrances.** The trick is to wobble the blotter under your nose; hold it at one end between your thumb and middle finger, and tap it lightly with your forefinger to make it vibrate. Whatever you do, don't ever feel pressured to make a decision because someone's breathing down your neck.

● **Once you've narrowed your choice down to one or two scents, try them on your skin.** Top American 'nose' Ann Gottlieb prefers the crook of the arm to the wrist, because even jewellery can distort a fragrance's smell. NB: Don't rub your wrists together after spritzing them; friction can alter the molecules of a fragrance, too.

● **Give the fragrance at least an hour to develop.** Fragrances traditionally have three 'levels' of notes – but where most of us go wrong is choosing on the basis of the first fleeting burst of a scent, or the middle notes (which unfurl after around 10 to 15 minutes). In fact, it's the base notes – which may not develop for an hour or two – which are ultimately what you'll live with. So walk away. Come back later, if you like the scent then.

● **If you're still in love with a scent after this, nip back another day and spray it all over.** It's the difference between wearing the dress rather than looking at it on the hanger.

● **Better still, ask for a sample and wear it for a few days.** Not all ranges include samples but it's worth trying. Get feedback from friends and loved ones, if it matters to you that they love what you smell like (we think it should).

● **Then, and only then – when you're truly happy – flex that credit card.** And if all this sounds laborious, just ask yourself: how many bottles have you bought, and fallen out of love with, almost faster than you can say eau de parfum?

EAU NATUREL

Switching to natural scents makes good sense, for some people. But new restrictions on the use of natural ingredients in perfume are putting 'natural perfumers' – and, indeed, the whole fragrance industry – under threat. Here's our rant…

As with cosmetics, there are different reasons women are drawn to 100 per cent natural fragrances. We may just love the idea that the ingredients in the bottle really did come from a Provençale rose harvest, rather than being synthesised in a lab – a feeling of being grounded in Nature when we use a perfume that's totally derived from plants, as it would have been for millennia.

Others are concerned about the cocktail of synthetic (artificial) chemicals in so many fragrances and fragranced products, some of which have been linked to a catalogue of health problems. These include headaches, respiratory problems, nausea, forgetfulness and loss of coordination; they may also act as hormone disrupters. For most people, however, it's unlikely that an occasional dab or spritz of scent will impact – and we like the idea of enjoying scent for 'special occasions', rather than splashing it on as an everyday commodity.

Ironically, another key health factor that may draw you to natural perfumes is the problem of sensitivity, which can manifest as rashes, itching, eczema, sensitivity to light, and so on. Artificial chemicals are recognised as culprits but many of the known 'allergens' in perfumes – which must now be labelled by international law – are naturals. You'll see warnings about limonene, geraniol and linalool among 26 potential allergens. Here's the thing: in their isolated form they can cause allergic reactions in susceptible people. But they also occur naturally in essential oils (much used in natural fragrances and fragranced products) where they do not have the same allergenic activity – and that is not taken into account by legislation.

A body called the International Fragrance Association (IFRA) sets the rules for perfume creators and manufacturers. Over the past 10 years, they've gradually reduced the levels at which several invaluable natural ingredients, such as oakmoss, vanilla and jasmine – which

Other than the allergens which must be listed by law, it's almost impossible to know what you're spraying, spritzing, dabbing or rolling on to your skin. The massive worth of the perfumery industry means that ingredients are Above Top Secret, as declaring them on the label would make it easy for anyone to produce a copycat No. 5 or Shalimar. In our recipe opposite, however, you know exactly what is in your Ravishing Rose Cologne.

are central to the magic of perfume creation – can be used. This has caused havoc in the perfume world and sent 'noses' into a tailspin. Some Very Famous Fragrances have had to be tweaked to meet the new guidelines. So, if you feel like your favourite fragrance has changed – yes, it may well have done.

Of course, we don't want people to suffer allergic reactions but some moves seem plain silly. An ingredient from citrus oil has been restricted – yet you get this all over your hands when you peel an orange and the zest bursts out. So what next: banning oranges? Jasmine, too, is restricted – yet we can brew and drink as many cups of jasmine tea a day as we'd like.

Happily, the cleverest people in the perfume world are figuring out 'workarounds', such as 'fractionation', a process that entails using a sort of centrifuge to separate the different components in a particular note (such as oakmoss), and then leave behind the 'safe', or non-allergenic part. That note is then different, though: as Guerlain's Thierry Wasser told us, 'fractionation leaves a hole'. When faced with that hole in oakmoss – the cornerstone of one of our favourite ever perfumes, Guerlain Mitsouko – Wasser had the idea of 'filling' the hole with a drop or two of celery. That sort of stroke of genius is why he is in-house nose at one of the most famous perfume houses in the world.

We do want the world of natural perfumery to have a future. Curiously, it's seldom the synthetic notes that are banned or the levels reduced. You might wonder if this whole process is driven by a sector of the perfume industry seeking to 'own' ingredients (like Monsanto wanting to 'own' the world's seed supply). And of course, they can't own or patent jasmine or bergamot, vanilla or oakmoss… crops that in many cases provide valuable incomes for communities in the developing world. If those livelihoods are threatened, that's important, too. And, in our book, a very good reason to dab naturally.

PURE DELIGHT

Alcohol is wonderful for extracting the fragrance from plants – as ancient perfumers knew. (And it's very sterile, ensuring that home-made colognes and scents don't go 'off'.) Alcohol is, in fact, still the main ingredient of most contemporary fragrances. Once you've experimented with the fragrances on these few pages, try similar recipes using the leaves and flowers of plants you love to create your own 'signature' scent, experimenting with essential oils to turbocharge the fragrance.

RAVISHING ROSE COLOGNE

- 100g (4oz) fresh, scented rose petals
- 50 drops rose essential oil
- 5 drops geranium essential oil
- 10 drops tincture of benzoin
- 600ml (1 pint) vodka
- 60ml (2fl oz) glycerine

Place the rose petals in a large glass container. In a separate jug, add the essential oils and the tincture of benzoin (which has a vanilla-ish fragrance) to the vodka and lastly add the glycerine. Pour over the rose petals. Shake daily for 3 weeks and distil into a beautiful bottle.

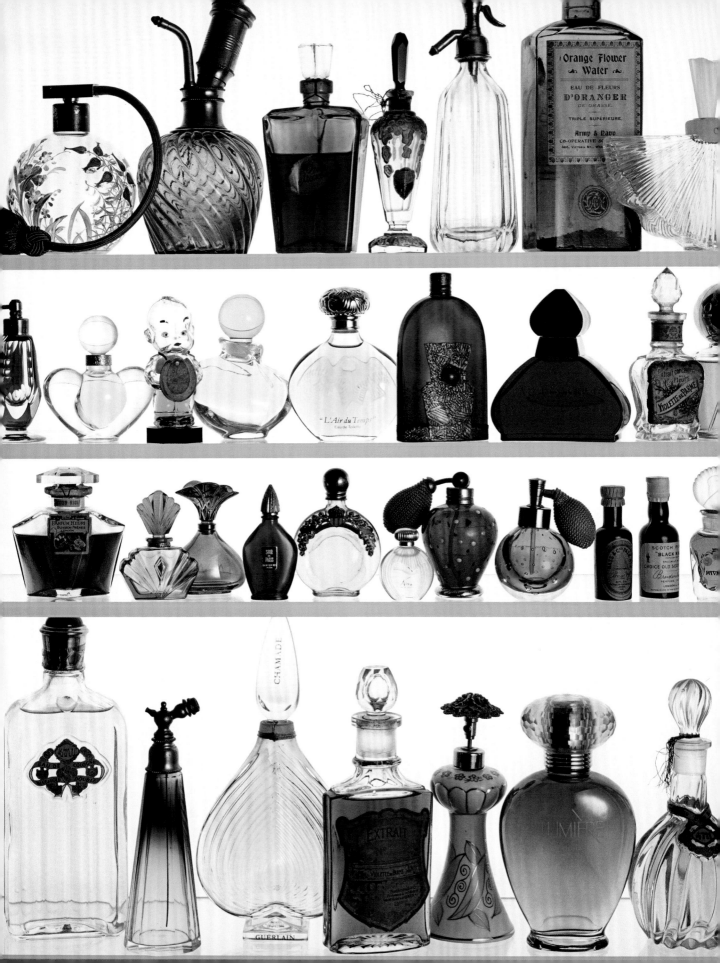

THE D-I-Y PERFUMER

Sometimes it's hard to find a scent that hits all the right notes, especially when it comes to naturalness. So why not create your own? Glenda Taylor is a leading aromatherapist and perfumer whose company Balm Balm specialises in blending unique fragrances – we're delighted that she has designed a selection of perfumes exclusively for *Beauty Bible*. You'll find a blend here for every occasion

According to Glenda: 'Essential oils are not recommended to apply directly on to the skin, so the blends featured here would work best in jojoba oil, or a very high-grade alcohol such as Absolut vodka. The blends give approximately 1ml of the fragrance ingredients, so add that to 10ml of jojoba oil or alcohol for eau de parfum.' (10ml is about a dessertspoonful, so increase the amounts in the same ratio, 1:10, if you want to make a little more.)

To put the strength into context, eau de parfum is usually a 7–15 per cent dilution; parfum itself can be anything from 15–40 per cent; while eau de toilette is 3–10 per cent.

Glenda continues, 'This recipe is much stronger than an aromatherapy blend as it's not intended for massage – just for pulse points. If you use jojoba oil, you will be creating what is known as a "perfumed oil", and this is absorbed very efficiently by the skin – so, again, use only on pulse points.'

There are now several brands of organic essential oils and we recommend you choose those to make your gorgeous perfumes. One supplier we like is Materia Aromatica which is certified by the Soil Association. NB: If you have any sensitivity to fragrance ingredients or essential oils, we don't recommend trying these. And beware of wearing any fragrance in the sun.

ROMANTIC
- 10 drops rose absolute essential oil ● 10 drops neroli
- 5 drops rose geranium

SENSUAL
- 3 drops ylang-ylang essential oil ● 7 drops jasmine
- 7 drops sandalwood ● 3 drops clary sage

or

- 10 drops rose absolute essential oil ● 10 drops frankincense
- 5 drops black pepper

UPLIFTING
- 10 drops grapefruit essential oil ● 10 drops lemon
- 3 drops rosemary ● 4 drops verbena

BREEZY
- 3 drops peppermint essential oil ● 15 drops bergamot
- 7 drops lime

SOOTHING
- 5 drops lavender essential oil ● 10 drops mandarin
- 5 drops petitgrain

or

- 10 drops frankincense essential oil ● 5 drops cedarwood
- 10 drops bergamot

CONCENTRATION BOOSTING
- 3 drops spearmint essential oil ● 12 drops grapefruit
- 10 drops bitter orange

MUM TO BE
- 10 drops mandarin essential oil ● 5 drops lime
- 10 drops lavender

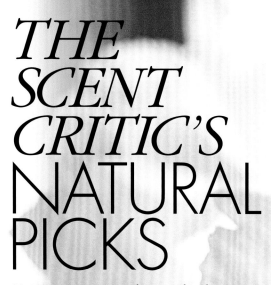

THE SCENT CRITIC'S NATURAL PICKS

Fragrance is Jo's thing. She has a scent blog, www.thescentcritic.com, and has also set up The Perfume Society with our friend, fragrance expert Lorna McKay. It's the first appreciation society that all perfume-lovers can subscribe to anywhere in the world (www.perfumesociety.org). So as someone who sniffs her way through thousands – literally thousands – of fragrances each year, who better to share her six all-time top natural scents…? (Look in our Directory for where to buy.)

4711 Eau de Cologne Did you know that one of the world's most famous eau de colognes is all-natural? It's zesty, so zesty: citrus-heavy, 4711 opens with tinglingly uplifting notes of bergamot, orange, neroli – and lemons so juicy they almost squirt straight out of the bottle into the eye. As the citrus softens, the aromatic heart of lavender and rosemary makes itself known. Like all colognes, it's short-lived – but the whole bliss of 4711 is that it invites you to keep splashing it on, to recapture the light freshness of the top notes throughout the day.

Bohemian Naturals: *Amber Rose* Perfume oils tend to last longer on the skin than liquids – and they've been having a bit of a 'moment' in perfumery, for just that reason. It's especially relevant with naturals, because many of the usual fixatives that 'tether' creations to the skin are synthetic. (These fixatives were often 'animalic' notes in the past – musk, castoreum, civet – but for obvious environmental reasons, those are a no-no now.) Bohemian Naturals was founded by natural perfume devotee Shannon Victoria, who moved from California to Edinburgh in search of adventure, and came up with a trio of scents. This is my favourite – a burst of zesty bergamot, giving way to hints of (yes) rose and amber, with tobacco leaf, too. It becomes warm and sultry on the skin: just bliss.

Neal's Yard Remedies: *Pure Essence Eau de Parfum No. 1 Frankincense* In a bottle that wouldn't look out of place next to Chanel No. 5, this may be a love-it-or-hate-it-scent for you: it all depends how you feel about frankincense – I adore its church-y potency. After the first whoosh of citrus – lime, bergamot, neroli and pink pepper – comes the heady frankincense, which then fuses with essential oils of patchouli and myrrh for a long-lasting (but not overpowering) sensual scent.

Honoré des Prés: *Chaman's Party* I'm a vetiver junkie – and this is a corker of a vetiver: pretty much that ingredient, pure and simple, from the first whoosh right through to the moment it fades into a Haitian sunset. (Haiti being the source for much of the world's vetiver – a particularly valuable crop for Haitians, post-earthquake.) Honoré des Prés is an exclusive French scent brand created by renowned perfumer Olivia Giacobetti, who's taken up the challenge of creating fabulous organic perfumes. This brilliantly captures vetiver's amazing earthy qualities: deep and dark, and blessed with excellent powers of endurance. For me, it's a love thing.

Strange Invisible Perfumes: *L'Invisible* SIP (as it's known) is an extraordinary fragrance line – though you may have to go to California to sniff it out. SIP is based on the too-cool-for-school Abbot Kinney Boulevard in Venice, Los Angeles, and is the creation of Alexandra Balahoutis, who calls herself a 'botanical perfumer'. She has a couple of dozen utterly sublime fragrances, based in organic grape alcohol, and wherever possible the ingredients are organically-certified and/or biodynamic, or at least wild-crafted. And this? An ethereal synergy of amber, moss, ylang-ylang and rose, described as the 'Little Black Dress' of the SIP collection. Gorgeous fresh/warm contrasts, and addictive on the skin.

Aftelier Perfumes: *Honey Blossom* Another California brand, from perfumer and author Mandy Aftel. (Her book *Essence and Alchemy* is a must-read for anyone interested in natural perfumery – or perfumery in any shape or form, actually.) This was a finalist in the US Fragrance Foundation's FiFi Awards, for Fragrance of the Year (Indie) – and no wonder: it's a lush, hypnotic floral garlanded with honeysuckle, almost drizzling with actual honey, thanks to notes of linden blossom and orange blossom absolute. Ambergris and benzoin then sneak in, giving delicious warmth. Again, you may need to source this perfume line when visiting the States – but for true natural scent-lovers, SIP and Aftelier Perfumes make it worth a California pilgrimage.

And one from Sarah, who loves Kai Perfume Oil, a warm, airy waft of tropical white flowers – led by gardenia – developed by the exotic Gaye Straza because she couldn't wear fragrance with synthetic chemicals. The first time Gaye wore it – on Manhattan's Madison Avenue – a beauty editor stopped her demanding to know where she could buy it. That led to a Kai range, with environmental fragrances, hair- and skincare – all heaven.

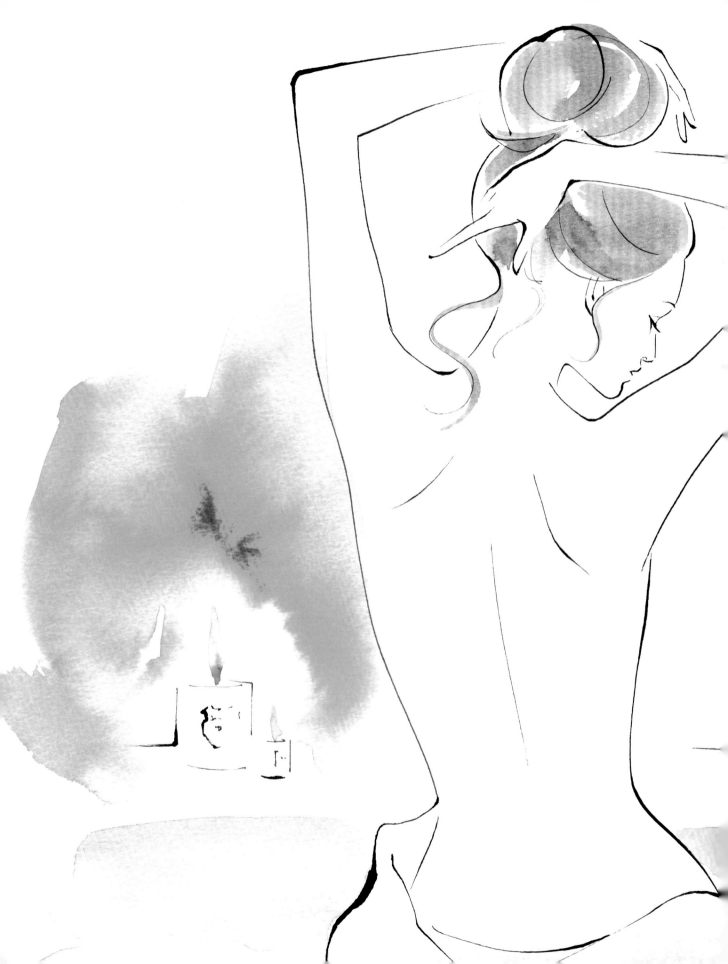

Dreamy
BATH AND BED

If you are anything like us, the rituals of bathing and caring for your body before bed are beauty's most pleasurable indulgences – and a signpost to restful slumber

SWEET ZZZZS

After decades of suspecting that lack of sleep accelerates skin ageing, scientists have finally proved what we knew from seeing our faces in the mirror every morning…

You know that look when you've had a good night's sleep? Plumper skin, wrinkles and lines ironed out to some extent, complexion (and eyes) brighter – not to mention your mood tends to be happier so you smile more, always a beautifier. Many experts hazarded that a major part of the complexion-enhancing effect of sleeping well was to do with nocturnal restoration and repair. But, until recently, no one had proved it.

Then, in 2013, research at University Hospitals Case Medical Center, Ohio (funded by cosmetics giant Estée Lauder) showed that 30 poor sleepers had more fine lines, uneven pigmentation and slacker, less elastic skin than a matched group of 30 good sleepers. 'Bad sleepers also recovered more slowly from sunburn, suggesting that you need sleep to repair skin damage, and their skin lost water 30 per cent faster than the good sleepers, so they were more prone to wrinkles and environmental damage,' our colleague Alice Hart-Davis reported in *The Times*.

Skin cells appear to operate on a 24-hour clock, protecting themselves during the day against the assault of environmental stressors – sunlight and pollution from outside and stress-provoked hormones inside – and then initiating repairs at night, when they can have a bit of peace and quiet.

But if you don't get enough sleep, your skin can't deal with the repairs. Plus the effect of sleep deprivation triggers the body into producing more stress hormones (adrenaline and cortisol), which have a profound effect on skin function. And if you are already stressed from your daytime occupations, that's a double whammy.

'There's a direct biochemical connection between psychological stress and the unwelcome signs of ageing, including lines, wrinkles, sags and brown spots. Stress also increases inflammation over the short term,' says Tom Mammone, executive director of research and development for Clinique Laboratories.

Inflammatory chemicals are linked to sensitivity, breakouts and other skin problems, and disrupt the skin barrier, weakening its defenses against UV rays and pollutants. Also, cortisol blocks the formation of collagen, the main protein responsible for keeping your skin toned and bouncy. The mantra? Less stress, more sleep – for your skin's sake.

HELP YOURSELF TO MORE BEAUTIFYING SLUMBER…

No argument, then: we need our sleep. But for about one in four people, particularly women, getting enough is tricky. Here are the natural strategies that help us and many others to slip into the land of Nod – and stay there

● **Avoid coffee as much as possible and always after tea time.** Don't drink any other caffeinated drink in the evening (tea, cocoa or cola) or eat chocolate (it contains caffeine and sugar).

● **Eat a light evening meal,** not too late; have a 10-minute stroll after.

● **Don't drink alcohol at night** or eat sweet puddings or hot sugary drinks, which agitate your brain.

● **Don't go to bed hungry either:** try a warm milky drink (almond milk is good, or full-fat organic) with grated nutmeg, cinnamon (about half a teaspoonful of each) and a small spoonful of Manuka honey.

● **Don't work or check your emails** or do anything that gets your brain whirring after 8pm (earlier if possible). You must give your brain time to wind down and switch off, especially if you are a worrier.

● **'Ground' your brain** by massaging a little oil into (washed) feet before bed, advises Ayurvedic doctor Thomas Mueller.

● **We also like detox foot patches,** which come in a version for sleep and work for us. They are based on traditional Chinese medicine and are used widely in Japan too, although Western doctors are sceptical. And we love soft, loose bed socks on a chilly night.

● **Keep your bedroom completely dark** – use an eye mask or blackout blinds if needed.

● **Make sure your bedroom is slightly cool,** around 16–18°C (60–64°F).

● **Decorate in soft pastels,** which are restful and less stimulating than bright colours.

● **Try pillow mists** scented with calming herbs such as lavender, or tuck a lavender bag in the pillowcase.

● **Banish electrical equipment** including TVs and computers from the bedroom; try turning off all electrics at the wall. (Sarah discovered that she is mildly electrosensitive – sleeping temporarily in her office with three computers, two phones and several chargers completely flattened her batteries.)

● **Invest in a good bed,** with a mattress that suits your body, and comfortable pillows to avoid neck ache. (We like soft feather ones, and carry them with us when we stay away.)

● **The sleep hormone melatonin is** switched on by darkness, off by light. So work with your natural rhythm by turning down lights as the evening goes on. Flooding our brains with electric light at night isn't natural. (See box below for new research.)

● **Aim to be in bed by 10pm at least two nights a week** so you won't get overtired and build up a sleep debt. In fact, you'll probably bound out of bed at 6am carolling along with the dawn chorus.

● **Have a warm bath with aromatherapy oils.** See Relaxing Bath Treats (page 200).Keep a large glass of water by your bed, and a notepad and pencil. Pop a few drops of Bach Rescue Remedy (flower essences) in the water; we also like Relaxing Essence by A. Vogel.

● **If you can't get to sleep, or wake in the small hours, have a strategy.** If you are worried or have a brilliant thought, scribble it down (don't turn the light on, though). Then lie flat, put on an eye mask if you have one (a lavender pillow is perfect, see page 98), put one hand on your chest, the other on your tummy and breathe slowly, following your breath. In your mind's eye, 'see' something you love (a place, a person, a pet); if worries intrude, return to your breath and visualisation.

● **Consider natural remedies:** homeopathic arnica helps calm your mind effectively. Herbal remedies include valerian, best combined with ashwagandha, according to Sebastian Pole from Pukka Herbs.

BLUE ALERT

Scientists now say that, at night, blue wavelengths – the type that light our computer screens and are also emitted by low-energy light bulbs – disrupt sleeping patterns by suppressing melatonin. They're fine in the daytime, boosting attention and concentration, but a no-no in the evening for poor sleepers.

● So avoid looking at bright screens for two or three hours before bed: simply turning down the brightness helps or try the free f.lux programme (www.justgetflux.com).

● Use pink- or red-tinted bulbs to read books (instead of tablets).

● If you work at night and/or use a lot of electronic devices, consider blue-blocking glasses. (Search for amber glasses online.)

● Expose yourself to lots of bright light during the day; this boosts your mood and alertness then, and helps you sleep well.

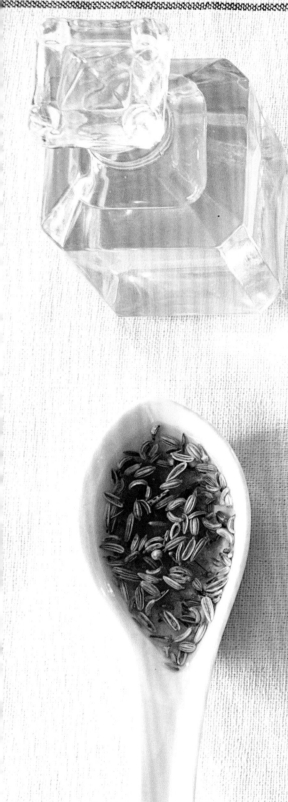

SMOOTH OPERATORS

Whether you choose a gentle or more vigorous scrub, these will leave your skin revitalised and baby soft

SUGAR-SWEET BODY SCRUB

A sugar scrub is a gentle alternative to the salt version – and as gardeners, we like it because it doesn't sting when we've scratched ourselves pruning the roses!

- 150g (5oz) golden granulated sugar, or white for a lighter-coloured scrub
- 25g (1oz) dried fennel seeds
- 375ml (12fl oz) sweet almond oil
- 20 drops sweet orange essential oil
- 5 drops ylang-ylang essential oil
- 5 drops patchouli essential oil

Mix the sugar and the fennel seeds in a bowl. Then pour into a large, sealable jar.
In a jug, add the essential oils to the sweet almond oil and pour over the sugar mix. If you need to, you can add more sweet almond oil to top up the jar. How much you need depends on the size of sugar granules.

You can vary the fragrance according to your favourite essential oils, adding a total of up to 50 drops of essential oil altogether (this particular blend is pretty warm and sexy).

Use scoopfuls in the shower or bath, and massage into skin in a circular motion. Delicious… Rinse or shower off.

LAVENDER AND SALT BODY SCRUB

- 150g (5oz) salt (use any grainy salt – Maldon, crystal, sea salt, kosher or Dead Sea salt)
- 100g (4oz) dried or fresh lavender flowers
- 375ml (13fl oz) sweet almond oil
- 25 drops lavender essential oil

Blend the dry ingredients and place in a sealable jar (preserving or pickling jars are perfect). Then pour the oil over them. Depending on the type of salt you use, you may need to add a little more oil to top up the jar. Use by the handful, applied in circular strokes everywhere except the face, which is way too fragile.

RELAXING BATH TREATS
our award winners

The simple act of having a warm bath before bedtime can gently aid the falling-asleep process: the body cools down naturally afterwards, regulating blood pressure and relaxing the brain. (Some experts advise running cool water over feet and legs to ensure this.) And infusing the water with oils known to have a soothing, calming effect turbo-charges that action. We're aromatherapy-bath-aholics ourselves, but any stressed, overtired woman – any woman, actually! – deserves to treat herself to one of these high-scorers, we think. (Take that as permission…)

GREEN & SPRING REPAIR & RESTORE BODY & BATH OIL
❋❋
SCORE: 8.67/10
Green & Spring's 'home' is the gorgeous Cotswold boutique hotel Cowley Manor, where this luxe sense-soothing range is incorporated into treatments at the C-Side Spa. You can recreate some of that blissful pampering at home with this oil, which features a blend of bergamot, lemon myrtle, orange, chamomile and lavender. We would say it's an 'adaptogenic' blend and find it perks us up when we're flagging, or calms us when we're frazzled. It also doubles as a body oil.
COMMENTS: 'Lovely natural fruity, floral aroma: I felt calmer just sniffing it' • 'skin felt lovely and smooth afterwards; knees and elbows were particularly improved after just one bath, and I didn't have to use moisturiser afterwards meaning I could get to bed quicker' • 'quite pricey but worth the cost and would make a lovely gift' • 'if I have a bath it's usually because I'm pooped, down in the dumps or stressed – all definitely applied the times I used this, yet I came out feeling like my own best friend, more confident and content with the world' • 'mmmm, a lovely fresh but calming fragrance, makes you feel human again' • 'this

AT A GLANCE

GREEN & SPRING REPAIR & RESTORE BODY & BATH OIL

NEOM TRANQUILLITY BATH FOAM

TISSERAND SIGNATURE BLEND RELAXING LUXURY BATH SOAK

AROMATHERAPY ASSOCIATES RELAX DEEP BATH & SHOWER OIL

AROMATHERAPY ASSOCIATES INNER STRENGTH BATH & SHOWER OIL

can only be 10/10 because I can't think of any way it could be improved' • 'I want more!'

NEOM TRANQUILLITY BATH FOAM
❋❋
SCORE: 8.57/10
If you prefer to bubble your troubles away (and isn't there just something so indulgent about a bath with bubbles?), start with this. Unlike many foaming baths, however, this avoids the use of notoriously irritating sodium lauryl sulphate in a much skin-friendlier formulation that incorporates aloe leaf, marsh mallow and sweet almond oil, together with a fragrant blend of English lavender, jasmine and sweet basil. Almost every tester reported better sleep.
COMMENTS: 'Lovely natural lavender smell; greatly improved sleep' • 'bubbles up brilliantly – most impressive for a natural bath foam' • 'bath was sparkling afterwards!' • 'love that I can still get the bubbles I love but without SLS/SLES' • 'went to bed early and slept through the night – a real improvement, and it was a treat to trial this product' • 'helped me nod off to sleep; a little goes a long way, too' • 'skin felt silky afterwards' • 'before bath: overtired, worried, slightly nauseous. Post-bath: gently tired, more relaxed, refreshed; I'd use the product every day if I could'.

TISSERAND SIGNATURE BLEND RELAXING LUXURY BATH SOAK

✳

SCORE: 8.56/10

This is definitely at the lower end of the price spectrum compared to the other winners, so for a 'beauty steal', look no further. The calming fragrance is based around lavender, bergamot and orange blossom, while extracts of linden flower (to soften skin) and melissa (for deep cleansing) also feature.

COMMENTS: 'Really like the lavender, bergamot, minty smell of this' • 'without a doubt, I felt miles better after this bath – I really did – much happier' • 'feels luxurious, smells nicer than other foam baths and creates lots of bubbles, too' • 'after my bath I had a really deep, undisturbed sleep' • 'had one of the best night's sleep for quite a while – I wasn't going over the day's events, which normally happens after a stressful day' • 'skin felt cleansed, soft, and no need for body lotion' • 'I closed my eyes and could imagine standing in a lavender field on a hot day in June'.

AROMATHERAPY ASSOCIATES RELAX DEEP BATH & SHOWER OIL

✳✳

SCORE: 8.4/10

We'd probably have had to give up work and retire if this oil – and the Inner Strength featured next – hadn't made it to the final line-up. But happily, the *Beauty Bible*'s testers clearly 'got' the exceptional relaxing power of these two bath oils, which are among our desert-island must-haves. Relax Deep blends vetiver, chamomile and sandalwood in such high quantities that it's like knockout drops. Forensic readers will know we've featured this wonder oil before, but it went to a new bunch of testers who appreciated its magic all over again.

COMMENTS: 'Followed the instructions and used it as a pre-shower treatment and it was absolutely fabulous: showered off easily but left skin feeling wonderful and filled my bathroom with the most amazing smell, which seemed to linger – I'd walk into the bathroom simply to inhale the gorgeous fragrance' • 'filled the whole bathroom with a zen-like fragrance' • 'a calming, relaxing smell and I did sleep better' • 'the only way to explain this is that it made me feel very happy (odd, I know!). I've now decided to use this every Friday to kick-start the weekend' • 'my daughter came home with a headache; I told her to use this. Half an hour later, the headache was gone – and she fell asleep as soon as her head hit the pillow. Will have to hide this' • 'a little goes a long way' • 'I would like to be bathed in this all the time'.

AROMATHERAPY ASSOCIATES INNER STRENGTH BATH & SHOWER OIL

✳✳

SCORE: 8.11/10

Inner Strength is something very special: Aromatherapy Associates founder Geraldine Howard created this blend to deliver some much-needed fortitude when she was undergoing cancer treatment. Most of us need fortification in today's busy world – and this does the job beautifully, fusing clary sage, frankincense, cardamom, rosemary, geranium and vetiver. It's new to our testers, new to this book – but will, we believe, become as much of a classic as Relax Deep. And 10 per cent of the proceeds will be donated to the Defence Against Cancer Foundation which is helping pioneer a new cancer vaccine treatment.

COMMENTS: 'It worked to soothe and get me to sleep and I really enjoyed my zeds after this' • 'I love this and will definitely buy it as my treat' • 'made my house smell gorgeous after just one bath' • 'luscious bath oil; I open this just to smell it and asked my mum to smell the wonderful oils – I'd recommend it 100 per cent to all women' • 'knackered and fed up before, but afterwards I was clearer-thinking and slept better, so I've used this a lot'.

WE LOVE

The Aromatherapy Associates blends included here feature in Jo's top-five beauty products ever. But she also loves Selexir Peace Bath – rich in magnesium chloride salts – and slooshes a good squirt of Life-Flo Magnesium Gel in the tub with almost any bath product. Another massive fave is This Works Deep Sleep Bath Soak. Selexir Peace Bath is Sarah's favourite in Dorset (brilliant for soothing aches after mucking out) as the eccentric plumbing can't cope with oils. Or it's Relax Deep, Ren Moroccan Rose Otto Bath Oil or her new 'addiction' Kneipp Sleep Well Herbal Bath with Valerian & Hops, a real steal, too.

SO SPA, SO GOOD

Create the Zen calm of a luxury spa in your own home with these fragrant, skin-pampering bath bags and tonics – just add candles and a glass of wine

PAMPERING BATH BAGS

With these bath treats you can experiment with different 'bulk' ingredients alongside the herbs below; use a total of around 50g (2oz) of herbs and/or other ingredients per bag.

Oatmeal is a very gentle ingredient and has a calming effect, but it's not the only skin-friendly possibility. Ground almonds or dried milk powder can also be added to the herbs and petals, or for a powdery sweet fragrance try dried orris root (from the root of the iris plant). You can even add polenta.

And don't only use the bags to fragrance the water; rub the muslin or cheesecloth over your skin to exfoliate, or apply the herbs topically to really maximise their benefits. Here are some other effective bath-bag combinations – have fun experimenting.

● Rose and lavender for a sensual soak. (Use fresh or dried lavender and rose petals.)

● Rosemary, bay, basil, thyme, sage and lemon verbena all invigorate a tired body and a weary mind.

● Peppermint and lovage are naturally deodorising and can be blissfully cooling in hot weather.

● Lime flowers, chamomile, lemon balm and valerian soothe and relax at bedtime.

● Grated ginger works wonderfully on aches and pains. Strawberry leaf, burdock and chamomile are also good.

● Peppermint, thyme, dandelion and sage are excellent for purifying blemished or oily skin on the body.

● Myrtle is good for cellulite and/or for toning slack skin.

ELDERBERRY BATH TONIC

Elderberry has a stimulating and tonic effect, and is soothing for inflammations, too.

● 110g (4oz) elderberry leaves and fruits
● 900ml (1½ pints) mineral, purified tap or rain water
● 10 drops rose essential oil
● 4 drops rose geranium essential oil

Add the water to the chopped leaves and berries in a pan and bring to the boil. Simmer for 5 minutes, then remove from the heat and allow to cool thoroughly.

Drop the essential oils into the bottom of a sterilised bottle, then strain the herb liquid through a funnel lined with muslin or kitchen towel into the bottle.

Add a cupful to the bath when you need a pick-me-up. Keep the bottle in the fridge.

HOW TO MAKE BATH BAGS

Trace a large circle – around 25cm (10in) across – onto muslin or cheesecloth, or any other sheer fabric, and cut out with scissors. Crush the herbs slightly to release their potency, then heap them in the middle of the bag and tie it up with a 45cm (18in) piece of ribbon. (Plain coloured raffia or rough string also look pretty.)

The bags can either be tossed in the tub – or, for best results, the ribbon should be tied around the tap so that the rushing water pours through the herbs, to fill the bathroom with fragrant steam. Once you're in the bath, let the bag soak in the water. After use, the bags can be untied and the contents left in the sun to dry, retied and used once or twice again. (On the second and third times, you can add 2–3 drops of essential oil; just be sure to choose one to match the herbs in your bag.)

TIP: Milk makes an ideal additive for itchy, scratchy or dry skin; add up to 1 cup of fresh (or dried) milk to your bath water. Milk is also great for dispersing essential oils: mix in 4–5 drops of your favourite fragrant oil into a cupful of milk (or cream) then swoosh into the water.

ROSE PETAL BATH OIL

This wonderfully luxurious oil is, quite simply, balm for the senses. The only downside is cleaning the tub afterwards: just swish with the shower and the petals will collect in the plughole, where they can be easily scooped out. Trust us, it's worth it.

- 125ml (4fl oz) rose water
- 1 tablespoon sweet almond oil
- 5 drops rose essential oil
- 75g (3oz) loosely packed rose petals (from any kind of rose bush, but this must, of course, be unsprayed – and scented roses are preferable)

In a bottle, combine the rose water with the sweet almond oil and then add the rose essential oil, drop by drop. Pour this under running taps and throw the rose petals into the bathwater. You can, of course, dry rose petals in summer to enjoy this bath all year round; the best roses to choose are Gallica roses (*Rosa gallica officinalis*), as these hold their fragrance even when dried.

UPLIFTING BATH TREATS
our award winners

Maybe you've got the blues. Or the 'blahs'. It's the sort of morning when you choke on your vitamins – or your get-up-and-go has got-up-and-gone. Can we suggest you follow our lead and rather than opt for a caffeine fix, why not try an uplifting bath or shower treat, instead? Essential oils truly have the power to make us feel calm, revived and our skin smooth. But as our testers found, not all uplifting bath goodies are created equal. (We trialled nearly 30 products in this section.) These five, however, will leave you feeling bathed in glory

SRANROM AWAKENING VITALITY BATH & MASSAGE OIL
✳✳
SCORE: 8.88/10

We can almost hear you saying this: 'Who...?' Well, Sranrom is an aromatherapeutic range 'for stressful living' which we believe deserves to be on more people's radar. (Jo swears by spritzing their aromatherapy mists in the *Beauty Bible* office when we can't knuckle down to the task in hand.) You say it 'sa-raan-rom' – a poetic Thai word used to describe feelings of pleasure, serenity and contentment – chosen as a name for their range by two young Thai career women. Here, they blend zingy lemongrass and kaffir lime in an exotic revitalising blend to slosh in the bath or massage into skin, to nourish it with aloe vera and moringa oil.

COMMENTS: 'I woke up feeling tired and achy, but once I opened the oil I experienced a gorgeous citrus scent which made me instantly want to smile. I just felt so awake after using it; muscles less tense – and I was ready to get up and go, and so much happier in myself' • 'a joy to use; skin felt softer and had a smoothness to it – didn't need to use a body cream' • 'loved the citrus, lemongrass scent; smells very natural, luxurious and expensive' • 'my limbs felt all

AT A GLANCE

SRANROM AWAKENING VITALITY BATH & MASSAGE OIL

LUCY ANNABELLA ORGANICS DATE NIGHT ORGANIC BATH MILK

ESPA RESTORATIVE BATH OIL

L'OCCITANE AROMACHOLOGY REVITALISING BATH & MASSAGE OIL

AROMATHERAPY ASSOCIATES REVIVE MORNING BATH & SHOWER OIL

refreshed and less tired after using this' • 'I was awake and energised after using this product' • 'my skin is normally tight after a bath, but it felt smooth and moisturised with this'.

LUCY ANNABELLA ORGANICS DATE NIGHT ORGANIC BATH MILK
✳✳✳
SCORE: 8.43/10

We're so delighted for Irish aromatherapist Colleen Harte that this 'hero' product from her range has so impressed our testers. It turns the waters milky, suffusing them with a sensual but awakening blend of patchouli, ylang-ylang, mandarin, palmarosa and nutmeg, in a skin-softening base of argan, coconut and soya oils. This 'organic luxe' range is gorgeously packaged, too. An all-round treat.

COMMENTS: 'Felt refreshed but relaxed; effect lasted most of the day' • 'put me in the right mood and gave me a real boost that was still with me by evening' • 'a really lovely bath milk. I have dry skin and always have to use body lotion, but with this there was no need – my skin was like pure silk' • 'I couldn't stop smelling the bottle – so uplifting' • 'the aroma is absolutely beautiful – a lovely, indulgent product' • 'I felt a bit more flirty – but don't know if that's because of the name!' • 'best bath oil I've used – this is going on my Christmas wish list' • 'frazzled before, then turned into a perky princess!' • 'the scent filled the whole house – my other half loved it, and the smell on my skin lasted for hours after I'd dried off'.

ESPA RESTORATIVE BATH OIL

❋

SCORE: 8.36/10

A real classic from the ESPA range that long ago was nicknamed by the press 'a hug in a bottle'. Because it's heavy on the lavender – which will 'adapt' to your needs, waking you up when tired or soothing you when frazzled – this bath oil could equally well have been trialled in our 'relaxing' category. But testers in need of oomph responded to the rebalancing effect delivered by sweet orange, geranium (and, of course, that lavender), in a sweet almond oil blend which helps skin regain its natural supple smoothness.

COMMENTS: 'Totally love this – it has an instant uplifting effect on the spirit' • 'did reinvigorate and have a reviving effect' • 'bath was easy to clean afterwards – some oils can leave a greasy tidemark around the tub' • 'skin still felt good next morning – and the smell is amazing: I felt like I had a spa in my bathroom!' • 'lifted my mood and made me feel happy' • 'made skin feel soft and look great'.

L'OCCITANE AROMACHOLOGY REVITALISING BATH & MASSAGE OIL

❋

SCORE: 8.29/10

Most of the high-scorers in this category are packaged in glass, which makes them unsuitable for travel. But L'Occitane's winning contender comes in a handy flip-top bottle, dispensing an aromatherapeutic, reviving blend of rosemary, mint and pine. (Men happily borrow this, we've found.) Use it to anoint your body – skin just loves the blend of apricot,

grapeseed, borage and sallow thorn oils – or, as our testers did, sloosh it into the bath.

COMMENTS: 'Very pleasant to use in the morning before a busy day and then in the evening to get into the spirit of going out' • 'gentle uplifting properties' • 'we used this as a massage oil, too, and found it sunk in beautifully (my husband was sceptical but liked the fact he didn't smell "girly" afterwards)' • 'skin very soft; didn't need moisturiser' • 'asked my sister to test this as I don't have a bath – her feedback was really positive, so much so that she's asked me to buy her another for her birthday'.

AROMATHERAPY ASSOCIATES REVIVE MORNING BATH & SHOWER OIL

❋ ❋

SCORE: 8.17/10

There is nothing – nothing on earth – we can do to influence the scores our testers give to products submitted to our trials. But we'd be lying if we didn't say we had our fingers crossed when we dispatched this long-term favourite of ours: the entire *Beauty Bible* team is devoted to Aromatherapy Associates oils. The 'refreshers' here are grapefruit, rosemary and juniper oil; eucalyptus and peppermint also feature. As the name suggests, it can enliven a shower – simply massage into your skin beforehand – or add a capful to the bath. That's truly all it takes – which is just one of the reasons our testers loved this as much as we do.

COMMENTS: 'Tired and lazy before my bath; felt uplifted and "lighter" after – great before an evening out' • 'expensive but worth it as you only use a small amount' • 'made me feel energised; I made the mistake of using it before going to bed one night and didn't get to sleep until 3am – so it really works!' • 'I always feel grumpy in the morning but less so with this' • 'it's my birthday next month and this will definitely be on the must-have list' • 'I'm a new mum – first baby – and this really helped on the days I could find time for a bath!'

WE LOVE

We've raved about them before. We'll rave about them again. The bath oils from Aromatherapy Associates (see Revive Morning, reviewed left), feature right at the top of our list of desert-island must-haves. (Along with This Works Energy Bank Bath & Shower Oil, which features a similarly powerful blend of essential oils.) We love the pretty packaging, too.

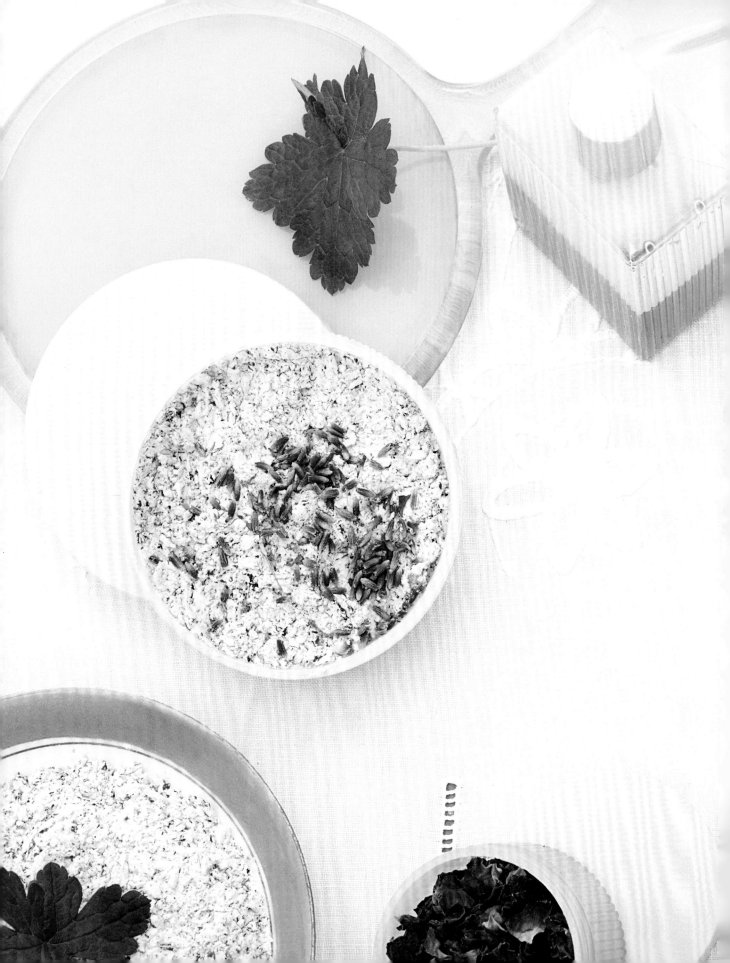

POWDER WOW

These body dusting powders look so pretty with their colourful flecks of rose, lavender and geranium – and smell heavenly, too. You'll wonder why you've never made your own before

ROSE PETAL AND LAVENDER DUSTING POWDER

A recent study found an increased risk of ovarian cancer in 20–30 per cent of women who used talcum powder for 'intimate personal hygiene'. The increased risk is tiny but we like to avoid it. Happily, we've found that botanical alternatives are just as effective.

- 110g (4oz) corn starch
- 55g (2oz) baking soda
- Approx. 25g (1oz) dried lavender flowers
- Approx. 25g (1oz) dried rose petals
- 2 drops lavender essential oil
- 2 drops rose essential oil

To make this recipe, put all the dry ingredients in a food processor and whizz until they produce a fine powder. (The lavender and rose petals will become tiny coloured flecks in the powder.)

Add the essential oils drop by drop and blend again; these enhance the fragrance. Then, using a sieve, shake the powder into a clean container, as if you were sifting flour, until it becomes a fine, soft texture.

Dust onto the body with a big fluffy powder puff (like your granny used to use). Alternatively, decant into a sugar shaker, and 'sift' onto skin after a bath.

ROSE GERANIUM BODY POWDER

- 75g (3oz) corn starch
- 12 fresh, scented geranium leaves, washed and dried (our favourite is called Attar of Roses)
- 1 drop rose essential oil
- 2 drops rose geranium essential oil

Put the corn starch in a large screw-top jar, and add the essential oils plus the whole geranium leaves. Screw the lid shut and shake to mix. Shake daily for a week, before removing the geranium leaves. Decant the fragrant powder into a sugar shaker or a clean and dry gift box, or vintage glass powder bowl.

> TIP: In summer, dust either of these body powders inside your shoes to prevent them from rubbing and giving you blisters.

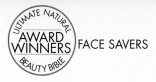
FACE SAVERS
our award winners

There are many different tricks for perking up your face in a flash. Gentle tapping movements (with fingertips) and/or facial massage are among our favourites – but products help, too, with skin-energising, plumping and radiance-enhancing ingredients designed to make you look like you've had eight hours' sleep even when it was closer to four... These winners are brilliant pre-party boosters, too

AROMATHERAPY ASSOCIATES INSTANT FIRMING SERUM
✺

SCORE: 8.25/10

A serum blended by the famous aromatherapy brand to restore firmness and radiance fast. It has long-term, age-defying powers but our testers were assessing it for speedy benefits. Key botanicals include tightening larch, marine algae (to protect against photo-ageing), anti-inflammatory pomegranate seed oil, and vanilla essential oil to lock in moisture. This is one of Sarah's secret weapons…

COMMENTS: 'Normally by 5pm I look quite tired, but I used this in the morning and when I looked in the mirror later, I had a nice glow (not shine)' • 'immediately after applying this my skin did feel and appear more radiant and soft' • 'made face look smooth and refreshed with an immediate firming effect' • 'a joy to use and worth every penny: skin looked brighter and clearer from first application, but not taut at all; I didn't believe in this type of product, till now' • 'love the natural (not girly) yummy smell'.

NOURISH RADIANCE REJUVENATING PEPTIDE SERUM
✺

SCORE: 8.14/10

Pauline Hili, the founder and formulator of Nourish, was for years in-house product creator at Neal's Yard Remedies; now she is flying solo with her own range. The serum is from Nourish's rose-based Radiance collection, and features skin-brightening bio-actives of Alpine foxberry (a new one to us), tonka bean (an

optical brightener), plus skin-plumping hyaluronic acid. Rose oil stimulates the production of collagen, according to Nourish, and also gives a divine scent, testers agreed. It can be used as both a hydrator and make-up primer.

COMMENTS: 'My face felt fresher and uplifted straight away; this isn't something I'd have considered at my age, but after trying it I can see how it makes a difference even to fairly young skin' • 'gives the complexion a nice lift and is lovely to use; with a 10-month-old baby I suffer from lack of sleep but this refreshes the skin so that even I could be fooled into believing I'd had a good night's sleep' • 'skin looked smoother, felt softer and make-up went on better' • 'made face feel lifted, smooth and younger looking; the benefits lasted for hours'.

AURELIA PROBIOTIC SKINCARE REVITALISE & GLOW SERUM
✺ ✺

SCORE: 7.63/10

Yet another winner in this book from the recently launched brand which has blown us away with their performance. This (like the two winners above) is a serum, combining baobab, omega 3, 6 and 9 fatty acids, firming kigelia Africana, hibiscus, a great whack of vitamin E – and it seduces with the blend of jasmine, plumeria, mandarin and tuberose which has bewitched testers in other categories.

COMMENTS: 'I feel 10 years younger when I've applied this; I would probably use it more than once a day if I could afford to' • 'made my face feel fresher instantly and appear more radiant, especially during our building work surrounded by dust!' • 'quick and easy to apply with a good effect on skin tone and the advantage of easier make-up application' • 'have finished the bottle and am going to buy another one' • 'thank you for giving me the opportunity to revitalise myself – and my complexion' • 'my skin was commented on by a work colleague today; when guessing my age she was 10 years out (too young) – so this must be doing something good!'

MELVITA ROSE EXTRAORDINARY WATER

✹ ✹✹

SCORE: 7.56/10

Now for something completely different, from a French organic brand: this has become a bit of a cult product with make-up artists and models alike. It's a 'hydrosol' – more akin to a toner – with a gel-like consistency that helps it to work like an instant, re-plumping skin drink. In Melvita's trials, 95 per cent of testers who used this rose treat found it delivered a firming action – just what a morning-after-the-night-before face often needs, we'd say!

COMMENTS: 'Loved this: I was surprised by the gel texture but it really glides onto skin and is very refreshing' • 'I used this during a hospital stay and my skin didn't suffer at all – it was radiant' • 'my face seemed to glow for a couple of hours after use; I've already bought more' • 'love everything about this: love that it's organic, love the consistency, love the fragrance, love that it makes my face look so fresh' • 'skin felt great after just the first use; it has a very pleasing smell, too'.

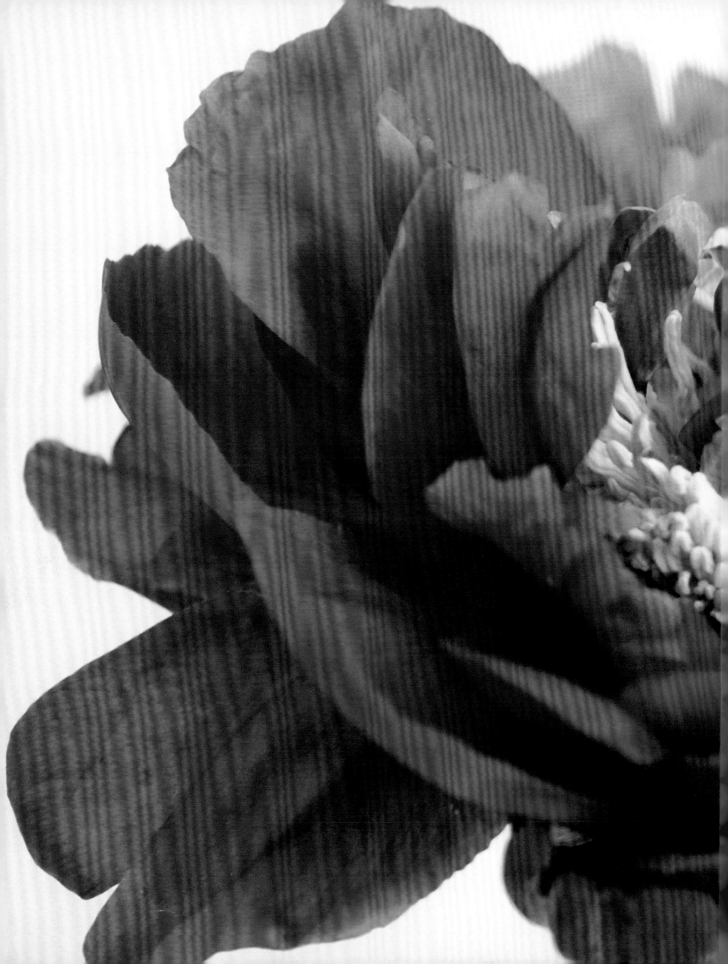

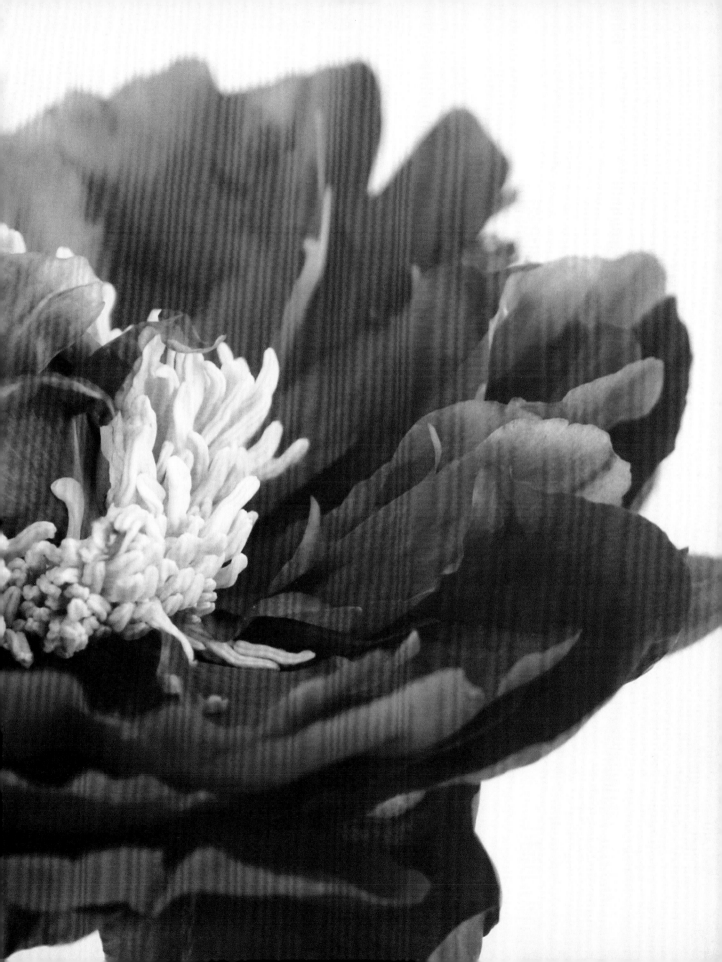

ESSENTIAL D-I-Y BEAUTY KIT

If you enjoy making a vinaigrette dressing or melting chocolate, you'll love cooking up your own cosmetics. While it's pretty simple, it does help to be organised. Find a list of useful equipment here, plus a guide to the easy techniques that will help you conjure up your homemade lotions and potions

EQUIPMENT CHECKLIST

- Kettle
- Heat-resistant jugs (if you use glass, make sure it's Pyrex, or a heatproof material)
- Heat-resistant bowls (see above)
- Stainless-steel or enamel saucepans (aluminium can stain)
- Double boiler (sometimes called a bain-marie) – this will be the most-used item in your equipment
- Measuring scales
- Measuring spoons (at least four from a quarter teaspoon to one tablespoon)
- Measuring cups (it's useful if they feature imperial, metric and US cup equivalents)
- Herb or coffee grinder
- Food processor or blender
- Pestle and mortar
- Hand whisk or hand-held blender (with rotating whisks)
- Wooden and metal spoons for stirring
- Sharp knives for cutting
- Vegetable peeler
- Grater (and a Microplane is an asset)
- Large sieve and smaller mesh tea strainer
- Muslin or cheesecloth – or plenty of paper towels for straining
- Funnel
- Sterilised bottles, jars and plastic containers in which to store and display your finished products
- Selection of different sizes of large glass containers in which to infuse oils and alcohol-based liquids such as fragrances and deodorants – these needn't be expensive, we find them at car-boot sales and in thrift stores

When you're making cosmetics, clear the workspace of any food before you start. Make sure you have plenty of elbow room and heatproof surfaces on which to place pans or hot jugs. (Bread boards or wooden trivets are ideal.) It's easiest to be organised and lay out everything you will need; and prepare any ingredients (slice, chop or grate), so that you have them all to hand.

BEAUTY COOKING TECHNIQUES

How to use a double boiler. If you put oils or beeswax directly in a pan and heat them, they'll get too hot. So, ingredients for making cosmetics – just as for melting chocolate – need to be insulated inside a double boiler (sometimes referred to as a bain-marie), and the easiest thing is to invest in one. A pan fits neatly inside a slightly larger one, and a small quantity of water is placed in the outer pan; when this boils, it gently melts the ingredients inside the inner pan without spoiling them. If you don't have a double boiler you can improvise with a saucepan and a smaller, Pyrex or heatproof ceramic bowl which fits snugly inside. Put about 2.5cm (1in) of boiling water in the bottom of the pan (it shouldn't touch the bowl) and place the bowl inside. The heat from the water will melt and infuse the ingredients inside the inner bowl. (NB: If you use the bowl and saucepan method, be careful not to be scalded by the steam, and also not to burn yourself when removing the inner bowl.)

SAFETY FIRST

Unlike the products you buy in a beauty hall or pharmacy, your home-made cosmetics aren't packed with preservatives. So it pays to follow some simple precautions that will maximise their bathroom shelf life and prevent them from going off or becoming contaminated.

Storage jars or bottles must be perfectly sterile. Before you use glass or metal containers, carefully scrub them, plus lids, with washing-up liquid to make sure there's nothing lurking in the crevices or rims. (Bottlebrushes of different sizes are very handy for this.) Next, put the containers in a large saucepan, cover with water and boil for 15 minutes. Or heat them in a 130°C (270°F) oven for 30 minutes. Dry thoroughly with a fresh cloth and stand upside-down on another clean towel until you use them – this is so they can't get dust or dirt inside.

Plastic containers need different treatment: once you know they are heatproof, place in a large saucepan, cover with water, bring slowly to the boil and heat for 2–3 minutes. Lift out with tongs and repeat as above.

Always allow home-made cosmetics to cool properly before sealing with a lid or cork, or you risk contamination from condensation.

Follow the storage guidelines in the recipes. Cosmetics will all last longer in a fridge but this is most important with water-based products where bugs breed far more readily than in oils or beeswax.

Always wash your hands thoroughly with soap before making or using cosmetics, to avoid transferring bacteria to your face, mouth or eyes. And replace lids, screw tops or corks to keep out bugs.

To avoid sensitivity reactions, do a patch test before applying creams to your face or large areas of the body. Apply a small amount on your inner arm, immediately below the elbow. Cover with sticking plaster (unless you're allergic to plasters), and leave for 24 hours. (Alternatively, apply it behind one ear.) If you experience any soreness, redness or irritation, your skin is reacting to an ingredient and you should avoid using the product on a wider scale.

How to make a tisane (or tea). Use one teaspoon of dried herb per 225ml (8fl oz) of boiling water (or one teabag per cup if, say, you're making a chamomile tisane). Ideally, cover the cup – a saucer is ideal – or the volatile oils will be lost into the air while the tea steams. Steep for 10–15 minutes.

How to make an infusion. Pour 600ml (1 pint) of boiling water over 25g (1oz) dried herbs and flowers and steep for several hours. (An infusion is stronger than a tisane so it steeps for longer.) Always make infusions in glass, stainless steel or enamel, never aluminium (as the herbs can leach out into the metal). Stored in the fridge, an infusion will keep for up to a week, as with a tisane.

How to make a decoction. Woody herbs and hard seeds need to be boiled for longer to extract their potency. For every 25g (1oz) of root, seed or bark, simmer in 600ml (1 pint) of water for up to an hour over a low flame on the stove. (Again, always use stainless-steel, glass or aluminium pans.) Then let the pan sit for at least another hour, to allow the goodness of the herbs to disperse fully into the water. (NB: As a rule of thumb, you should use approximately half the quantity of dried herbs as you would fresh in a decoction or tisane.) You can also do this in a double boiler if you're making a decoction using oils.

How to macerate oils. All herbs should be chopped or ground and, for maceration, dried herbs perform better than fresh. Submerge the herbs totally in oil, pushing them down if necessary, otherwise mould may occur; tap the jar to see if you can get rid of any air bubbles that the plants may have trapped. (Do not wash the herbs, even if they seem a little dusty.) Stand the jar in a warm, sunny place for about 10 days to 3 weeks; you may want to stir or shake gently daily. After the oils have macerated for long enough, strain them through a piece of muslin or a double layer of kitchen paper, pressing down with the back of a wooden spoon or with your fingers, to squeeze the last of the goodness out of the herbs. (Macerated oils generally last from 6 months to a year.)

DECODING ORGANIC

How much can you trust the labels on your natural beauty buys? Due to a lack of regulation the word 'organic' can be used to describe less-than-wholesome products… but there are logos and terms to look out for that help guarantee naturalness

Your skin is the largest organ of your body and what you put on it can be absorbed in tiny amounts. So, like many other 'green beauties', we want to know that what goes on our body – like the food we put in it – is as clean, pure and wholesome as it can be.

There's a problem, however, at a regulatory level. Unlike organic food, there are no legal standards for organic beauty products. The result can be confusing for consumers.

To true organic producers, the word means a system of producing ingredients sustainably, without agricultural chemicals and a long list of other synthetics which are widely used in the cosmetics industry. It means allowing those processes to be tracked and traced, all the way from the field where the ingredient grew, through to when the final product is packaged.

To some less-scrupulous marketing departments, however, it means an opportunity to jump on a potentially lucrative bandwagon. Some companies label a product as 'organic' even when it contains as little as one per cent organic ingredients – a waft of organic lavender or rosemary, say – plus a long list of chemicals that might be linked to sensitivity or graver problems.

In order to give consumers some assurance, five leading European organic certification bodies have combined to create the COSMOS standard (Cosmetic Organic Standard). The five charter members are the Soil Association (Great Britain), Ecocert (France), Cosmebio (France), BDIH (Germany), and ICEA (Italy).

Under COSMOS, there are two types of certified-organic beauty product:

Over 95 per cent organic: a product can only be called 'organic' in the product name where at least 95 per cent of the ingredients (excluding water) are organic.

70–95 per cent organic: some products require higher quantities of preservatives, which reduces their organic content. Provided at least 70 per cent of the ingredients (excluding water)

are organic the product can be certified as such with COSMOS. However, these products cannot include the word 'organic' in the product name, and must state the percentage of organic ingredients in the product description.

Each of the bodies which contribute to the COSMOS standard, however, has its own (and sometimes slightly different) organic standard, which may in some cases be higher than the COSMOS standard. And the USA has its own organic certification, USDA, which offers the same sort of field-to-jar organic reassurance. Yes, it's confusing! But if you'd like to delve deeper, you can find details of the websites for all these organisations in our Directory (see page 216). And we say: if you care about whether your beauty products are organic, the simplest way to be sure is to look out for one of these logos (see left).

Other words and labels to look out for when natural-beauty shopping include the following:

Biodynamic: this term refers to a type of farming based on organic principles where specific steps are taken by farmers to optimise the health of soil and plants, such as planting by phases of the moon. (Remember that the moon has the power to move tides so it makes sense it can affect plant growth, too.) Weleda and Dr.Hauschka are the best-known biodynamic ranges.

The word **natural** is, for obvious reasons, the umbrella term used to describe natural cosmetics. But do bear in mind that it has no legal status, so when you see it on labels it's no guarantee of the purity of what's in the jar and tube. There are a couple of organisations that certify naturalness: the German **BDIH**, plus **NATRUE** whose logo (appearing on more and more natural products we notice) is a guarantee that the materials used in beauty products are plant derived; ingredients allowed include minerals, plus some nature-identical preservatives. Not permitted are synthetic dyes, colourants or fragrances, silicones, petroleum products, or any ingredient produced via 'ethoxylation', such as sodium laureth sulphate.

Beauty
WITHOUT FEAR

If the thought of testing cosmetics on animals upsets you as much as it does us and many others – every single woman we polled in a *Beauty Bible* survey voted against the practice – we have some good news… but there is still a long way to go

After a long-standing campaign by BUAV (the trading name for The Campaign to End Animal Testing) a ban came into force in spring 2013 on animal testing for cosmetics and their ingredients in the European Union. (A testing ban on finished cosmetic products had been in place for some years.) Companies can use alternative methods of testing, for instance skin irritation can be assessed on Reconstituted Human Epidermis using skin donated from cosmetic surgery. According to an official communication from the European Commission, this 2013 ban applies to the sale and marketing of all cosmetic products placed on the EU market, 'thus to those produced in the Union and to imported cosmetic products alike'.

However, companies can still carry out tests on animals outside the EU on cosmetics that will be sold outside the Union.

It's not just cosmetics which are animal-tested – the cleaning materials you use may also go through this process. Cruelty-Free International (C-FI), an arm of BUAV, is calling for the British government, and others worldwide, to ban testing on animals for household products, both for finished items and their ingredients.

Some brands have already signed up to this and display the Leaping Bunny logo, supplied by C-FI. Products bearing the Leaping Bunny are certified cruelty free according to rigorous standards. (For more about the Leaping Bunny logo criteria, visit www.gocrueltyfree.org.)

But there are no restrictions on animal testing for cosmetics or household products in other parts of the world, including the USA and Asia. The Chinese government requires all cosmetics to be submitted for animal testing in its laboratories.

A number of companies, such as The Body Shop, refuse to sell cosmetics in China until they can do so without animal testing. However, in late 2013, the Chinese government undertook to review its regulations for cosmetics testing. C-FI is submitting proposals towards enabling companies to market cosmetics in China without testing on animals.

There is also some progress on animal testing for Botox (which may extend to other fillers). According to the European Coalition to End Animal Experiments (ECEAE), of which BUAV is a member, hundreds of mice die to make each batch of botulinum toxin. However, US company Allergan, has received an EU-wide approval for an alternative test method. ECEAE hopes that 2014 will see the other two companies that make Botox, Ipsen and Merz Pharma, cease using the LD (Lethal Dose) 50 test. Ipsen has confirmed its intention to do so.

Animals should not suffer so that people can look good (you can read more details on www.crueltyfreeinternational.org). According to C-FI, 80 per cent of the world still allows animal testing. C-FI is calling on governments around the world to ban animal testing for cosmetics. Please sign their petitions and support them in every way you can.

DIRECTORY

Where to get ingredients for recipes

G. BALDWIN & CO
171/3 Walworth Road, London
SE17 1RW
tel: 020 7252 5550 www.baldwins.co.uk
Baldwins, who supplied many of the raw ingredients for the photography for this book, offers a good selection of jars and bottles, as well as aromatherapy supplies, herbs, waxes and oils. They ship worldwide.

JEKKA'S HERB FARM
Rose Cottage, Shellards Lane,
Alveston, Bristol BS35 3SY
www.jekkasherbfarm.com
If you want to grow your own herbal and plant ingredients, this is a superb resource.

NEAL'S YARD REMEDIES
tel: 0161 831 7875
www.nealsyardremedies.com
A fantastic source for home beauty supplies, which offers the widest range of organically certified base oils, essential oils, dried herbs and other ingredients such as wax and clay. They also provided many ingredients for the book. As well as having distributors in various countries, they ship worldwide.

Organic and Natural Certification bodies

BDIH
www.kontrollierte-naturkosmetik.de/e/index_e.htm
COSMEBIO
www.cosmebio.org/en/
ECOCERT
www.ecocert.com/en
ICEA
www.icea.info/en/
NATRUE
www.natrue.org
SOIL ASSOCIATION
www.soilassociation.org

A

4711 eau de cologne tel: 0845 609 0055

AD Skin Synergy tel: 01495 325284
www.adskinsynergy.com

AEOS tel: 01507 533581
www.aeos.net

Aesop tel: 020 7407 4994
www.aesop.com

Aftelier Perfumes www.aftelier.com

A'kin tel: 0845 456 0639
www.mypure.co.uk

Antipodes
www.antipodesnature.com

Apicare tel: 0800 0141 923
www.simplymanuka.co.uk

Argan 5+ www.boots.com

Aromatherapy Associates
tel: 020 7838 1117
www.aromatherapyassociates.com

Aurelia tel: 020 3623 7208
www.aureliaskincare.com

Aveda tel: 0800 0542 979
www.aveda.co.uk

B

Balance Me tel: 020 7593 1070
www.balanceme.co.uk

Barefoot Botanicals tel: 01273 325666
www.barefoot-botanicals.com

BareMinerals tel: 0800 6523 362
www.bareminerals.co.uk

Beauty Bible Lip Balm tel: 0800 3898 195
www.victoriahealth.com

Beeswax tel: 0845 2623 145
www.nealsyardremedies.com

Bellàpierre tel: 020 8993 0077
www.bellapierre.co.uk

Bodytox tel: 0800 3898 195
www.victoriahealth.com

Bohemian Naturals
www.bohemiannaturals.com

Bourjois www.bourjois.co.uk

British Association of Skin Camouflage (NHS and private practice) tel: 01254 703 107
www.skin-camouflage.net

Burt's Bees tel: 0808 2341 423
www.burtsbees.co.uk

By Terry tel: 020 8740 2085
www.uk.spacenk.com

C

Castile Liquid Soap tel: 0845 0725 825
www.drbronner.co.uk

Caudalie tel: 020 7720 7111
www.uk.caudalie.com

Chanel No.5 www.chanel.com/en_GB/

Changing Faces
tel: 0300 012 0275
(for support and advice)
tel: 0300 012 0276
(for the Skin Camouflage Service)
www.changingfaces.org.uk

Cinq Mondes
tel: 01483 450 830
www.cinqmondes.com

Circaroma
tel: 0800 3898 195
www.victoriahealth.com

Clarisonic tel: 0800 0286 874
www.clarisonic.co.uk

Covermark
www.extrememakeup.co.uk

Crabtree & Evelyn
tel: 0800 1114 406
www.crabtree-evelyn.co.uk

D

Darphin tel: 0800 0746 905
www.darphin.co.uk

Decléor tel: 020 7313 8787
www.decleor.co.uk

Dermacolor
www.extrememakeup.co.uk

DLux 1000
Spray by Better You
tel: 0800 3898 195
www.victoriahealth.com

Doll Face tel: 07946 327 818
www.amazon.co.uk

Dr.Hauschka tel: 01386 791 022
www.drhauschka.com

Dr.Organic tel: 0870 606 6605
www.hollandandbarrett.com

DynoMins tel: 0800 3898 195
www.victoriahealth.com

E

Ecotools www.ecotools.com

Elemental Herbology tel: 020 8968 4477
www.elementalherbology.com

Elemis tel: 0117 316 1818
www.timetospa.co.uk

Eminence Organic tel: 01527 834 904
www.theskinsmith.co.uk

Emma Hardie tel: 020 7307 2380
www.emmahardie.com

ESPA tel: 01252 352 230
www.espaskincare.com

Essential Care tel: 01638 716593
www.essential-care.co.uk

Eve Snow tel: 020 8359 1160
www.evesnow.com

Evolve tel: 0844 991 0061
www.evolvebeauty.co.uk

Eye Logic tel: 0800 3898 195
www.victoriahealth.com

F

Face Matters www.facematters-skincare.com

FitFlops tel: 0845 359 9884
www.fitflop.co.uk

Food intolerance testing: YorkTest
Laboratories www.yorktest.com
tel: 0800 1300 580

Fresh Therapies tel: 023 8073 9595
www.freshtherapies.com

G

Gielly Green tel: 020 7034 3060
www.giellygreen.co.uk

Goldfaden MD tel: 020 8740 2085
www.uk.spacenk.com

Green People tel: 01403 740 350
www.greenpeople.co.uk

Green & Spring tel: 020 8964 0949
www.greenandspring.com

Guerlain tel: 0845 643 0119
www.feelunique.com

H

Honoré des Prés www.honoredespres.com

I

Inika www.inikacosmetics.co.uk

Inlight tel: 01326 281114

www.inlight-online.co.uk

Intelligent Nutrients tel: 01737 222 563
www.intelligentnutrients.co.uk

J

Jane Iredale tel: 020 8450 2020
www.janeiredale.co.uk

Jason tel: 08450 725 825
www.jasonnaturalcare.co.uk

John Frieda www.boots.com

John Masters
tel: 01874 610667
www.johnmasters.co.uk

Jurlique tel: 020 7297 2222
www.jurlique.co.uk

JustBe www.justbebotanicals.co.uk

K

Kai tel: 08456 529 521
www.cultbeauty.co.uk

Keromask tel: 01276 415741
www.keromask.com

Kneipp tel: 0800 3898 195
www.victoriahealth.com

Korres tel: 01179 270430
www.bathandunwind.com

Kure Bazaar tel: 0800 123 400
www.selfridges.com

L

Lanolips www.lanolips.com/uk/

Lavera tel: 01557 870266
www.pravera.co.uk

LifeFlo Magnesium Gel
tel: 0800 3898 195
www.victoriahealth.com

Lifetime Vitamins Clarify Blemish Formula
tel: 0800 3898 195
www.victoriahealth.com

Living Nature tel: 0845 643 0119
www.feelunique.com

Liz Earle tel: 01983 813913
http://uk.lizearle.com

L'Occitane tel: 020 7907 0301
www.loccitane.com

Louise Galvin tel: 020 7835 0453
www.louisegalvin.com

Love Your Skin tel: 0800 032 4871
www.lys-london.com

Lucy Annabella Organics
tel: 028 8747 0000
www.lucyannabella.com

M

Dr Rabia Malik, MRCGP
Cosmetic doctor
tel: 020 3086 7715
www.drrabiamalik.com

Manuka Doctor tel: 014556 18887
www.manukadoctor.co.uk

Mary Elizabeth
www.maryelizabethbodycare.com

Materia Aromatica tel: 01548 831671
www.materiaaromatica.com

Mega Probiotic ND tel: 0800 3898 195
www.victoriahealth.com

Melvita tel: 0800 1387 045
www.uk.melvita.com

MICRO Pedi www.boots.com

MV Organic Skincare
tel: 08456 529 521
www.cultbeauty.co.uk

N

Nail Magic tel: 0800 3898 195
www.victoriahealth.com
Natio tel: 0844 561 6161
www.debenhams.com

NATorigin tel: 0845 838 6724
www.natorigin.co.uk

Neal's Yard Remedies tel: 0845 262 3145
www.nealsyardremedies.com

NEOM tel: 0870 460 4677
www.neomorganics.com

Nourish tel: 020 7622 0688
www.nourishskinrange.com

NutriWorks Patch It
www.amazon.co.uk

O

Ogario tel: 0844 556 4393
www.ogariolondon.com

Ojon tel: 0800 088 4165
www.ojon.co.uk

One Love Organics
tel: 0845 5199 120
www.oneloveorganics.eu

OPI tel: 01923 240 010
www.opiuk.com

Ora Naturals tel: 020 8658 4860
www.oranaturals.co.uk

Organic Glam tel: 0844 800 8399
www.theorganicpharmacy.com

Origins tel: 0800 054 2888
www.origins.co.uk

OSKIA tel: 01600 710 710
www.oskiaskincare.com

Outback Gold tel: 020 7893 8333
www.urbanretreat.co.uk

P

Phylia de M tel: 0800 3898 195
www.victoriahealth.com

Phyto tel: 0845 643 0119
www.feelunique.com

Poppy King tel: 020 8740 2085
www.uk.spacenk.com

Power of Krill tel: 0800 3898 195
www.victoriahealth.com

Pure Lochside tel: 0800 021 4245
www.purelochside.com

Pür Minerals
tel: 0845 609 0200
www.marksandspencer.com

R

Relaxing Essence by A.Vogel
tel: 0845 608 5858
www.avogel.co.uk

REN tel: 020 7724 2900
www.renskincare.com

S

Selexir tel: 0800 3898 195
www.victoriahealth.com

Shiffa tel: 0800 123 400
www.selfridges.com

Skin Camouflage Network (NHS and private practice)
www.skincamouflagenetwork.org.uk

Solgar Vegetal Silica
tel: 0800 3898 195
www.victoriahealth.com

Spatone
www.boots.com

Sranrom
www.sranrom.co.uk

Strange Invisible Perfumes
www.siperfumes.com

St. Tropez tel: 020 7845 6330
www.st-tropez.com

Sun Chlorella A
tel: 0800 3898 195
www.victoriahealth.com

Super Digestive Enzymes
tel: 0800 3898 195
www.victoriahealth.com

Suti www.suti.co.uk

T

Dr Nigma Talib, ND
Naturopathic doctor
tel: 020 7792 8073
www.healthydoc.com

TanOrganic tel: 0870 820 0073
www.tanorganic.com

The Body Shop
tel: 0800 0929 090
www.thebodyshop.co.uk

The Eye Doctor
tel: 0800 3898 195
www.victoriahealth.com

The Organic Pharmacy
tel: 0844 800 8399
www.theorganicpharmacy.com

The Perfume Society
www.perfumesociety.org

The Scent Critic
www.thescentcritic.com

This Works tel: 020 8543 3544
www.thisworks.com

Tisserand tel: 01273 325 666
www.tisserand.com

Trilogy tel: 0845 643 0119
www.feelunique.com

Tweezerman
tel: 0845 262 1731
www.tweezerman.co.uk

U

UNE
www.unebeauty.com/en/

V

Veil tel: 01207 279 432
www.veilcovercream.com

Viridian tel: 01327 87 8050
www.viridian-nutrition.com

W

Weleda tel: 0115 9448222
www.weleda.co.uk

Wild About Beauty
www.wildaboutbeauty.com

Y

Yes to Carrots
tel: 0845 643 0119
www.feelunique.com

Bookshelf
ESSENCE & ALCHEMY
by Mandy Aftel

GI DIET
by Antony Worrall Thompson

HEALING WITHOUT FREUD OR PROZAC
by David Servan-Schreiber

SOLVE YOUR FOOD INTOLERANCE
by Dr John Hunter

THE BEAUTY DETOX SOLUTION
by Kimberly Snyder

All available at www.amazon.co.uk

INDEX

A

acne 82–85
AD skin synergy 74, 75
after-sun care 48, 158–161
age-related macular degeneration (AMD) 95
ageing: and cellulite 119
  stress and 196
  sun and 147
A'kin 96
alcohol 189, 197
allergies 10
  and dark circles under eyes 93
  parabens 153
  perfumes 188
  to hair colours 178
aloe vera: after-sun care 159, 161
  and rosacea 87
  starflower mask for dry skin 73
animal testing 215
Antipodes 20, 36
Apicare 57
apples: apple juice dandruff blitzer 176
  apple skin-clearing treatment 84
  apple zit-blaster 84
Argan 5+ 128–129
Aromatherapy Associates 200, 201, 204, 205, 208
Aurelia 52, 56, 60, 74, 97, 208
Aveda 16, 22, 36, 38, 45, 169, 172–173, 174, 175

B

Balance Me 90, 91
balms 39, 50
banana mask, for hair 176
bareMinerals 19, 20, 21, 28, 38, 43, 82, 83, 90
barrier creams 137
bath bags 202
baths 197, 200–205
Beauty Bible lip balm 39
bedrooms 197
beds 197
beetroot lip tint 41
Bellápierre 29, 43
bikini waxes 183
biodynamic products 214
bloating 112
blondes: hair brightener 180
  make-up 14
blushers 41, 42–43
body butter bliss 108
bodycare 100–123

after-sun care 158–161
body brushing 119
body butters 114–115
body washes 104–105
dusting powders 207
lotions 110
moisturisers 108–109
oils 116
scrubs 106–107, 198–199
self-tanners 148–151, 152
sun protection 156–157
borage, starflower mask for dry skin 73
Botox 215
bottles, sterilising 213
Brazilian waxes 183
breast cancer 153
breathing techniques 87
bronzers 45
brows 27, 183
brunettes, make-up 15
brushes 22–23
buffing nails 126, 133
Burt's Bees 104, 105

C

caffeine 87, 112, 197
calendula skin salve 51
cancer 146, 152, 153
carrots, vita-carrot mask for mature skin 72
Castile shampoo, herb-boosted 170
Caudalíe 116
cellulite 118–122
chamomile: chamomile and rhubarb hair brightener 180
  chamomile eye bag banisher 98
Chanel, Coco 146
chlorella 127
cider vinegar 112, 161
Cinq Mondes 116
Circaroma 56, 138, 139
citrus peel, as deodorant 123
clay mask, for oily hair 176
cleansers 52–55
  geranium cleansing balm 55
  milk, cucumber and mint cleanser 55
cocoa butter, body butter bliss 108
collagen 118–119, 196
colognes 189, 193
colour, lipstick 33
colour types, make-up for 14–15
coloured skin, make-up 15
colouring hair 178–179
computers, and insomnia 197
concealers 24–25
conditioners: haircare 168–169
  sage lash conditioner 31

confidence 64–65
contact lenses 94
cortisol 87, 196
cosmetics, making 212–213
cotton wool pads 23
cow's milk: and acne 82
  and hair 164
Crawford, Cindy 64
cress and oatmeal skin buffers 69
cucumber: after-sun care 161
  cucumber body lotion 109
  cucumber mask for sensitive skin 72
  cucumber refreshing gel 99
  milk, cucumber and mint cleanser 55
  refreshing eyes with 98
curly hair 164
cuticles 128–130, 133, 142

D

dairy products 112, 119
daisy rating 7
damaged hair, herbs for 170
dandruff 164
  apple juice dandruff blitzer 176
dark circles, under eyes 93
Darphin 96, 97
day creams 56
decoctions 213
Delevingne, Cara 64
deodorants 123
DHA (dihydroxyacetone) 150, 152–153
diet: and bloating 112
  and cellulite 119
  and dark circles under eyes 93
  and eye problems 95
  food intolerances 86–87, 93
  and haircare 164
  and nails 127
  and rosacea 86–87
  vitamin D deficiency 146
digestive problems 86,127
Doll Face 45
double boiler 212
Dr. Hauschka 36, 52, 53, 70, 71, 78, 90, 104, 105, 126, 128, 129, 158, 159, 214
Dr. Organic 106, 107, 114, 115, 140, 142, 158–159
dry eyes 93–94
dry hair: hair mask for 176
  herbs for 170
dry skin: facial oils 77
  on feet 142
  starflower mask for dry skin 73
dusting powders 207
dyes, hair 178–179

For Amy Eason, the loveliest and most efficient right-hand we could possibly wish for, ever.

Our very best thanks to the following:
Jessie Lawrence (the so-efficient 'Tester Coordinator'), Sacha Burrows,
Dave Edmunds and to Lily Evans (who helped Jo on the original recipes).

All the PRs and brands who provided products for our trials, and our
thousands of diligent testers.

Our friends and colleagues, notably Sue Peart and Catherine Fenton at
YOU magazine, Gill Sinclair and Shabir Daya at
Victoria Health, and – as ever – Kay McCauley, our agent.

Our fantastic team on this book: designer Jane Berry,
photographer Claire Richardson, picture researcher Sally Cole,
copy editors Alice Butler and Liz Murray, and also to Vicky Orchard at Kyle Books.

Finally, thanks to our husbands: Craig Sams – the original 'Mr. Natural', who puts up
with tens of thousands of products every year coming in and out of his and Jo's house...
And to Sarah's husband Alex Allan who never complains about having to forage his
way through the beauty jungle in our shared office and helps with
proof-reading and all the rest.

First published in Great Britain in 2014
by Kyle Books an imprint of
Kyle Cathie Limited
67–69 Whitfield Street
London W1T 4HF
general.enquiries@kylebooks.com
www.kylebooks.com

10 9 8 7 6 5 4 3 2 1

ISBN: 978 0 85783 222 1

A CIP catalogue record for this title is
available from the British Library

Sarah Stacey and Josephine Fairley are
hereby identified as the authors of this
work in accordance with Section 77 of
the Copyright, Designs and Patents
Act 1988.

Editor: Vicky Orchard
Design and styling: Jane Berry
Photography: Claire Richardson
Production: Lisa Pinnell

Colour reproduction by ALTA London
Printed and bound in China by C&C
Offset Printing Company Ltd